Imaging for Students

SECOND EDITION

David A. Lisle FRACR

Consultant Radiologist, Holy Spirit Hospital, Brisbane; Visiting
Radiologist, Royal Children's Hospital; Lecturer in Radiology
at the Queensland University of Technology; Clinical Lecturer
in Radiology at the University of Queensland Medical School,
Brisbane, Australia

with a contribution from

Andrew Russell FANZCA

Consultant Anaesthetist, Holy Spirit and Princess Alexandra
Hospitals, Brisbane, Australia

A member of the Hodder Headline Group
LONDON
Distributed in the United States of America by
Oxford University Press Inc., New York

First published in Great Britain in 2001 by
Arnold, a member of the Hodder Headline Group,
338 Euston Road, London NW1 3BH
http://www.hoddereducation.com

Distributed in the United States of America by
Oxford University Press, Inc.,
198 Madison Avenue, New York, NY10016
Oxford is a registered trademark of Oxford University Press

Whilst the advice and information in this book are believed to be true and
accurate at the date of going to press, neither the author[s] nor the publisher
can accept any legal responsibility or liability for any errors or omissions
that may be made. In particular (but without limiting the generality of the
preceding disclaimer) every effort has been made to check drug dosages;
however it is still possible that errors have been missed. Furthermore,
dosage schedules are constantly being revised and new side-effects
recognized. For these reasons the reader is strongly urged to consult the
drug companies printed instructions before administering any of the drugs
recommended in this book.

British Library Cataloguing in Publication Data
A catalogue record for this book is available from the British Library

Library of Congress Cataloging-in-Publication Data
A catalog record for this book is available from the Library of Congress

ISBN-10: 0 340 76231 4
ISBN-13: 978 0 340 76231 8

5 6 7 8 9 10

Composition by Scribe Design, Gillingham, Kent
Printed and bound by Replika Press Pvt. Ltd., India

What do you think about this book? Or any other Hodder Education title?
Please send your comments to www.hoddereducation.co.uk

If one tells the truth, one is sure, sooner or later, to be found out.

OSCAR WILDE (1856–1900)

To my wife Lyn and my daughter Victoria

Contents

Preface

In the four years since the publication of the first edition of this book, the development of imaging technology has continued at a frenetic pace. Ultrasound is used increasingly in the investigation of vascular and musculoskeletal disorders. In many centres, CT is the first imaging investigation of choice in pulmonary embolism, and in a host of abdominal disorders including renal colic, acute appendicitis, and acute diverticulitis. The applications of MRI continue to grow. Functional, as well as anatomical, information may now be obtained with implications especially for the imaging of a diverse range of neurological disorders. Interventional radiology continues to develop as a subspecialty, with a wide range of vascular, biliary, renal, and neurological disorders now routinely managed non-surgically.

Given the above, it is hard enough these days for practising radiologists to keep up with their own specialty. How then does the medical student, struggling to learn so much in so short a time, attain the knowledge essential to a rational use of imaging in clinical practice? My answer would be to give priority to the 'basics'. In my opinion, by the time that he or she graduates from medical school, a student should be able to do the following:

- Interpret X-rays to diagnose common conditions such as pneumonia, cardiac failure, intestinal obstruction, fractures and dislocations.

- Order more sophisticated tests rationally to sort out a particular clinical problem.
- Have a broad understanding of the advantages, disadvantages, and possible side-effects of the various imaging modalities.

I have tried to set this book out accordingly. The first five chapters give a brief overview of the various imaging modalities. Chapter 6 outlines the hazards and risks associated with medical imaging. As in the first edition an anaesthetist colleague, Dr Andrew Russell, has written the section on contrast media reactions and their management. Chapters 7 to 16 then deal with imaging under broad clinical headings. In each section I have tried to emphasize the plain film findings. Where further imaging is required, I have tried to indicate the modality of choice and a suggested plan of investigation. Where radiological procedures are required, I have tried to set out the common indications as well as brief notes on patient preparation, method, postprocedure care, contraindications, and complications. Although this adds to the length of the book, I feel that it is important for students to understand at least the basics of what the patient is going through. Where appropriate, a small amount of clinical information is given to try to assist in the planning of imaging investigation.

David A. Lisle
Brisbane, June 2000

Acknowledgements

Many people have assisted me in the writing of this book. I would like to thank the following for donating images: Dr John Earwaker, Dr John Ratcliffe, Dr Jane Reasbeck and Dr David Simpson.

Once again, my good friend Andrew Russell has kindly contributed the section on contrast media reactions.

Thanks also to Fiona Goodgame and Nick Dunton at Arnold publishers for their continued trust and support. Finally, I must thank my wife Lyn and daughter Victoria for their continued forbearance.

1   Conventional radiography

Conventional radiography (X-rays; plain films)

X-rays are a form of electromagnetic radiation; their frequency and energy are much greater than visible light. X-rays are produced in an X-ray tube by focusing a beam of high-energy electrons on to a tungsten target. They are able to pass through a patient and on to X-ray film thus producing an image (*Fig. 1.1*).

In passing through a patient the X-ray beam is decreased according to the density and atomic number of the various tissues in a process known as

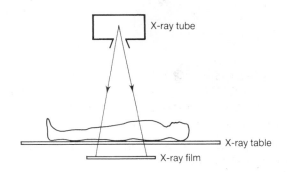

Figure 1.1 *Conventional radiography.*

attenuation. X-rays turn X-ray film black. Therefore the less dense a material, the more X-rays get through and

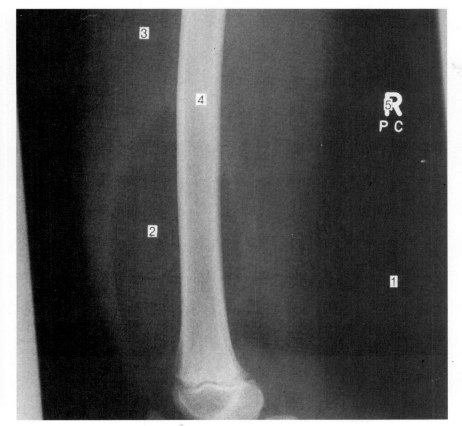

Figure 1.2 *The 5 principal radiographic densities. This plain film of a benign lipoma in a child's thigh demonstrates nicely the 5 basic radiographic densities:*
1. air
2. fat
3. soft tissue
4. bone
5. metal.

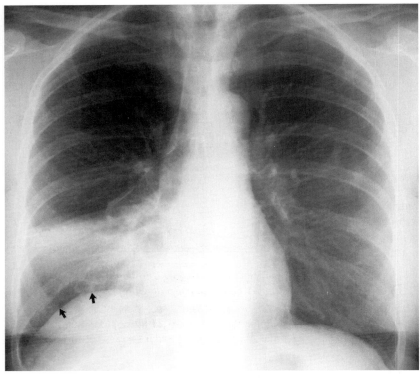

a

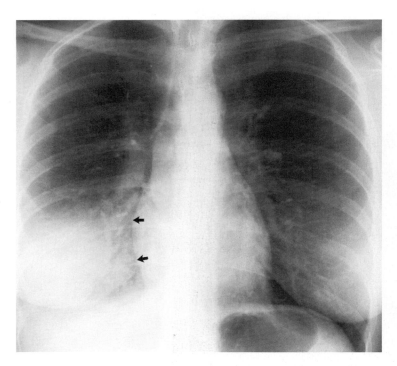

. b

Figure 1.3 *Abnormal chest X-ray.*
(a) Right middle lobe consolidation. The right heart border is not visualized. This is due to right middle lobe consolidation. The consolidated lung is of soft tissue density as is the heart. The silhouette of the right heart border is therefore lost. Note that the right diaphragm is still seen, indicating normal aeration of the right lower lobe (arrows). (b) Right lower lobe consolidation. In this case there is consolidation in the right lower lobe with loss of visualization of the right diaphragm. The right heart border can still be seen (arrows). Compare this appearance with that of right middle lobe consolidation.

the blacker the film, i.e. materials of low density appear darker than objects of high density.

Five principal densities are recognized on plain X-ray films. They are listed here in order of increasing density:

1. Air/gas: black, e.g. lungs, bowel and stomach.

2. Fat: dark grey, e.g. subcutaneous tissue layer, retroperitoneal fat.

3. Soft tissues/water: light grey, e.g. solid organs, heart, blood vessels, muscle and fluid-filled organs such as bladder.

4. Bone: off-white.

5. Contrast material/metal: bright white (*Fig. 1.2*).

An object will be seen with conventional radiography if its borders lie beside tissue of different density. For example, the heart border is seen because it lies against aerated lung, which is less dense. When lung consolidation occurs, such as in pneumonia, the lung density approaches that of soft tissue. Consolidated lung lying against the heart border will therefore cause non-visualization of that border. A good example is consolidation or collapse of the right middle lobe causing loss of definition of the right heart border (*Fig. 1.3*). Similarly, the psoas muscle margin is seen on a plain abdominal film owing to the lower density of fat lying against it. Retroperitoneal fluid or soft tissue mass lead to loss of visualization of the psoas margin (*Fig. 1.4*). These comments apply to all radiographically visible anatomical interfaces in the body.

Conventional tomography

Conventional tomography or sectional radiography may be used where an object is obscured by overlying or underlying structures. A good example is during intravenous pyelogram (IVP) where overlying bowel loops may obscure the kidneys.

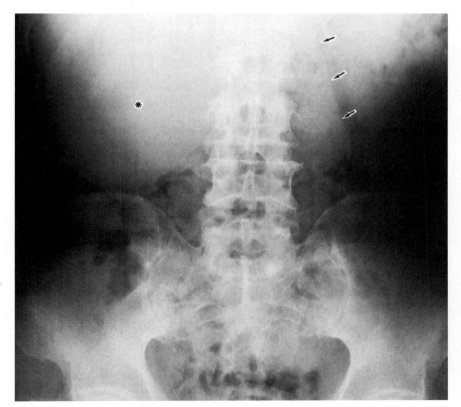

Figure 1.4 *Retroperitoneal mass.*
The left psoas margin is well defined (arrows). The right psoas margin is lost due to a large renal cell carcinoma (*).

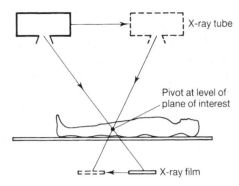

Figure 1.5 *Conventional tomography.*
The X-ray tube and X-ray film move about a pivot, the level of which is set at the desired plane of interest.

With conventional tomography, the X-ray tube and X-ray film move about a pivot set at a desired level of interest (*Fig. 1.5*). The motion of tube and film blurs objects above and below the plane of pivot, while objects in the plane of interest are seen in sharper relief (*Fig. 1.6*).

Conventional tomography is used less in modern practice since the advent of cross-sectional imaging techniques (ultrasound, CT, MRI), though it still finds application in IVP as above, and in some complex orthopaedic problems.

Fluoroscopy

Fluoroscopy refers to the technique of examination of the anatomy and motion of internal structures by a constant stream of X-rays. The term 'fluoroscopy' is derived from the ability of X-rays to cause fluorescence.

Uses of fluoroscopy include:

- Barium studies of the gastrointestinal tract.

- Angiography and interventional radiology.

- General surgery: operative cholangiography, colonoscopy, etc.

- Orthopaedic surgery: reduction and fixation of fractures, joint replacements, etc.

- Airway screening in children for tracheomalacia, and diaphragm screening.

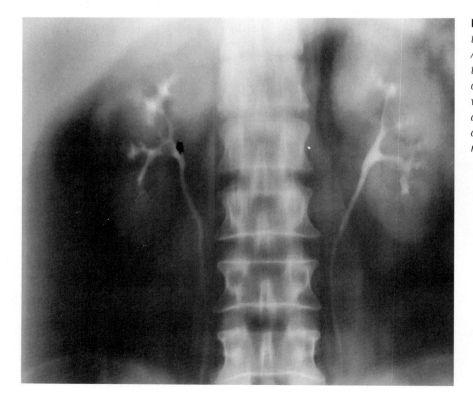

Figure 1.6 *Conventional tomography.*
A tomogram at the level of the kidneys 'removes' overlying bowel loops from view. Note that the spine is also blurred. A calculus is clearly seen in the right renal pelvis (arrow).

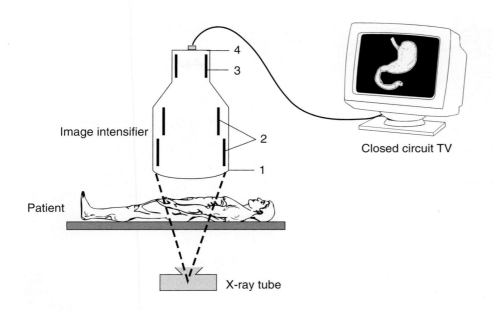

Figure 1.7
Fluoroscopy.
Note the components of the image intensifier:
1. *input fluorescent screen and photocathode*
2. *electrostatic lens*
3. *accelerating anode*
4. *output fluorescent screen.*

The original fluoroscopes were rather primitive and consisted of an X-ray tube, fluorescent screen and X-ray table. The radiologist directly viewed the image on the fluorescent screen. The images were very faint; examinations were performed in a darkened room by a radiologist with dark-adapted vision. Dark adaptation was achieved by wearing red goggles for 30 min.

Fluoroscopy was revolutionized in the 1950s by the development of the image intensifier. An image intensifier consists of the following:

- Vacuum tube.

- Input fluorescent screen.

- Photocathode.

- Accelerating anode.

- Electrostatic focusing lens.

- Output fluorescent screen.

The fluoroscopic image is produced in the following way:

- X-ray beam passes through the patient and enters the image intensifier vacuum tube.

- X-rays strike the input fluorescent screen and produce light photons.

- Light photons strike the photocathode producing electrons.

- Electrons are drawn away from the photocathode by the accelerating anode and focused by the electrostatic lens.

- Focused electrons strike the output fluorescent screen producing the fluoroscopic image (*Fig. 1.7*).

The fluoroscopic image is usually viewed via a closed circuit television chain. Images may be recorded in a number of ways:

- X-ray 'spot' films performed during screening.

- Light image from output fluorescent screen recorded by photospot or cine camera.

- Electronic image from television camera recorded in digital format on magnetic tape, magnetic disc or optical disc.

Digital subtraction angiography (DSA)

Digital subtraction is a process whereby a computer removes unwanted information from a radiographic image. It is particularly useful for angiography and the technique is referred to as DSA.

First, an image is taken of the relevant area prior to

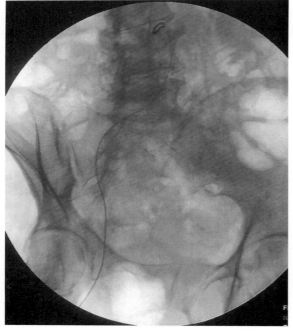

a

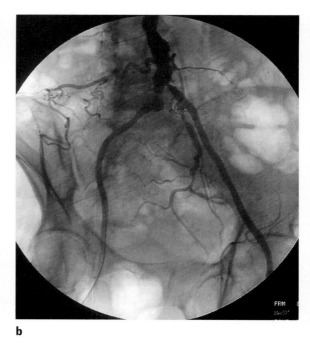

b

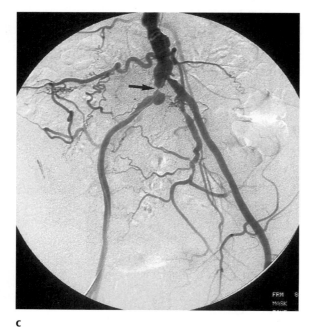

c

Figure 1.8 *Digital subtraction angiography.*
(a) Mask. Immediately prior to contrast injection a preliminary digitized image known as the 'mask' is performed. Note:
- *pelvic bones*
- *bowel gas*
- *arterial catheter.*

(b) Contrast image. Contrast is injected through the catheter producing opacification of the arteries.

(c) Subtracted image. The computer subtracts the 'mask' from the contrast image leaving an image of contrast-filled blood vessels unobscured by overlying bone and bowel. Note a tight localized stenosis of the right common iliac artery (arrow).

injection of contrast. This is called the 'mask'. Images are then taken with contrast in the blood vessels, and the computer then subtracts the 'mask' leaving an image of the contrast-filled blood vessels, unobscured by overlying bone, bowel, etc. (*Fig. 1.8*).

Patient preparation

- Sedation may be required for nervous patients.
- Anaesthetic cover may be needed for children and for agitated patients, and where there is a high risk of contrast reaction.

Method

The great majority of arteriography is done via a femoral artery puncture. Occasionally, if the femoral route cannot be used due to previous surgery or extreme tortuosity of the iliac arteries, the axillary or brachial arteries may be punctured. Catheter insertion is performed by the Seldinger technique as follows:

- The artery is punctured with a needle.
- A wire is threaded through the needle into the artery.
- The needle is removed leaving the wire in the artery.
- A catheter is inserted over the wire into the artery.

Depending on which artery is to be studied, variously shaped catheters are used. Indeed a bewildering array of catheters and wires has left few arteries in the body free from the prying eyes of radiologists.

Postprocedure care

- Bed rest for several hours.
- Observe puncture site for bleeding/swelling and apply direct pressure if either of these is seen.

Complications

- Due to contrast material: see Chapter 6.
- Due to arterial puncture:

    (i)   Haematoma at the puncture site.

    (ii) False aneurysm formation.

    (iii) Damage to brachial plexus with axillary or brachial artery puncture.

    (iv) Arterial dissection.

    (v)   Embolism due to dislodgement of atheromatous plaques.

It must be noted that newer techniques for examining arteries are being rapidly developed and accepted. These include ultrasound with Doppler, CT angiography (CTA), and magnetic resonance angiography (MRA). With the development of these techniques, the role of diagnostic arteriography will no doubt be reduced. The development of a vast array of interventional techniques, however, will ensure a steady increase in the therapeutic role of angiography.

2 Ultrasound (US)

Physics and terminology

Ultrasound (US) imaging uses ultra-high-frequency sound waves to produce cross-sectional images of the body. The basic component of the US probe is the *piezoelectric crystal*. Excitation of this crystal by electrical signals causes it to emit ultra-high-frequency sound waves: this is the *piezoelectric effect*. Sound waves are reflected back to the crystal by the various tissues of the body. These sound waves act on the piezoelectric crystal in the ultrasound probe to produce an electric signal, again by the piezoelectric effect. Analysis of this electric signal by a computer produces a cross-sectional image (*Fig. 2.1*).

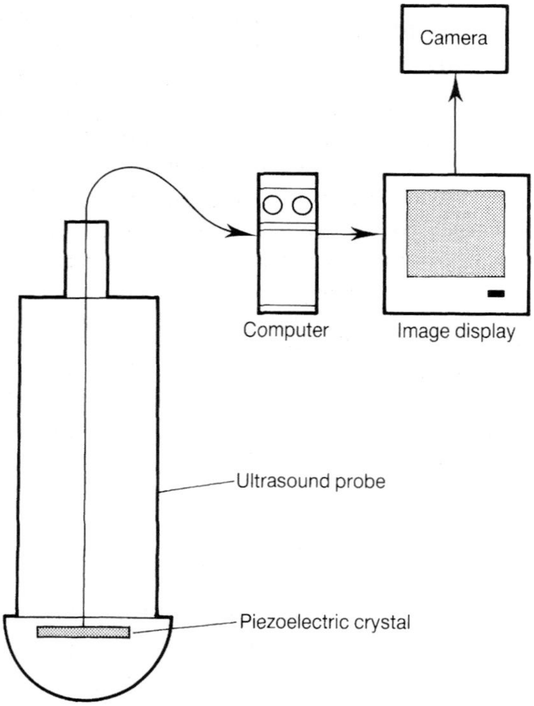

Assorted body tissues produce various degrees of sound wave reflection and are said to be of different echogenicity. A tissue of high echogenicity reflects more sound than a tissue of low echogenicity. The terms *hyperechoic* and *hypoechoic* are used to describe tissues of high and low echogenicity respectively. In producing an image hyperechoic tissues are shown as white or light grey, compared with hypoechoic tissues which are seen as dark grey. Examples of hyperechoic tissues include fat-containing masses and liver haemangiomas; lymphoma and fibroadenoma of the breast are examples of hypoechoic tissues.

Pure fluid reflects virtually no sound and is said to be anechoic. Fluid is seen on US images as black. Furthermore, because virtually all sound is transmitted through a fluid-containing area, tissues distal to such an area receive more sound and hence appear lighter. This effect is known as *acoustic enhancement* and is

Figure 2.1 *Ultrasound (US).*
The piezoelectric crystal in the US probe is used to both transmit and receive the US waves. The returned signal is analysed by computer and displayed as an image.

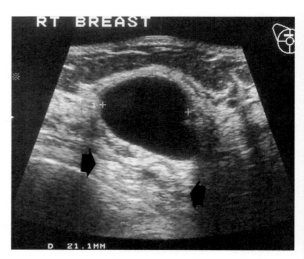

Figure 2.2 *Acoustic enhancement – simple cyst.*
A well-defined area of increased echogenicity or brightness is seen deep to a simple cyst of the breast. This is an area of acoustic enhancement (arrows).

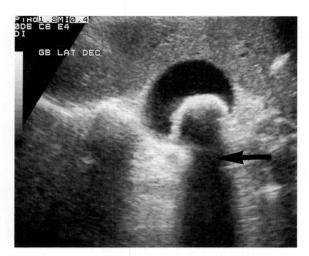

Figure 2.3 *Acoustic shadow – gallstone. Prominent acoustic shadow (arrow) deep to a large gallstone.*

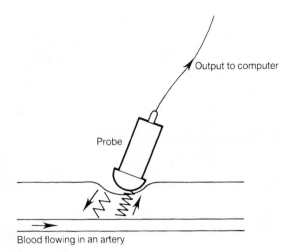

Blood flowing in an artery

Figure 2.4 *Doppler US. Blood flow is toward the ultrasound probe. As such the returning signal is of higher frequency. The frequency shift is analysed by computer and displayed as a graph.*

seen in tissues distal to the gallbladder, the urinary bladder and simple cysts (*Fig. 2.2*). The reverse effect occurs with areas of sharply increased echogenicity where distal tissues receive little sound and are thus perceived as black. This phenomenon is known as *acoustic shadow* and is seen distal to gas-containing areas, as well as gallstones, renal stones, and other areas of calcification (*Fig. 2.3*).

Further developments

Doppler US

Anyone who has heard a police or ambulance siren speed past will be familiar with the Doppler effect, which describes the influence of a moving object on sound waves. An object travelling towards the listener causes sound waves to be compressed giving a higher frequency; an object travelling away from the listener gives a lower frequency.

The Doppler effect has been applied to US imaging. Flowing blood causes an alteration to the frequency of sound waves returning to the US probe. This frequency change or shift is calculated allowing quantitation of blood flow (*Fig. 2.4*).

Colour Doppler is an extension of these principles, in that blood flowing towards the transducer is coloured red, blood flowing away from the transducer is coloured blue. The colours are superimposed on the cross-sectional image allowing instant assessment of direction of flow. Colour Doppler is particularly useful in echocardiography and for identifying very small vessels such as the calf veins, or arcuate arteries in the kidneys. It is also used to confirm blood flow within organs (e.g. testis to exclude torsion) and to assess the vascularity of tumours.

The combination of conventional two-dimensional US imaging with Doppler US is known as Duplex US (*Fig. 2.5*). As outlined in following chapters, Duplex US is an important technique in the examination of arteries and veins.

Intracavitary scanning

An assortment of probes is now available for imaging various body cavities and organs, the most widely used and accepted being transvaginal scanning. This technique allows more accurate assessment of gynaecological problems and of early pregnancy up to about 12 weeks' gestation. Transrectal probes are used to assess the prostate gland (*Fig. 2.6*). US crystals can be attached to endoscopes for

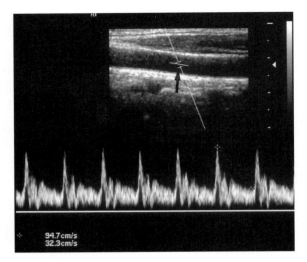

Figure 2.5 *Duplex US.*
Duplex US refers to a combination of two things: real-time imaging plus pulsed wave Doppler. The area of interest is identified on the real-time image. The Doppler sample gate is set at the appropriate level (arrow). Frequency shifts are displayed as a graph. By knowing the angle between the blood vessel and the US beam the computer is able to calculate velocities from the frequency shifts so that velocities are directly measured off the graph. In this case peak systolic and end diastolic velocities are displayed.

assessment of tumours of the upper gastrointestinal tract. To date, this technique has found greatest application for staging of oesophageal tumours. Echocardiography can also be performed via an endoscopic probe sited in the oesophagus. This removes the problem of overlying ribs and lung, which can obscure the heart when performing conventional echocardiography. Tiny US probes have also been developed for attachment to arterial catheters. These probes provide very accurate cross-sectional images of the arterial wall and, although expensive at present, are under continuing development.

High-frequency scanning

The use of high-frequency probes has opened up the area of musculoskeletal ultrasound (*Fig. 2.7*). This technique has found greatest application in the shoulder joint, specifically in the assessment of the rotator cuff. Most muscles and tendons of the body can also be examined for rupture, inflammation, tumour, etc. In general surgery, high-frequency US has increased the accuracy of small parts imaging, e.g. thyroid and parathyroid. Intraoperative US also uses high-frequency probes directly applied to the organ of interest, e.g. liver and pancreas.

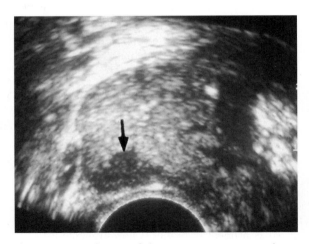

Figure 2.6 *Carcinoma of the prostrate – transrectal ultrasound (TRUS).*
A small carcinoma of the prostrate is seen on TRUS as a focal hypoechoic mass in the peripheral zone (arrow). Note that the adjacent capsule is smooth and that the tumour is confined to the prostrate gland, i.e. stage A. Diagnosis was confirmed by TRUS-guided biopsy.

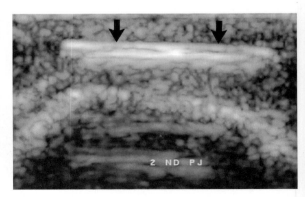

Figure 2.7 *Musculoskeletal US: foreign body.*
High-frequency US is an excellent modality for showing foreign bodies not seen on X-ray. This example shows a piece of wood (arrows) in the soft tissues of the index finger, adjacent to the proximal interphalangeal joint.

Uses and advantages

The advantages of US are as follows:

- Lack of ionizing radiation.
- Relative low cost.
- Portability of equipment.

US scanning is applicable to the solid organs of the body. Initially, studies were directed to the liver, kidneys, spleen and pancreas and to the pelvic organs. Higher-frequency, smaller probes led to the use of US in diseases of the thyroid, breast and testes, as well as the musculoskeletal system as above. The lack of ionizing radiation is a particular advantage in the assessment of pregnancy and in paediatrics. Used in conjunction with Doppler, US is now used in a wide variety of cardiovascular applications including echocardiography; assessment of carotid, renal, mesenteric and peripheral arteries for stenosis; and assessment of deep veins for thrombosis or incompetence.

Disadvantages and limitations

US cannot penetrate gas or bone. Hence, lesions lying behind or within gas or bone cannot be visualized. Therefore US is not used for pulmonary conditions, and bowel gas may obscure structures deep in the abdomen such as the pancreas or renal arteries. Bone lesions are not usually amenable to assessment with US. Similarly, the intracranial contents cannot be examined due to the overlying skull vault. The two exceptions to this are:

- An infant where the fontanelle is still open and provides a 'window'.
- Intraoperative localization of brain lesions during craniotomy.

3 Computed tomography (CT)

Physics and terminology

Computed tomography (CT) is an imaging technique whereby cross-sectional images are obtained with the use of X-rays. The patient passes through a gantry that rotates around at the level of interest. The gantry has an X-ray tube on one side and a set of detectors on the other. Information from the detectors is analysed by computer and displayed as an image (*Fig. 3.1*). Owing to the use of computer analysis, a much greater array of densities can be displayed than on conventional X-ray films. This allows differentiation of solid organs from each other and from pathological processes such as tumour or fluid collections. It also makes CT extremely sensitive to the presence of minute amounts of fat, calcium or contrast material.

As with plain radiography, high-density objects cause more attenuation of the X-ray beam and are therefore displayed as lighter grey than objects of lower density. White and light grey objects are therefore said to be of 'high attenuation'; dark grey and black objects are said to be of 'low attenuation'. Furthermore, the image information can be manipulated by the computer to display the various tissues of the body. This is called 'altering the window settings'. For example, in chest CT where a wide range of tissue densities is present, a good image of the mediastinal structures shows no lung details. By setting a lung window the lung parenchyma is seen in remarkable detail, though the mediastinal structures are poorly differentiated (*Fig. 3.2*). This technique can also be used to accentuate a subtle difference in tissue density. For example, the use of 'liver windows' allows greater differentiation of tumours whose tissue density closely approximates that of surrounding normal liver tissue.

Intravenous contrast is used in CT for a number of reasons, as follows:

- Differentiation of normal blood vessels from abnormal masses, e.g. hilar vessels versus lymph nodes.

- To make an abnormality more apparent, e.g. liver metastases.

- To demonstrate the vascular nature of a mass and thus aid in characterization (*Fig. 3.3*).

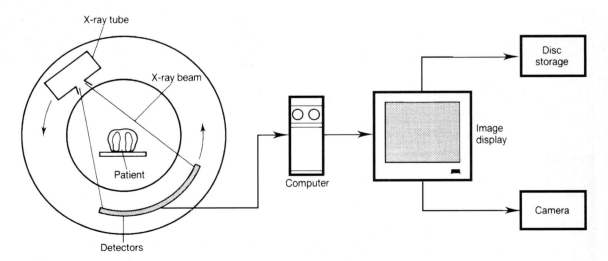

Figure 3.1 *Computed tomography – CT.*

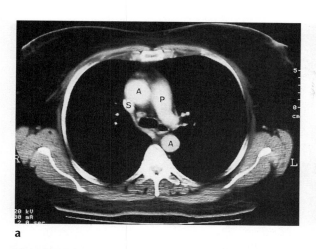
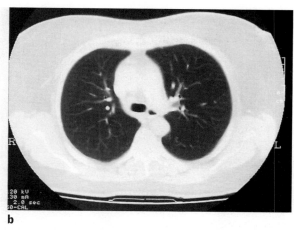

a   b

Figure 3.2 *CT windows.*

(a) Mediastinal window. Note that mediastinal anatomy is well shown; no lung detail can be seen. Note also the following structures:
- *aorta (A)*
- *superior vena cava (S)*
- *pulmonary artery (P).*

(b) Lung window. Note that the vascular anatomy of the lungs is now well seen.

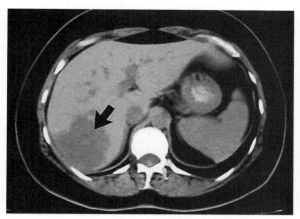

a

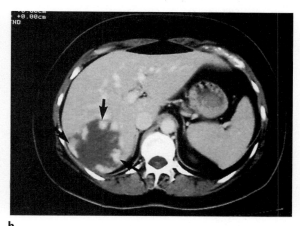

b

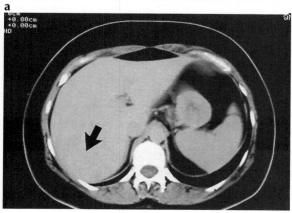

c

Figure 3.3 *Contrast CT – liver haemangioma.*

(a) Precontrast scan. Note:
- *large mass in the right lobe of the liver (arrow)*
- *low attenuation compared with surrounding normal liver.*

(b) Immediate postcontrast scan. Note:
- *contrast in aorta, inferior vena cava and portal vein branches*
- *dense contrast enhancement of the periphery of the mass (arrows).*

(c) 50-min postcontrast scan. The mass is now uniformly enhanced (arrow), so its density is equal to that of normal liver tissue. This is a typical enhancement pattern for haemangioma of the liver.

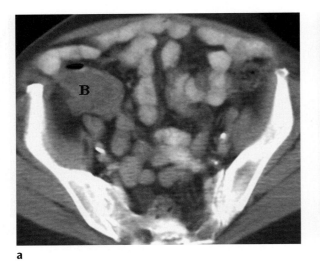
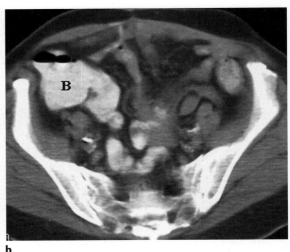

a   b

Figure 3.4 *CT: oral contrast and opacification of the bowel.*
(a) Bowel loops (B) may mimic a mass or abdominal fluid collection on CT. (b) Oral contrast causes opacification of bowel loops (B), thus differentiating them from masses and fluid collections.

Oral contrast is also used for abdomen CT to allow differentiation of normal enhancing bowel loops from abnormal masses or fluid collections (*Fig. 3.4*). For detailed examination of the pelvis, rectal contrast and a vaginal tampon will aid in the differentiation of these structures from pathology.

Further developments

Helical (spiral) CT

CT scanners have now been developed which allow continuous acquisition of data as the patient passes through the gantry. These machines differ from conventional scanners in that the tube and detectors rotate without stops as the patient passes through on the scanning table. In this way, a volumetric set of data is obtained which has a helical configuration (*Fig. 3.5*). This remarkable advance has been due to a number of factors:

- Better X-ray tube technology.

- Better detector technology.

- More sophisticated computer software allowing calculation of the complex data.

- Development of slip-ring technology.

The X-ray tube and detectors rotate on a number of

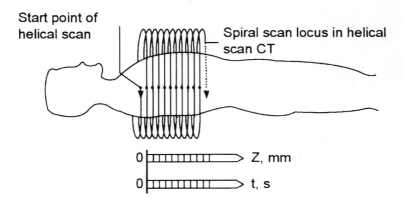

Figure 3.5 *Spiral CT.*
A schematic diagram to show the scanning method of spiral CT. 'Z' represents the Z-plane, i.e. the direction of passage of the patient through the scanner; 't, s' equals time in seconds. Obviously the scanner spins in a circle. The spiral 'shape' of acquired data is due to movement of the patient through the spinning gantry. (Courtesy of GE Medical Systems Australia Pty Ltd.)

slip rings; these are metal rings, which have three functions:

- Supply of high-voltage electricity to the X-ray tube.
- Supply of low-voltage electricity for various control mechanisms.
- Transfer of digital data from the detectors to the computer.

The major advantages of helical scanning over conventional scanning are:

- Increased speed of examination.
- Rapid examination at optimal levels of intravenous contrast concentration.
- Images can be retrospectively reconstructed at any desired level.
- The continuous volumetric nature of data allows accurate high-quality 3D reconstruction.

3D reconstruction techniques have many applications including:

- Planning of cranial and facial reconstruction surgery.
- Repair of fractures in complex areas, e.g. acetabulum.
- CT angiography.

Uses and advantages

The first CT scanners developed, due to their small size, were used only for examination of the head and its contents. With the development of larger scanners, CT is now applied to all areas of the body. CT is the modality of choice for the mediastinum and for many pulmonary conditions. It is also the method of choice for examination of the retroperitoneum and for many disorders of the solid abdominal and pelvic organs. It is excellent in the delineation of bony pathology and it has been used extensively for spinal diseases despite some limitations, as outlined below.

Limitations and disadvantages

Disadvantages of CT relate to its use of ionizing radiation, hazards of intravenous contrast, lack of portability of equipment, and its relatively high cost. A number of areas of the body are imaged relatively poorly with CT. These include the pituitary fossa and the posterior intracranial fossa where artefact from adjacent bony structures obscures normal anatomy. Magnetic resonance imaging (MRI) is the modality of choice for these areas. In the spine, despite its excellent soft tissue contrast capabilities, CT is unable to differentiate spinal cord and nerve roots from surrounding cerebrospinal fluid (CSF). For this reason, MRI is the imaging modality of choice in the spine.

CT imaging is usually limited to the transverse (axial) plane. Exceptions relate to areas of the body that can be tilted in the gantry, e.g. the head or ankles to give coronal scans. Helical scanning allows reconstructive imaging in any plane.

4 Scintigraphy

Physics and terminology

Scintigraphy refers to the use of gamma radiation to form images following the injection of various radio-pharmaceuticals. The key word to understanding scintigraphy is 'radio-pharmaceutical'.

'Radio' refers to the radionuclide, i.e. the emitter of gamma rays. The most commonly used radionuclide in clinical practice is technetium, written in this text as ^{99m}Tc, where 99 is the atomic mass, and the small 'm' stands for 'metastable'. Metastable means that the technetium atom has two basic energy states: high and low. As the technetium passes from the high-energy state to the low-energy state, it emits a packet of energy in the form of a gamma ray which has an energy of 140 keV (*Fig. 4.1*). The gamma rays are detected by a gamma camera that converts the absorbed energy of the radiation to an electric signal. This signal is analysed by a computer and displayed as an image (*Fig. 4.2*). Other commonly used radionuclides include gallium citrate (^{67}Ga), thallium (^{201}Tl), indium (^{111}In) and iodine (^{131}I).

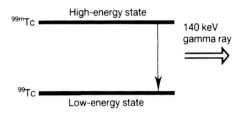

Figure 4.1 *Gamma ray production. The metastable atom ^{99m}Tc in passing from the high-energy state releases gamma radiation which has a peak energy of 140 keV. This makes it very suitable for use in imaging. ^{99m}Tc has a half-life of about 6 h.*

'Pharmaceutical' refers to the compound to which the radionuclide is bound. This compound will depend on the area to be examined. For example, sulphur colloid is taken up by the reticulo-endothelial cells of the liver and spleen and is therefore used in imaging these organs. For some applications a pharmaceutical is not required. An example would be the use of free technetium (^{99m}Tc), referred to as pertechnetate, for thyroid scanning (*Table 4.1*).

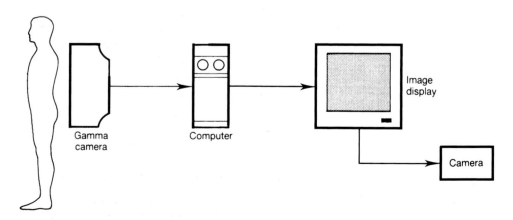

Figure 4.2 *Scintigraphy.*

Table 4.1 *The common radiopharmaceuticals and their applications*

Organ	Radiopharmaceutical	Clinical application
Kidneys	^{99m}Tc-DTPA ^{99m}Tc-MAG3 ^{99m}Tc-DMSA ^{99m}Tc in saline passed into bladder by catheter	Renal function, anatomy, drainage of collecting systems Renal cortical scars Monitoring of vesico-ureteric reflux
Bone	^{99m}Tc-MDP or HDP	Bone metastases, activity of bone lesions, stress fractures
Lungs	Ventilation: ^{99m}Tc–DTPA aerosol Perfusion: ^{99m}Tc-MAA	Pulmonary embolism
Liver/spleen	^{99m}Tc-colloid	Liver/spleen masses
Bile ducts/gallbladder	^{99m}Tc-IDA	Acute cholecystitis, biliary obstruction, biliary atresia, postliver transplant
Thyroid	^{99m}Tc	Thyroid function, thyroiditis, function of thyroid masses, location of aberrant thyroid tissue
Gated cardiac study	Stannous pyrophosphate to reduce Hb then ^{99m}Tc which binds reduced Hb and thus red blood cells	Left ventricular ejection fraction, localized wall motion defects
Gastrointestinal bleeding studies	^{99m}Tc-labelled red blood cells as above	Acute gastrointestinal bleeding
Myocardium	^{201}Tl ^{99m}Tc-sestamibi	Cardiac ischaemia/infarction
Parathyroid	^{99m}Tc-sestamibi	Hyperparathyroidism
Adrenal medulla	^{131}I-MIBG	Localization of phaeochromocytoma, staging of neuroblastoma
CSF	^{111}In-DTPA	Differentiation of communicating hydrocephalus from cerebral atrophy

DTPA, diethylenetriamine pentaacetic acid.
MIBG, metaiodobenzylguanidine.

Areas of high uptake of pharmaceutical and therefore of the radionuclide to which it is bound show resultant high emission of gamma rays, These areas are referred to as 'hot'. Areas of low uptake are referred to as photon-deficient or 'cold'.

Uses and advantages

The main advantages of scintigraphy are:

- Highly sensitive. For example, early osteomyelitis may not be visible on plain films for 7–10 days, while scintigraphy will be positive at the time of presentation.

- Functional information is provided as well as anatomical information. For example, diethylenetriamine pentaacetic acid (DTPA) renal scans provide information on renal function, as well as renal size and drainage of the collecting systems.

Gallium (^{67}Ga) scanning is used in a number of clinical situations. Gallium is bound to plasma proteins, most strongly to transferrin. It is also taken up by white blood cells. Scanning is performed at 24, 48 and occasionally 72 h postinjection. The three most common indications for gallium scanning are:

- To localize occult infection usually in a patient with pyrexia of unknown origin or suspected abdominal abscess not localized by CT or US (see *Fig. 7.33*).

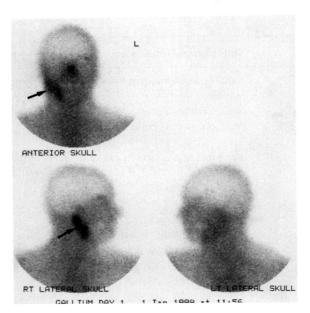

Figure 4.3 *Lymphoma – gallium scan.*
Recurrent non-Hodgkin's lymphoma of the right cervical lymph nodes is well shown as an oval-shaped area of gallium uptake in the right side of the neck.

- To confirm or deny that an abnormality seen on other studies such as plain films is due to infection.

- In staging and follow-up of lymphoma (*Fig. 4.3*), although this role is usually performed by CT.

Limitations and disadvantages

The main disadvantage of scintigraphy is its non-specificity. To take a common example, an isolated 'hot spot' on a bone scan could be due to infection, trauma, or neoplasia and correlation with clinical history and other imaging studies is of paramount importance. On the other hand, multiple 'hot spots' on the bone scan of an elderly man being staged for prostatic carcinoma are easily diagnosed as skeletal metastases.

Furthermore, given the high sensitivity of bone scans, a normal study in such a patient virtually excludes skeletal metastatic disease. Other disadvantages relate

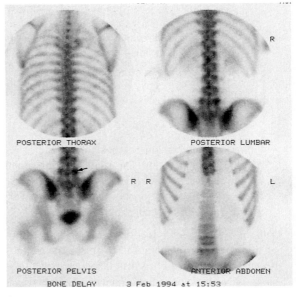

a

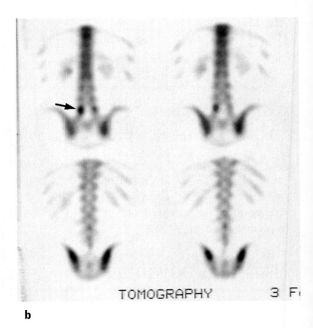

b

Figure 4.4 *Single photon emission computed tomography (SPECT) scan – pars interarticularis defect.*
(a) Conventional bone scan. There is a subtle area of increased uptake of radiopharmaceuticals in the region of the right pars interarticularis of L5 (arrow). (b) SPECT scan. SPECT scans in the coronal plane give a much better demonstration of the 'hot spot' in L5 indicating a pars interarticularis defect (arrow).

to the use of ionizing radiation, the cost of equipment, and the extra care required in handling radioactive materials.

Further developments

SPECT (single photon emission computed tomography)

This is a technique whereby the computer is programmed to analyse data coming from a single depth within the patient. In this way, cross-sectional scans analogous to plain tomography are obtained. This technique allows greater sensitivity in the detection of subtle lesions overlain by other active structures. A common example is the detection of pars interarticularis defects in the lower spine (*Fig. 4.4*). The main applications of SPECT are in bone scanning, ^{201}Tl cardiac scanning, and in cerebral perfusion studies.

PET (positron emission tomography)

PET is a relatively new imaging technique that is gaining increasing acceptance, particularly in the fields of oncology and cardiology. PET requires radionuclides that decay by positron emission. Positron emission occurs when a proton-rich unstable isotope transforms protons from its nucleus into neutrons and positrons. Positron-emitting isotopes are produced in a cyclotron.

PET is based on similar principles to other fields of scintigraphy whereby a radionuclide is attached to a biological compound to form a radiopharmaceutical, which is injected into the patient. The most commonly used radionuclide in PET scanning is FDG, i.e. fluorodeoxyglucose, which is 2-deoxyglucose labelled with the positron-emitter fluorine-18. Positrons emitted from the fluorine-18 in FDG collide with negatively charged electrons. The mass of both particles is converted into two 511 keV photons, i.e. high-energy gamma rays, which are emitted at 180° to each other. This event is known as *annihilation*.

The PET camera consists of a ring of detectors that register the annihilations. An area of high concentration of FDG will have a large number of annihilations and will be shown on the resulting image as a 'hot spot'.

The current roles of PET imaging may be summarized as follows:

- Oncology:

    (i) Differentiate benign and malignant masses, e.g. solitary pulmonary nodule.

    (ii) Primary tumour staging, especially for breast carcinoma, melanoma, non-small cell carcinoma of the lung and Hodgkin's disease.

    (iii) Detect tumour recurrence, especially in areas where changes from surgery or radiotherapy make CT difficult to interpret, e.g. colorectal carcinoma.

- Cardiac:

    (i) Non-invasive assessment of coronary artery disease, i.e. differentiation of viable from non-viable myocardium.

- Central nervous system:

    (i) Characterization of dementia disorders.

    (ii) Localization of seizure focus in epilepsy.

5   Magnetic resonance imaging (MRI)

Physics and terminology

Over the past 10 years, magnetic resonance imaging (MRI) has become accepted as a powerful imaging tool. It uses the magnetic properties of the hydrogen atom to produce images. The physics of MRI is extremely complex and a full discussion would require a much larger book than this (and another author!). The following is a brief summary of the physical principles behind MRI.

The nucleus of the hydrogen atom is a single proton. Being a spinning, charged particle, it has magnetic properties and, for the sake of discussion, may be thought of as a small bar magnet with north and south poles (*Fig. 5.1*). The first step in MRI is the application of a strong, external magnetic field. For this purpose, the patient is placed within a large magnet, either a permanent or superconductive magnet. The hydrogen atoms within the patient align in a direction either parallel or antiparallel to the strong external field. A greater proportion aligns in the parallel direction, so that the net vector of their alignment, and therefore the net magnetic vector, will be in the direction of the external field (*Fig. 5.2*).

Though aligned in a strong magnetic field, the hydrogen nuclei do not lie motionless. Each nucleus spins around the line of the field in a motion known as *precession* (*Fig. 5.3*). The frequency of precession is an inherent property of the hydrogen atom in a given magnetic field and is known as the *Larmor frequency*. The Larmor frequency therefore changes in proportion to magnetic field strength. It is of the order of 10 MHz (megahertz), a frequency in the same part of the electromagnetic spectrum as radio waves.

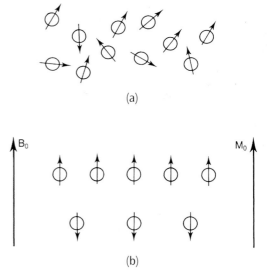

Figure 5.2 *Effect of application of a strong external magnetic field.*
In (a), the hydrogen atoms are randomly aligned in the normal resting state. In (b), a strong external magnetic field, B_0, is applied. The atoms align either parallel or antiparallel to this field. The majority align parallel so their net magnetic vector, M_0, is in the same direction as the external field, B_0.

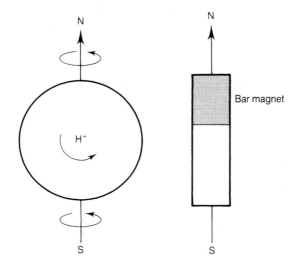

Figure 5.1 *The spinning hydrogen atom.*
The hydrogen atom, being a spinning charged particle, has a small magnetic field, analogous to a bar magnet.

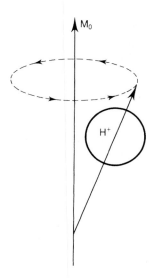

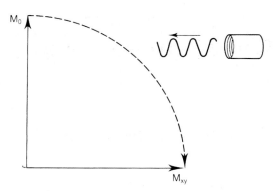

Figure 5.4 *Application of the RF pulse.*
Application of a pulsed magnetic field at 90° to the original field and at the Larmor frequency causes the net magnetic vector of the hydrogen atoms, M_0, to rotate through 90° on to the xy plane.

Figure 5.3 *Precession.*
The hydrogen atom spins around the line of the magnetic field in a motion called precession at a frequency called the Larmor frequency.

A second magnetic field is now applied at right angles to the original external field. This second magnetic field is applied at the same frequency as the Larmor frequency and is known as the *radiofrequency pulse* (RF pulse). A second magnetic coil, the RF coil, applies the RF pulse. The RF pulse causes the net magnetization vector of the hydrogen atoms to turn towards the transverse plane, i.e. a plane at right angles to the

direction of the original, strong external field (*Fig. 5.4*). As such, the RF pulse adds energy to the system. Following cessation of the RF pulse, the extra energy is dissipated to the surrounding chemical lattice in a process known as T1 *relaxation*. In addition, the RF pulse brings the precessing protons into phase, i.e. their spins are now in synchrony. The process of dephasing, which occurs due to tiny inhomogeneities in the nuclear magnetic environment, is known as T2 *relaxation*.

The component of the net magnetization vector in the transverse plane induces a current in magnetic coils

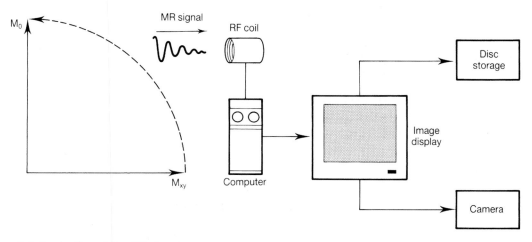

Figure 5.5 *Production of the MR signal.*
When the RF pulse is switched off, the net magnetization vector returns to its original direction and emits a signal that is received by the RF coil. This signal is analysed by computer to produce an image.

known as *radiofrequency, or RF receiver coils.* This current is known as the *MR signal* and is the basis for formation of an image. Note that the MR signal can be produced only when the precession of the spinning protons is in phase. Complex computer analysis of the MR signal from the RF receiver coils is used to produce an MR image (*Fig. 5.5*).

Whereas CT depends on tissue density and ultrasound on tissue echogenicity, much of the complexity of MRI arises from the fact that the MR signal depends on many varied properties of substances being examined. These properties include:

- Proton density.
- The chemical environment of the hydrogen atoms, e.g. whether in free water or bound by fat.
- Flow: blood vessels or CSF.
- Magnetic susceptibility.
- T1 relaxation time.
- T2 relaxation time.

By altering the duration and amplitude of the RF pulse, as well as the timing and repetition of its application, various sequences have been developed to use and accentuate these various properties. The most common types of images produced have been:

- TI-weighted: excellent anatomical definition, though with lower sensitivity to pathology.
- T2-weighted: highly sensitive to the presence of pathology.

Numerous other image sequences are now used. A common example is fat suppression sequences that are excellent for demonstrating pathology in areas containing a lot of fat, e.g. the orbits and bone marrow. Inversion recovery sequences are used increasingly in the investigation of CNS and skeletal disorders. Short T1-inverted recovery (STIR) sequences give excellent delineation of subtle bone marrow disorders such as oedema and infiltration. Fluid-attenuated inversion recovery (FLAIR) sequences are commonly used to image the brain and are particularly useful for demyelinating disorders such as multiple sclerosis.

Note that in viewing MRI images, white or light grey areas are referred to as 'high signal'; dark grey or black areas are referred to as 'low signal'. On certain sequences flowing blood is seen as a black area referred to as a 'flow void'.

Uses and advantages

The main advantages of MRI are as follows:

Excellent soft tissue contrast

As explained above, MRI uses many varied properties of matter in the generation of an image.

Lack of artefact from adjacent bones

This makes MRI the imaging modality of choice in areas such as the posterior fossa and pituitary fossa where the quality of CT images is degraded by artefact (*Fig. 5.6*).

Multiplanar capabilities

MRI is able to obtain images in any plane. The sagittal plane is particularly useful for the spine and this property, combined with the excellent soft tissue contrast, makes MRI the modality of choice for imaging of spinal disorders. Multiple planes are also useful in the musculoskeletal system, e.g. sagittal and coronal planes for the knee, and coronal and oblique planes for the shoulder.

Lack of ionizing radiation

In summary, MRI is the imaging modality of choice for most brain and spine disorders. It has also found wide acceptance in the assessment of musculoskeletal disorders. Although excellent for visualization of the heart, echocardiography is more widely used as it produces functional as well as anatomical information. MRI has not displaced other modalities such as CT, ultrasound and endoscopy in the imaging of most thoracic and abdominal disorders.

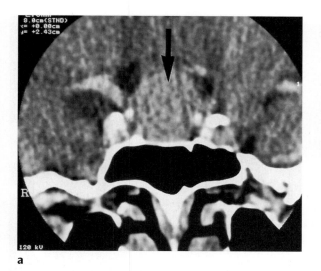
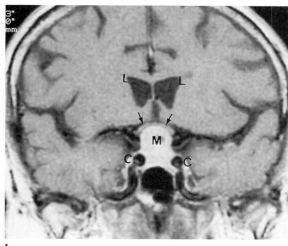

a   b

Figure 5.6 *Pituitary adenoma.*
(a) CT. CT in the coronal plane demonstrates a mass arising from the pituitary fossa (arrow). (b) MRI T1-weighted image with contrast. Anatomical detail is much better than with CT. Note:

- *mass arising from the pituitary fossa (M)*
- *compressed optic chiasm (arrows)*
- *carotid arteries on either side (C)*
- *lateral ventricles (L).*

Limitations and disadvantages

Cost

The equipment for MRI is very expensive. Running and maintenance costs are also high. Potential benefits to patient care must be carefully weighed against these costs when ordering MRI scans.

Artefacts

Although free of artefacts from bony structures, a wide variety of artefacts does occur in MRI.

Metal foreign objects

See Chapter 6.

Reduced sensitivity for certain substances

MRI is less sensitive than CT in the detection of small amounts of calcification and in the detection of acute haemorrhage. As such, CT is still the imaging modality of choice for the assessment of acute subarachnoid haemorrhage and for acute head injury.

Fine bone detail

MRI is unable to provide the degree of bone detail possible with CT, although it is more sensitive in the detection of infiltrative disorders of bone marrow.

Further developments

Contrast material

Gadolinium (Gd) is a paramagnetic substance that causes increased signal on T1-weighted images.

Unbound gadolinium is highly toxic. For this reason, binding agents are required for *in vivo* use. The most common of these is diethylenetriamine pentaacetic acid (DTPA). Gd-DTPA is non-toxic and used in a dose of 0.1 mmol per kilogram.

The main indications for the use of Gd-DTPA are as follows:

Brain

- Multiple lesions, e.g. metastases, multiple sclerosis.
- Selected tumours, e.g. acoustic neuroma, meningioma (*Fig. 5.7*).
- Tumour residuum/recurrence following treatment.

Spine

- Metastases: intraspinal, CSF.
- Tumour recurrence.
- Postoperative to differentiate fibrosis from recurrent disc protrusion.
- Infection.
- Selected tumours, e.g. neurofibroma.

Musculoskeletal system

- Soft tissue tumours.
- Intra-articular Gd-DTPA in subtle shoulder disorders.

Magnetic resonance angiography (MRA)

With varying sequences, flowing blood can be shown as either signal void (i.e. black), or increased signal (i.e. white). Computer reconstruction techniques allow the display of blood vessels in 3D, and allow viewing of the blood vessels from any angle. Indications would include:

- Imaging of the carotid arteries for stroke and transient ischaemic attack (TIA).
- Aneurysm and arteriovenous malformation (AVM).
- Imaging of the peripheral vessels for claudication.

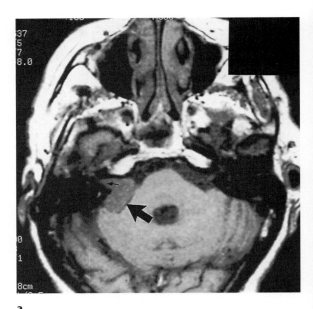

a

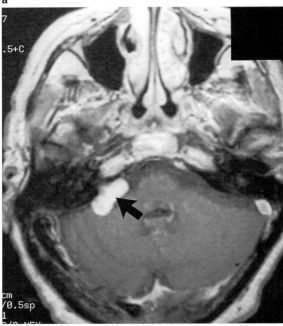

b

Figure 5.7 *MRI with contrast – acoustic neuroma. (a) T1-weighted scan, axial plane. Right cerebellopontine angle mass (large arrow). The mass shows lateral extension into the internal auditory meatus (small arrow), typical of acoustic neuroma. (b) T1-weighted scan with contrast, axial plane. The cerebellopontine angle mass shows quite marked enhancement (arrow).*

Echoplanar imaging (EPI)

Echoplanar imaging (EPI) is an ultrafast MRI technique that has resulted from improvements in hardware, software and instrumentation, as well as the development of newer imaging sequences. The ability to apply large magnetic field gradients extremely rapidly with reduced data sampling times means that artefacts due to motion are markedly reduced. With EPI, the visualization of physiological events is now possible and this has led to new functional applications including BOLD imaging, diffusion and perfusion-weighted imaging, and spectroscopy.

Blood oxygen-level-dependent (BOLD) imaging

BOLD imaging is a non-invasive functional MRI (fMRI) technique used for localizing regional brain signal intensity changes in response to task performance. It does not require injection of contrast. Rather, BOLD imaging depends on regional changes in concentration of deoxyhaemoglobin, and is therefore a tool to investigate regional cerebral physiology in response to a variety of stimuli. BOLD fMRI may be used prior to surgery for brain tumour or AVM, as a prognostic indicator of the degree of postsurgical deficit.

Diffusion-weighted imaging (DWI)

Diffusion refers to the random motion (Brownian motion) of all molecules, which is driven by thermal energy. MRI may be made sensitive to diffusion by the addition of balanced gradient pulses to spin echo sequences. With diffusion-weighted imaging, signal loss occurs in areas of high diffusion rates. In acute stroke there is reduced diffusion and therefore relatively increased signal. Signal changes visible on DWI have been shown to occur almost instantly following an ischaemic event, and certainly much earlier than with any other imaging technique (see *Fig. 14.15*). DWI may also be used to characterize certain cerebral masses, e.g. epidermoid cyst.

Because of the tiny distances involved in molecular diffusion, DWI is inherently extremely sensitive to motion. Ultrashort imaging times are therefore mandatory and DWI can only be performed on a machine capable of echoplanar imaging.

Perfusion-weighted imaging (PWI)

PWI is a technique whereby cerebral tissue perfusion may be measured following injection of contrast agents. Dynamic imaging is performed during first passage of a contrast bolus. Various measurements may be made including cerebral blood flow and transit time, and maps of relative cerebral blood flow may be generated. PWI will therefore detect areas of reduced perfusion.

MR spectroscopy (MRS)

MRS uses different frequencies to identify certain molecules in a selected volume of tissue, known as a voxel. An area of interest is selected by conventional MRI imaging, followed by spectroscopic analysis. Following data analysis, a spectrographic graph of certain metabolites is drawn. Metabolites of interest include the following:

- Lipid.

- Lactate.

- NAA (n-acetyl-aspartate). This is a neuronal marker, with reduced concentration in focal brain lesions such as abscess and infarct.

- Choline. Choline is a marker of membrane synthesis with increased concentration in neoplasm and reduced concentration in stroke and dementia.

- Creatinine (Cr). Cr is an end-product of anaerobic glycolysis with increased concentration in infection and tumour.

- Myoinositol. Early research indicates an increased concentration of myoinositol in Alzhiemer's disease.

Possible uses of MRS include imaging of dementias, and characterization of changes seen on conventional MRI in relation to cerebral neoplasm as follows:

- Recurrent tumour vs radiation necrosis.

- Recurrent tumour vs normal postoperative changes.

- Tumour infiltration vs oedema.

Multivoxel MRS is a developing field in which multiple spectra may be obtained in a single acquisition. This will allow thorough lesion characterization and mapping.

6   Hazards and precautions in medical imaging

This chapter deals with the hazards and risks associated with the field of medical imaging. It is important for the referring doctor to have a working knowledge of these factors when considering whether to order an imaging investigation. The chapter is divided into the following topics:

- Contrast media reactions
- Radiation hazards
- Protection in radiological practice
- MRI safety issues

The first of these sections has been written by an anaesthetist colleague, Dr Andrew Russell.

Contrast media reactions
Andrew Russell

Immediate generalized reactions are presently classified as anaphylactoid though more recent work suggests an IgE mechanism is involved in a substantial number of severe reactions. Clinically these reactions are indistinguishable from anaphylaxis. Other mechanisms that may be implicated particularly in more minor incidents are:

- Direct histamine release from mast cells and basophils.
- Complement activation.
- Disruption of the vascular endothelium and consequent recruitment of other chemical mediators such as kinins.

Risk factors

- Previous adverse reaction to contrast (10–30 fold).
- Allergic history including asthma (4-fold).
- Conventional high osmolar media > lower osmolar non-ionic media.
- Intravenous > intra-arterial > injection into body cavities such as thecal sac or joints > oral.
- Anxious patient.
- Patient on beta-blocker medication.
- Fatal reactions are more likely in elderly, debilitated patients.

Clinical features

Minor reaction (5–8%)

- Rash, flushed.
- Rhinitis, cough.
- Mild urticaria, pruritis.
- Nausea, vomiting.

Major reaction (0.1%)

- Commonest manifestation is cardiovascular collapse.
- Bronchospasm, pulmonary oedema.
- Angioedema, laryngeal oedema.
- Vomiting, gastrointestinal cramps.
- Death (0.01–0.04%).

Treatment

Minor reaction

- Cease administration of contrast.

- Reassure patient.
- Establish intravenous access.
- Oral or parenteral antihistamines.

Major reaction

There are three essential points to remember:

- Oxygen.
- Adrenaline.
- Fluids.

Detailed protocol for treatment of a major reaction

Death is most likely to occur during or within 5 min of injection. Hence resuscitation must be rapid and effective.

- Call for help.
- ABC:

  (i) Secure airway and maintain oxygenation.

  (ii) Secure iv access with large bore cannula (18-gauge minimum).

  (iii) If pulseless, commence external heart massage.

  (iv) Institute regular monitoring of the patient including oxygen saturation, blood pressure, pulse rate, ECG, and commence recording of observations and drugs given.

  (v) Remember simple manoeuvres such as Trendelenberg position for hypotension.

- Adrenaline:

  (i) The drug of choice and the preferred route of administration is iv.

  (ii) The dose is 3–5 mL of 1:10 000 and repeat as needed or commence an infusion 0.3–0.5 mL of 1:1000 s/c or imi if very early in the course of reaction, if no iv access or unmonitored cardiac patient due to risk of arrhythmias.

  (iii) If iv access is lost during resuscitation then the administration of adrenaline should not be delayed until iv access is established.

- Fluids:

  (i) May need 1–2 L and colloid solutions are more effective than crystalloid in severe cases.

- Ensure regular reassessment of adequacy of resuscitation of patient and once stable continue observation in hospital for at least 12 h as late deterioration may occur.

- Investigation. Severity of reaction correlates with the level of mast cell tryptase and serum histamine though the rise in histamine is very transient, peaking at 2 h.

- Follow-up. The nature of the reaction and the response to treatment should be accurately documented. The patient is given a letter, and advised to wear a warning device such as a Medi-alert bracelet should future administration of contrast be necessary.

Cardiovascular collapse

If blood pressure remains low, central venous pressure measurement may be helpful. Rarely, severe hypotension may not respond to adrenaline and may necessitate the use of other inotropes such as noradrenaline and dopamine. Intravenous H2 blockers may also be helpful in cases of prolonged profound hypotension.

Bronchospasm

If severe, this is the most difficult feature to treat. Adrenaline is the drug of first choice. If inadequate response consider:

- Continuous nebulized and iv infusion of beta agonists.
- Aminophylline if no response to above.
- Steroids, though response not immediate.
- Intubation and intermittent positive-pressure ventilation (IPPV) may be necessary.
- If conventional treatment has failed, an inhalational anaesthetic or ketamine may be life saving.

Pulmonary oedema

The oedema that occurs during anaphylaxis is a membrane type and is associated with a volume deficit. Treatment is positive end expiratory pressure (PEEP) and cautious fluid replacement with colloid, *not* morphine and diuretics.

Angioedema, laryngeal oedema

Early intubation is the treatment of choice. Following the administration of adrenaline the oedema does not progress. To prevent a recurrence an H1 antihistamine should be given.

Prevention of allergic reaction in high-risk patients

Recheck with patient about previous reactions to contrast material and other risk factors. Does the patient really need contrast material? Document the reason on the chart. Advise patient of risk of exposure to contrast material. Reduce likelihood of reaction:

- Use non-ionic, low osmolality contrast.

- Cease or replace beta-blocker medication.

- Use a pretreatment regime:
  (i)   Premedicate, e.g. Temazepam 10–20 mg 1 h prior to procedure.
  (ii)   Prednisone 50 mg po 13,7,1 h precontrast.
  (iii) Diphenhydramine 50 mg orally.

- If procedure is urgent:
  (i)   Hydrocortisone 200 mg iv immediately and then 4-hourly till procedure.
  (ii)   Diphenhydramine 50 mg imi.

- Do not presume a pretreated patient cannot experience a severe reaction. These precautions will not prevent all reactions.

- Ensure staff are skilled in the treatment of severe reactions and the appropriate resuscitation equipment is immediately available.

- Secure iv access with large-bore cannula and commence monitoring (blood pressure, ECG, oxygen saturation).

- Document on the chart and in patient letter the response to contrast on this occasion.

Pretesting with a small dose of contrast has been shown to be ineffective and dangerous.

Further reading

Anderson JA. Allergic reactions to drugs and biological agents. *JAMA* 1992; **268**: 2845–2857.

Brasch RC. The case strengthens for allergy to contrast media. *Radiology* 1998; **209**: 35–36.

Bush WH, Swanson DP. Acute reactions to intravascular contrast media. *AJR* 1991; **157**: 1153–1161.

Desforges JF. Anaphylaxis. *NEJM* 1991; **324**: 1785–1790.

Fisher MM. Acute life threatening reactions to contrast media. *Aust Radiol* 1978; **22**: 365–367.

Fisher MM. Treating anaphylaxis with sympathomimetic drugs. *BMJ* 1992; **305**: 1107–1108.

Fisher MM, Baldo BA. Respiratory complications of anaphylaxis. *Ballière's Clinical Anaesthesiology* 1993; **7**: 867–872.

Greenberger PA, Patterson R. The prevention of immediate generalized reactions to contrast media. *J Allergy Clinical Immunology* 1991; **67**: 91–97.

Lang DM. Increased risk for anaphylactoid reaction from contrast media in patients on beta blockers or with asthma. *Ann Int Med* 1991; **115**: 270–276.

Larouche D. Mechanisms of severe immediate reactions to iodinated contrast media. *Radiology* 1998; **209**: 183–190.

Liberman P. Anaphylactoid reactions to radiocontrast materials. *Ann Allergy* 1991; **67**: 91–97.

Marik PE. Allergic reactions to oral contrast agent. *AJR* 1997; **168**: 1623.

Ridley LJ. Allergic reaction to oral iodinated contrast agents. *Aust Radiol* 1998; **42**: 114–117.

Stellato C. Pathophysiology of contrast media anaphylactoid reactions. *Allergy* 1998; **53**: 1133–1140.

Radiation hazards

The International Commission on Radiological Protection (ICRP) was set up in 1928. It consists of expert delegates from many countries and its recommendations are accepted as worldwide standards. This section is a summary of numerous ICRP publications and recommendations on radiation hazards and protection, as well as recommendations of the National Health and Medical Research Council of Australia.

Radiation hazards occur as a result of damage to cells caused by radiation. This damage takes many forms:

- Cell death.

- Mitotic inhibition (temporary/permanent).

- Chromosome damage/genetic damage leading to mutations.

- Actively dividing cells are particularly sensitive (i.e. bone marrow, lymph glands, gonads).

The nature and degree of cell damage vary according to:

- Radiation dose.

- Dose rate.

- Irradiated volume.

- Type of radiation.

In general, two types of effects are seen as a result of radiation damage:

Stochastic effects

- Probability of effect, not severity, regarded as a function of dose.

- No dose threshold below which an effect will not theoretically occur.

- Due to modified cell, e.g. somatic cell leading to cancers; reproduction cell leading to hereditary effect.

Deterministic effects

- Severity of effects varies with dose.

- Dose threshold may exist below which the effect will not occur.

- Due to cell death, deterministic effects occur when cell loss is sufficient to impair organ function (e.g. radiation burns, cataracts and decreased fertility).

Units of radiation dose

Absorbed dose

- Absorbed dose refers to the amount of energy imparted by ionizing radiation in a given mass of matter.

- The SI unit is joules per kilogram (i.e. $J\,kg^{-1}$) and is referred to as the Gray (Gy): $1\,Gy = 1.0\,J\,kg^{-1}$.

Dose equivalent

- The concept of dose equivalent takes into account the fact that some kinds of radiation can produce more damage in tissue than others, even though the absorbed dose may be the same.

- Weighting factors are used for various radiation types, as outlined in Table 6.1 below.

Table 6.1 *Weighting factors for calculation of equivalent dose*

Type of radiation	Weighting factor
Photons i.e. X-rays and gamma rays	1
Electrons	1
Neutrons	5–20 depending on energy
Protons	5
Alpha particles	20

Equivalent dose = weighting factor $\times$ absorbed dose.
The SI unit is joules per kilogram (i.e. $J\,kg^{-1}$) and is referred to as the Sievert (Sv): $1\,Sv = 1.0\,J\,kg^{-1}$.

Examples of typical doses to an adult patient for some common X-ray procedures are given in Tables 6.2 and 6.3.

Table 6.2 *Dose per film (mGy = 0.001 Gy)*

Examination	Skin	Bone marrow	Ovary
Abdomen AP	4.9	0.48	0.84
Chest PA	0.2	0.042	0.002
Pelvis AP	4.0	0.530	0.75
IVP	5.2	0.47	0.53
Lumbar spine lateral	20.7	0.79	1.36

Table 6.3 *Examples of typical doses to an adult patient from some common nuclear medicine studies*

Study	Total body dose equivalent (mSv)
Thyroid scan ^{99m}Tc	11.6
Bone scan ^{99m}Tc-MDP	5.2
Lung scan ^{99m}Tc-MAA	1.8
Gallium scan ^{67}Ga	20.3

Total average intake from natural background radioactivity, including cosmic and terrestrial radiation, is 1–2 mSv per year.

In considering the concept of detriment caused by radiation exposure, four factors are considered:

- Probability of developing a fatal cancer.

- Probability of developing a non-fatal cancer.

- Probability of severe hereditary effects.

- Length of life lost if harm occurs.

Based heavily on studies of Japanese survivors of atomic bomb attacks, ICRP-calculated probability coefficients for stochastic effects in the general population are as follows:

Detriment (10–2/Sv)

Fatal cancer:	5.0
Non-fatal cancer:	1.0
Severe hereditary effects:	1.3
Total	7.3

For example, if 100 people are exposed to 1 Sv of radiation, five will theoretically develop a fatal cancer.

A dose of 5–6 Sv over a short time period leads to acute radiation sickness and death.

Protection in radiological practice

Aims and principles of radiation protection are:

- To prevent deterministic effects.

- To limit the probability of stochastic effects by keeping all justifiable exposure *as low as is reasonably achievable* (ALARA principle): this includes keeping as low as possible doses to individuals, the number of people exposed, and the likelihood of others being exposed.

- No practice is adopted unless its introduction produces a benefit that outweighs its detriment, i.e. positive net benefit.

With these aims and principles in mind, the following guidelines are used for radiographic procedures.

Protection of patient

- Each exposure justified on a case-by-case basis.

- Minimize number of X-ray films taken. Minimize screening time.

- Focus beam accurately to area of interest.

- Only trained personnel to operate equipment. Good equipment to be used including rare earth screens, adequate filtration of X-ray beams, etc.

- Minimize the use of mobile equipment. Use ultrasound or MRI where possible. Quality assurance programmes in each department, including correct installation, calibration and regular testing of equipment.

Paediatrics

- Special attention to minimizing number of exposures, screening times, and the use of well-focused beams.

- Use of restraining devices and/or sedation. Gonad shields.

- If parents are required in the room, they should wear lead coats and not be directly exposed to radiation.

Women of reproductive age

- Minimize radiation exposure of abdomen and pelvis.

- Consider any woman of reproductive age whose period is overdue to be pregnant.

- Ask all females of reproductive age if they could be pregnant.

- Post multilingual signs in prominent places asking patients to notify the radiographer of possible pregnancy.

Pregnancy

- As organogenesis is unlikely to be occurring in an embryo in the first 4 weeks following the last menstrual period, this is not considered a critical period for radiation exposure.

- Organogenesis commences soon after the time of

the first missed period and continues for the next 3–4 months; hence during this time the foetus is considered to be radiosensitive.

- Examination of the abdomen or pelvis should be delayed if possible to a time when foetal sensitivity is reduced, i.e. post-24 weeks' gestation (or ideally until the baby is born).

- Where possible, US or MRI should be used.

- Exposure to remote areas (e.g. chest, skull and limbs) may be undertaken with minimal foetal exposure at any time during pregnancy.

- Lead aprons draped over the abdomen are more reassuring than of practical value.

- Nuclear medicine studies are best avoided if possible during pregnancy.

- For nuclear medicine studies in the postpartum period, it is advised that breast-feeding be ceased and breast milk discarded for 2 days following the injection of radionuclide.

Protection of staff (including medical students!)

- Only necessary staff to be present in a room where X-ray procedures are being performed: TV monitors placed outside the screening room usually mean that students may observe procedures at a safe distance.

- Staff to wear protective clothing (e.g. lead aprons).

- At no time should staff be directly irradiated by the primary beam: lead gloves must be worn if the hands may be irradiated (e.g. in immobilizing patients or performing stress views).

- All X-ray rooms should have lead lining in their walls, ceilings and floors.

MRI safety issues

MRI involves the use of a strong static magnetic field, rapidly switching magnetic gradient fields, and radiofrequency (RF) fields. At the time of writing there is no evidence of direct deleterious biological effects

from any of these sources. However, a number of potential hazards associated with MRI do exist. These predominantly relate to the interaction of the magnetic fields with metallic materials and electronic devices.

The field from the MRI unit can be described in terms of two spatial regions. Region 1 refers to the area around the isocentre of the magnetic field within the bore of the magnet. Ferromagnetic objects within region 1 experience rotational forces or torque. Region 2 refers to the field outside the bore of the magnet. The strength of this field decreases with distance from the magnet. Metal objects within region 2 experience rotational and translational forces, i.e. objects are pulled toward the magnet. Reports exist of objects such as spanners, oxygen cylinders and drip poles becoming missiles; the hazards to personnel are obvious. The most widely used safety standard is the '5 Gauss line'. This is the line around the magnet in both horizontal and vertical planes beyond which the magnetic field strength is less than 5 Gauss (0.0005 T). Physical barriers and prominent signs should be used to prevent entry within the 5 Gauss line of any person not screened as below and not accompanied by a trained technician.

More importantly, ferromagnetic materials within the patient could potentially be moved by the magnetic field causing tissue damage. The two most common problems are:

- Metal fragments in the eye.

- Intracerebral aneurysm clips.

Patients at risk for metal fragments in the eye, e.g. those with a past history of penetrating eye injury or possible occupational exposure, should be screened prior to entering the MRI room with plain films of the orbits. MRI compatible aneurysm clips are now being manufactured. MRI should not be performed until the safety of an individual device has been established.

The presence of electrically active implants, i.e. cardiac pacemakers, cochlear implants and neurostimulators, is a contraindication to MRI unless the safety of an individual device is proven.

Other causes for concern in MRI include:

High auditory noise levels

Earplugs should be provided to all patients undergoing MRI examinations.

Claustrophobia

Although 'open' magnets are available on the market, the majority of MRI machines are in the shape of a tunnel and claustrophobia remains a major issue affecting a significant number of patients. Sedation is therefore a common procedure, used in up to 10% of cases. Adequate monitoring of the sedated patient by properly trained staff using MRI-compatible equipment is mandatory.

Allergy to injected contrast materials

Although rare, anaphylactoid reactions to gadolinium compounds have been reported. For treatment see above.

RF burns

Rare reports exist of RF burns associated with inductive heating of conducting leads placed against the patient's skin. Where possible, MRI-compatible instruments should be used, e.g. pulse oximeters. Care should be taken to separate conducting leads such as ECG leads from the patient's skin.

Peripheral nerve stimulation

Rapidly switching magnetic fields can stimulate muscles and peripheral nerves. Guidelines are used in MRI to limit the rate of gradient field switching to well below the threshold for nerve stimulation.

Pregnancy

There is no evidence of any adverse effects of MRI in pregnancy.

Management of risk

There are two basic measures involved in reduction and management of risk in MRI:

- Education programme.
- Screening of staff and patients.

Education programme

An education programme covering the risks as outlined above should be given to all medical staff associated with MRI including doctors, nurses, radiographers and other technologists. Other staff who may enter the scanning room such as engineers, cleaners and security staff should be included.

Screening of staff and patients

A standard questionnaire should cover any relevant factors such as:

- Previous surgical history;
- The presence of metal foreign bodies including aneurysm clips, etc.
- The presence of cochlear implants and cardiac pacemakers.
- Any possible occupational exposure to metal fragments.
- Any other factors such as previous allergic reaction.

Where clips or implants are present, safety of individual devices must be confirmed prior to the patient entering the MRI room. Where there is possible occupational exposure to metal fragments, a radiograph of the orbits should be performed.

7 Respiratory system

Chest X-ray

Projections performed

A standard chest X-ray (CXR) examination consists of two projections, as follows.

PA erect

The patient stands with his or her anterior chest wall up against the X-ray film. The X-ray tube lies behind the patient so that X-rays pass through in a posterior to anterior (PA) direction.

Reasons for performing the film PA:

- Accurate assessment of cardiac size due to minimal magnification.
- Scapulae able to be rotated out of the way.

Reasons for performing the film erect:

- Physiological representation of blood vessels of mediastinum and lung; in the supine position mediastinal veins and upper lobe vessels may be distended leading to misinterpretation, e.g. overdiagnosis of widened mediastinum on supine CXR.
- Gas passes upwards: pneumothorax is more easily diagnosed, as is free gas beneath the diaphragm.
- Fluid passes downwards, therefore pleural effusion is more easily diagnosed.

Lateral

Reasons for performing a lateral CXR:

- Further view of lungs, especially those areas obscured on the PA film, e.g. posterior segments of lower lobes, areas behind the hila, left lower lobe, which lies behind the heart on the PA.
- Further assessment of cardiac configuration.

- Further anatomical localization of lesions.
- More sensitive for pleural effusions.
- Good view of thoracic spine.

In general, the use of two views, PA and lateral, is advocated in the assessment of most chest conditions.

Exceptions where a PA film alone would suffice are:

- 'Screening' in young people, e.g. for insurance or diving medicals.
- Large-population screening programmes, e.g. for TB.
- Follow-up of known conditions seen well on the PA, e.g. pneumonia following antibiotics, metastases following chemotherapy, pneumothorax following drainage.

Other projections that may be used instead of, or as well as, the two standard views are outlined below.

AP/supine X-ray

- Where the patient is too ill to stand, i.e. ICU, CCU, trauma, very elderly patients.
- Note that the mediastinum will appear wider on an AP supine film due to venous distension and magnification.
- This may lead to an incorrect diagnosis of widened mediastinum which may be a trap, e.g. in a chest trauma patient where aortic rupture needs to be excluded.

Expiratory film

- Suspected pneumothorax.
- Suspected bronchial obstruction with air trapping (e.g. inhaled foreign body in a child).

Decubitus film

- Radiograph performed with the patient lying on his/her side.

- Used occasionally in patients too ill to stand to exclude pleural effusion or pneumothorax.

Lordotic view

- Radiograph taken with the patient leaning backwards against the X-ray film and the X-ray tube is angled up.

- Shows the apical region, which may be obscured by overlying ribs and clavicle on the PA film.

- Used less since the advent of CT.

Oblique views

- Used to show the ribs or sternum.

Technical assessment

Prior to making diagnostic pronouncements, pause briefly to assess the technical quality of the PA film; the following factors should be considered:

Ensure patient properly centred on film

The radiograph should include the lung apices and both costophrenic angles.

Rotation

The easiest way to ensure that there is no rotation is to check that the spinous processes of the upper thoracic vertebrae lie midway between the medial ends of the clavicles.

Ensure adequate inspiration

The diaphragms should lie at the level of the 5th or 6th ribs anteriorly. A straight trachea should be seen in children.

Ensure proper exposure

The lower thoracic vertebral bodies should be faintly discernible through the heart. Blood vessels to the left lower lobe should be seen through the heart. Most dedicated departments use 'high kilovolt (kV)' techniques for chest radiography. The lungs and mediastinal outlines are shown superbly with this technique.

Diagnostic assessment of the CXR

A teacher of mine once said that the best aid to viewing CXRs would be a 1 metre cage strapped to the chest of the viewer! Most medical students to whom I show CXRs peer closely at the film, as if the answer is written in tiny letters on the patient's lungs. The best tip I can give is to stand back a bit when viewing radiographs. If you don't believe me, try this small experiment: stand 1 metre away from a CXR and assess it as directed below. Now move as close to the film as you like and see if any further information presents itself. In the majority of cases it won't.

When starting to look at radiographs try to use a system. This will help you avoid missing relevant findings. A systematic approach to analysis of the CXR should include identification and assessment of the following:

PA film

Heart

- Position.

- Size.

- Configuration.

Mediastinum

- Trachea.

- Aorta.

- Pulmonary arteries.

- Superior vena cava (SVC).

- Azygos vein.

Lungs

Divide each lung into thirds, first from top to bottom, then from the hilum to the periphery. Look at top, middle and lower thirds, followed by medial, central and lateral thirds. Assess the vascular pattern: compare upper lobe vessels to lower lobe vessels. Look particularly at difficult areas where lesions are easily missed:

- Behind the heart.

- Behind each hilum.

- Behind the diaphragms.

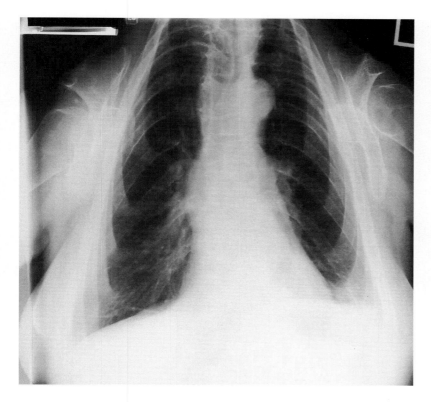

Figure 7.1 *Absent clavicles – cleidocranial dysplasia.*
This film illustrates the benefit of using a systematic approach in viewing radiographs. A gross finding such as absent clavicles can be surprisingly easy to miss. As such, this sort of case is a favourite with certain examiners.

- Lung apices.

Check the lung contours for signs of blurring or loss of definition:

- Cardiac borders.
- Mediastinal margins.
- Diaphragms.

Bones

- Ribs.
- Clavicles (*Fig. 7.1*).
- Scapulae/humeri.
- Sternum on the lateral film.
- Thoracic vertebral bodies.

Other

In female patients, check the breast shadows for evidence of previous mastectomy. Check below the diaphragm for free gas and to ensure that the stomach bubble is in correct position. Check the axillae and lower neck for masses.

Lateral film

Heart

- Size.
- Configuration.

Mediastinum

- Trachea.
- Right and left pulmonary arteries.

Lungs

- Retrosternal airspace.
- Retrocardiac airspace.
- Identify both hemidiaphragms.
- Posterior costophrenic angles: very small pleura effusions are seen with greater sensitivity than the PA film.

Bones

- Sternum and thoracic spine.

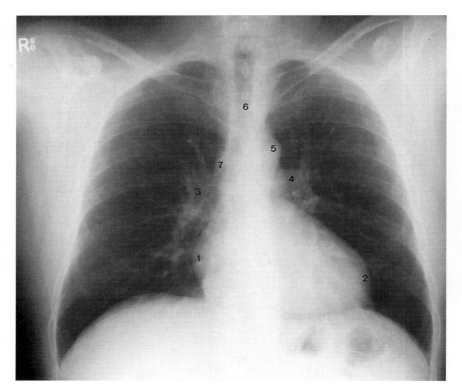

Figure 7.2 *Normal PA chest X-ray.*

Identify the following structures: 1, right heart border; 2, left heart border; 3, right hilum; 4, left hilum; 5, aortic knuckle; 6, trachea; 7, azygos vein.

- The lower thoracic vertebral bodies should appear blacker than upper ones. Increased apparent density of the lower vertebral bodies may be the only sign of consolidation in the posterior basal segments of the lower lobes. This area is difficult to see on the PA film due to overlying diaphragm.

Radiographic anatomy

The PA view (*Fig. 7.2*)

The trachea is well seen in the midline, as is its division into right and left main bronchi. A thin line on the right margin of the trachea is noted. This is termed the right paratracheal stripe. It is an important line to look for on the PA view as it may be lost or thickened in the presence of lymphadenopathy. The right paratracheal stripe is continuous inferiorly with a small convex opacity, which sits in the concavity formed by the junction of the trachea and right main bronchus. This opacity is formed by the azygos vein, seen 'end-on' as it loops forwards over the right main bronchus to enter the SVC. The SVC is often seen as a straight line, contin-

uous inferiorly with the right heart border. The right heart border is formed by the right atrium, outlined by the aerated right middle lobe. The right hilum lies approximately midway between the diaphragm and lung apex. It is formed by the right main bronchus and right pulmonary artery, and their lobar divisions.

The left mediastinal border can be thought of as three convexities. The most superior of these, sometimes termed the aortic knuckle, is formed by the aortic arch. The descending aorta can be traced downwards from this convexity. It forms a line to the left of the spine. This line may be obscured by a posterior mediastinal mass, or by pathology in the left lower lobe. The second convexity is quite variable and is formed by the main pulmonary artery. Posterior to this and extending laterally is the left hilum. It consists of the left main bronchus and left pulmonary artery and their main lobar divisions. The largest and most inferior convexity is the left heart border. The left heart border is formed by the left ventricle, except in cases where the right ventricle is enlarged. The left atrial appendage lies on the upper left cardiac border; it is not seen unless enlarged.

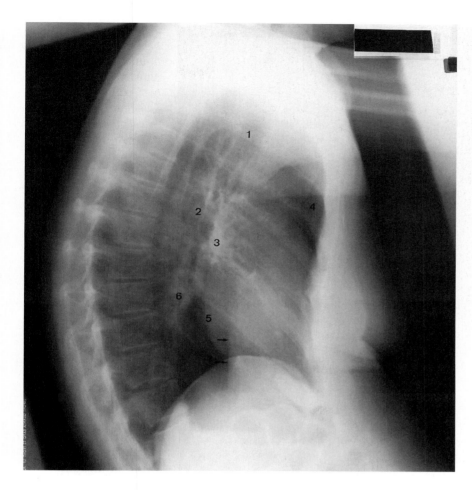

Figure 7.3 *Normal lateral chest X-ray.*
Identify the following structures: 1, trachea; 2, left pulmonary artery; 3, right pulmonary artery; 4, retrosternal airspace; 5, posterior heart border; 6, lower lobe arteries. Arrows point to the inferior vena cava (IVC).

The lateral view (*Fig. 7.3*)

The lateral view is usually performed with the patient's arms held out horizontally. The humeral heads may be seen as round opacities projected over the lung apices. They should not be mistaken for abnormal masses. The trachea is seen as an air-filled structure in the upper chest, midway between the anterior and posterior chest walls. The posterior aspect of the aortic arch forms a convexity posterior to the trachea. The trachea can be followed inferiorly to the carina where the right and left main bronchi may be seen end on as round lucencies. The left main pulmonary artery forms an opacity posterior and slightly superior to the carina. The right pulmonary artery forms an opacity anterior and slightly inferior to the carina.

On the lateral view, the posterior cardiac border is formed by the left atrium superiorly and the left ventricle inferiorly. The right ventricle forms the anterior cardiac border. The main pulmonary artery forms a convex opacity continuous with the right upper cardiac border.

Interpretations of CXRs

The lungs may be divided into two compartments:

- The alveoli or airspaces.

- The interstitium, i.e. supporting soft tissues between the airspaces.

The trachea divides into right and left bronchi. Each bronchus divides into lobar and segmental bronchi, and by repeated branching into smaller bronchi and bronchioles. The branching bronchi and bronchioles, accompanying arteries, veins and lymphatics, plus

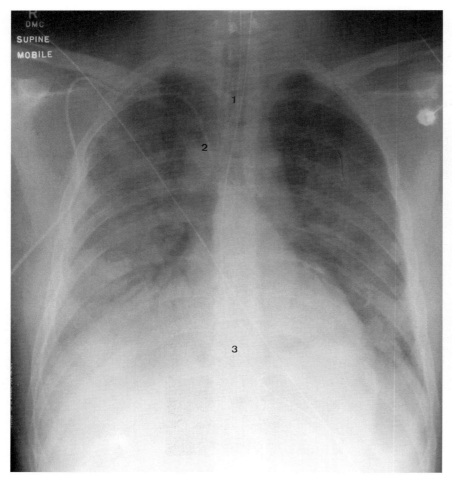

Figure 7.4 *Air bronchograms – pulmonary oedema.*
Air-filled bronchi are seen outlined by surrounding fluid-filled alveoli. Note:
- *endotracheal tube (1)*
- *central venous catheter (2)*
- *nasogastric tube (3)*
- *cardiac monitoring leads.*

supporting connective tissue form the interstitium of the lung. The most distal small bronchioles are called terminal bronchioles. The lung distal to each terminal bronchiole is termed the lung acinus. The lung acinus consists of multiple generations of tiny respiratory bronchioles and alveolar ducts. The alveoli or airspaces arise from the respiratory bronchioles and alveolar ducts.

Disease processes may involve the alveoli or the interstitium, or both. One of the most important factors in interpreting CXRs is the ability to differentiate alveolar from interstitial shadowing.

Alveolar processes

Signs of alveolar shadowing:

- Opacity tends to appear rapidly after the onset of symptoms.

- Fluffy, ill-defined areas of opacification.

- Areas of consolidation tend to coalesce.

- Two patterns of distribution tend to occur: segmental or lobar distribution and 'bats wing' distribution, i.e. bilateral opacification spreading from the hilar regions into the lungs with relative sparing of the peripheral lung fields, signifying extensive alveolar disease (e.g. pulmonary oedema).

- Air bronchograms (*Fig. 7.4*): air-filled bronchi are able to be seen as they are outlined by surrounding consolidated lung: air bronchograms are not seen in pleural or mediastinal processes.

Causes of alveolar shadowing:

- Alveolar shadowing may be due to oedema fluid, inflammatory fluid, blood or protein; they all have the same density on X-ray.

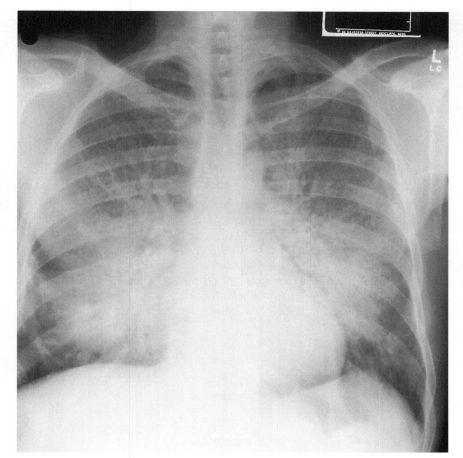

Figure 7.5 *'Bat's wing' pattern: congestive cardiac failure.*
Note extensive bilateral alveolar shadowing in keeping with pulmonary oedema.

- Definite diagnosis may often be made where the CXR findings are correlated with the clinical signs and symptoms.

- Common alveolar processes are listed below.

Segmental/lobar alveolar pattern:

- Pneumonia.

- Segmental/lobar collapse.

- Pulmonary infarct.

- Alveolar cell carcinoma.

- Contusion (associated with rib fractures, pneumo-thorax, and other signs of trauma).

'Bat's wing' pattern (*Fig. 7.5*):

Acute

Pulmonary oedema:

- Cardiac failure.

- Adult respiratory distress syndrome (ARDS).

- Fluid overload.

- Drownings and other causes of aspiration.

- Head injury or other causes of raised intracranial pressure.

- Drugs and poisons (e.g. snake venom, heroin OD).

- Hypoproteinaemia (e.g. liver disease).

- Blood transfusion reaction.

- Pneumonia: often 'unusual' etiology; pneumocystis carinii (AIDS); TB; viral pneumonias; mycoplasma.

- Pulmonary haemorrhage: Goodpasture's syndrome; anticoagulants; bleeding diathesis: haemophilia, disseminated intravascular coagulation (DIC); extensive contusion.

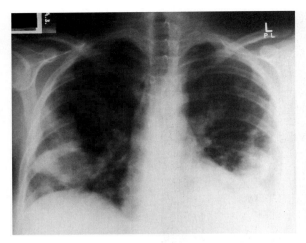

Figure 7.6 *Reversed 'bat's wing' consolidation – lymphomatoid granulomatosis.*
Note predominantly peripheral distribution of consolidation with relative sparing of the perihilar regions. This is a typical distribution of changes in eosinophilic lung disease for which there is a wide differential diagnosis.

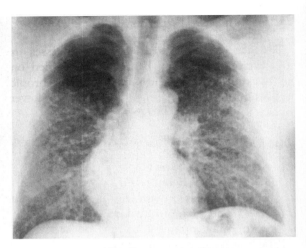

Figure 7.7 *Interstitial disease – sarcoidosis.*
Note numerous small, well-defined nodules with associated linear markings throughout both lungs. This pattern indicates an interstitial disease process, in this case, sarcoidosis.

Chronic

- 'Atypical pneumonia': TB, fungi.

- Lymphoma/leukaemia.

- Sarcoidosis: interstitial form much more common.

- Pulmonary alveolar proteinosis.

- Alveolar cell carcinoma: localized form more common.

'Reversed bat's wing' pattern (*Fig. 7.6*):

- Refers to processes that produce widespread alveolar opacification peripherally with relative sparing of the central zones.

- Loffler's syndrome.

- Eosinophilic pneumonias.

- Fat embolism: occurs 1–2 days following major trauma, particularly with fractures of the large bones of the lower limbs.

Interstitial processes

Three types of pattern are seen in interstitial processes: linear, nodular and honeycomb pattern.

These may occur separately or together in the same patient, i.e. considerable overlap in appearances may be seen.

Linear pattern:

- Network of fine lines running through the lungs.

- Lines are due to thickened connective tissue septae and may be further classified as below.
  (i)   Kerley A lines: long, thin lines in the upper lobes.
  (ii) Kerley B lines: short, thin lines predominantly in the lower zones extending 1–2 cm horizontally inwards from the lung surface.
  (iii) Kerley C lines: diffuse linear pattern through the entire lung.

Nodular pattern (*Fig. 7.7*):

- Interstitial nodules are small (1–5 mm), well defined and not associated with air bronchograms.

- Tend to be very numerous and distributed evenly throughout the lungs.

Honeycomb pattern (*Fig. 7.8*):

- Represents the end-stage of many interstitial

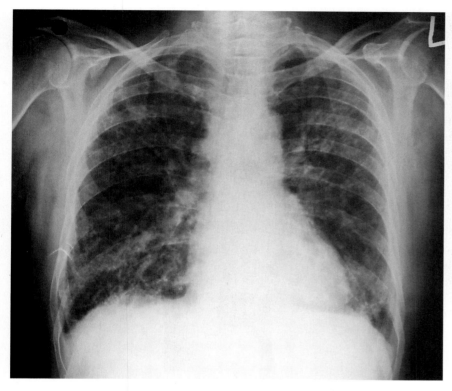

Figure 7.8 *Honeycomb lung.*
Note:
- *loss of normal lung architecture*
- *coarse linear interstitial markings with small air-filled cystic spaces.*

processes and implies extensive destruction of pulmonary tissue.

- Lung parenchyma replaced by cysts that range in size from tiny up to 2 cm in diameter.

- Cysts have very thin walls.

- Normal pulmonary vasculature cannot be seen.

- Frequently complicated by pneumothorax.

The list of interstitial disease processes is extensive. Diseases may be roughly classified on the basis of whether they are acute or chronic, or distribution in the lungs, i.e. upper or lower zones.

Acute

- Interstitial oedema.

- Kerley B lines (*Fig. 7.9*).

- Associated with cardiac enlargement and pleural effusions.

- May progress to, or be associated with, an alveolar pattern.

- Acute interstitial pneumonia – usually viral.

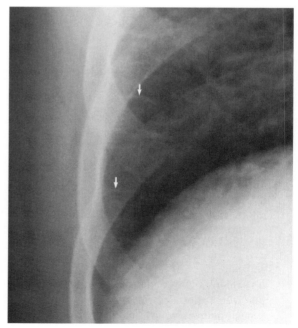

Figure 7.9 *Kerley B lines – interstitial oedema.*
Short, horizontal lines extending to the pleural surface (arrows).

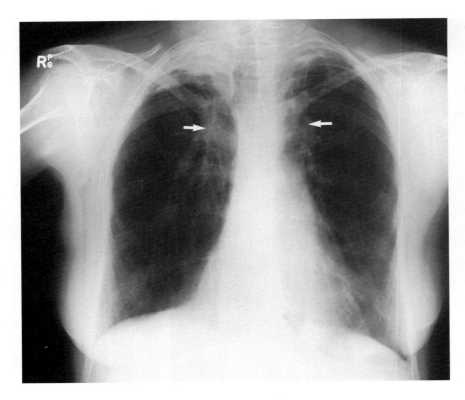

Figure 7.10 *Bilateral upper-zone fibrosis. Note loss of volume in both upper zones with elevation of both hila (arrows). Differential diagnosis includes: TB, sarcoidosis, radiotherapy and silicosis.*

Intermediate

Lymphangitis carcinomatosa

• Prominent linear and nodular shadowing with Kerley B lines.

• Often associated with mediastinal/hilar lymphadenopathy.

Chronic, upper zones (*Fig. 7.10*)

• TB:
  (i)   Upper lobe fibrosis with loss of volume.
  (ii) Associated calcification in cavities.
  (iii) Acute miliary form gives a widespread fine nodular pattern.

• Sarcoidosis:
  (i)   Nodular form dominates.
  (ii) Often associated with hilar lymphadenopathy, though pulmonary involvement alone occurs in 25% of cases.

• Silicosis:
  (i)   Nodular and linear pattern.
  (ii) Associated with hilar lymph node calcification and enlargement.
  (iii) May be associated with large confluent masses, i.e. progressive massive fibrosis (PMF).

• Extrinsic allergic alveolitis.

• Bronchopulmonary aspergillosis.

• Histiocytosis-X.

Chronic, lower zones

• Fibrosing alveolitis.

• Asbestosis:
  (i)   May be associated with pleural plaques and calcification particularly of the diaphragmatic pleura.

• Rheumatoid disease:
  (i)   Associated with pleural effusions.
  (ii) Rheumatoid nodules.

• Other connective tissue disorders:
  (i)   Systematic lupus erythematosis (SLE).
  (ii) Systemic sclerosis.
  (iii) Dermatomyositis/polymyositis.

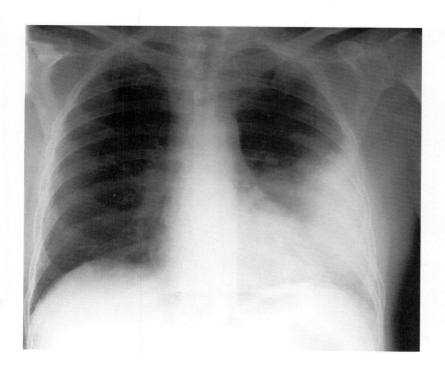

Figure 7.11 *Consolidation of the lingula.*
There is extensive consolidation in the lower left lung. Loss of definition of the left heart border localizes this to the lingula.

Honeycomb lung

• End-stage of all diseases listed above.

• Tuberous sclerosis.

• Amyloidosis.

• Neurofibromatosis.

• Cystic fibrosis.

Localization of lung lesions

Silhouette sign

Remember that in Chapter 1 it was stated that an object would be seen with conventional radiography if its borders lie beside tissue of different density. This especially applies in the chest where diaphragms, heart and mediastinal outlines are well seen due to their lying adjacent to aerated lung. Should a part of lung lying against any of these structures become non-aerated due to collapse, consolidation or a mass, then the outline of that structure will no longer be seen. This is known as the 'silhouette' sign and is one of the most important principles in chest radiography (Table 7.1).

Lung lesions adjacent to fissures

Straight margins occur in the lungs at the pulmonary

Table 7.1 *Examples of the silhouette sign*

Part of lung that is non-aerated	Border that is obscured
Right middle lobe (*Fig. 1.3*)	Right heart border
Left lingula (*Fig. 7.11*)	Left heart border
Right lower lobe (*Fig. 1.3*)	Right diaphragm
Left lower lobe (*Fig. 7.12*)	Left diaphragm
	Descending aorta
Right upper lobe	Right border of ascending aorta
	Right mediastinal margin
Left upper lobe	Aortic knuckle*
	Upper left cardiac border

*Note that in severe collapse of the left upper lobe, the apical segment of the left lower lobe may be pulled upwards and forwards enough such that aerated lung lies beside the aortic knuckle. The aortic knuckle will therefore be seen in this situation.

fissures. If an area of consolidation or collapse has a straight margin, that margin must abut a fissure and this can help in localization, as below:

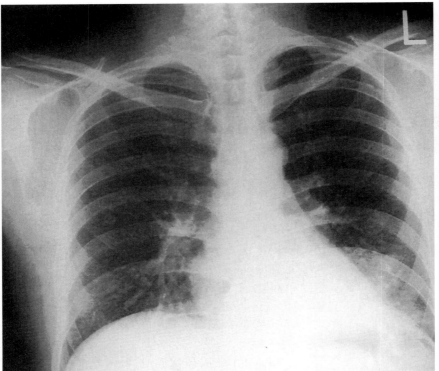

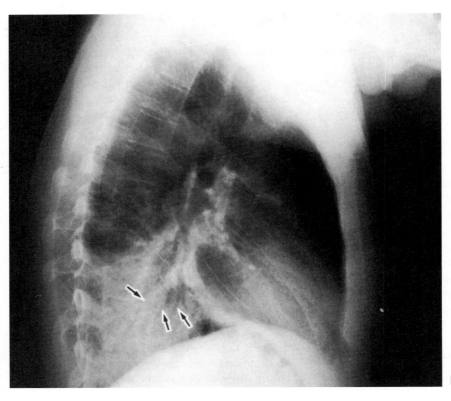

Figure 7.12 *Left lower lobe pneumonia.*
(a) PA film. Increased density of left lower hemithorax. Loss of definition of left diaphragm.
(b) Lateral film. Increased density of lower thoracic vertebral bodies. Loss of definition of left diaphragm posteriorly. Air bronchiograms (arrows).

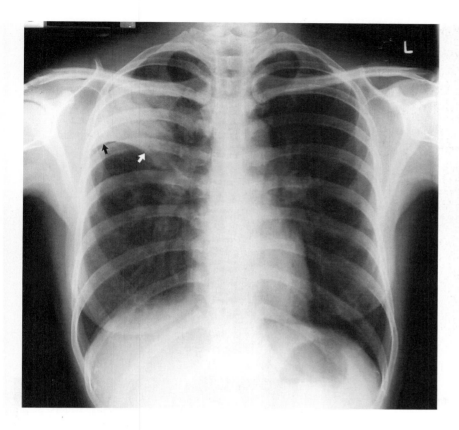

Figure 7.13 *Right upper lobe consolidation.*
Note:
- *opacity in the right upper lung with a well-defined lower margin (arrows) due to the horizontal fissure*
- *upward bowing of the horizontal fissure indicates some loss of volume in the right upper lobe.*

- Right upper lobe:
  (i)   Abuts horizontal fissure inferiorly on PA film (*Fig. 7.13*).
  (ii) Abuts oblique fissure posteriorly on lateral film.
- Right middle lobe:
  (i)   Abuts horizontal fissure superiorly on PA film.
  (ii) Abuts oblique fissure posteriorly on lateral film.
- Right lower lobe:
  (i)   Abuts oblique fissure anteriorly on lateral film.
  (ii) Collapse causes rotation and visualization of the oblique fissure on the PA film.
- Left upper lobe:
  (i)   Abuts oblique fissure posteriorly on lateral film.
- Left lower lobe:
  (i)   Abuts oblique fissure anteriorly on lateral film.
  (ii) Collapse causes rotation and visualization of the oblique fissure on the PA film.

Patterns of pulmonary collapse

General signs of lobar collapse

- Decreased lung volume.
- Displacement of pulmonary fissures.
- Local increase in density due to non-aerated lung.
- Elevation of hemidiaphragm.
- Displacement of hila.
- Displacement of mediastinum.
- Compensatory overinflation of adjacent lobes.

Specific signs of lobar collapse

- Right upper lobe – collapses upwards and anteriorly (*Fig. 7.14*):
  (i)   Decreased volume of right lung.
  (ii)   Elevation of horizontal fissure.
  (iii) Increased density of right upper zone.
  (iv)   Loss of definition of right mediastinal margins.
  (v)   Elevation of right hilum.
  (vi)   Tracheal deviation to the right.

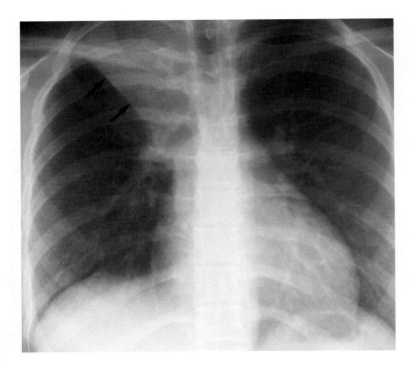

Figure 7.14 *Right upper lobe collapse.*
Note the following features:
- *reduced volume of the right lung*
- *elevation of the right hilum*
- *elevation of the horizontal fissure (arrows)*
- *loss of definition of the right side of the superior mediastinum.*

- Right middle lobe:
  (i)   Increased density in right midzone with loss of definition of the right cardiac border.
  (ii) Lateral film: triangular opacity projected over the heart.

- Right lower lobe – collapses downwards and posteriorly (*Fig. 7.15*):
  (i)   Decreased volume of right lung.
  (ii)   Triangular opacity at the right base medially.
  (iii) Loss of definition of the right hemidiaphragm.
  (iv)   Heart border not obscured.
  (v)   Elevation of right hemidiaphragm.
  (vi)   Depression of right hilum.
  (vii) Non-visualization of the right lower lobe artery.
  (viii) Lateral film: increased apparent density of lower thoracic vertebral bodies.

- Left upper lobe – collapses upwards and anteriorly (*Fig. 7.16*):
  (i)   Decreased volume of left lung.
  (ii)   Increased density of left upper zone.
  (iii) Loss of definition of left upper cardiac border and left mediastinal margin; in severe left upper lobe collapse the aortic knuckle may be well outlined by elevated apical segment of the left lower lobe.

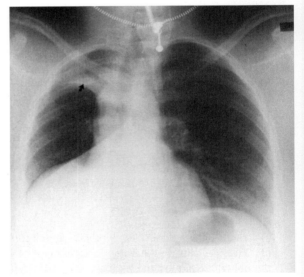

Figure 7.15 *Right lower lobe collapse.*
Note the following:
- *loss of volume of the right lung*
- *triangular opacity at the right base*
- *loss of definition of the right diaphragm.*
There is also collapse of the right upper lobe (arrow):
- *elevation of the horizontal fissure*
- *opacity abutting the right mediastinum*
- *tracheal deviation to the right.*

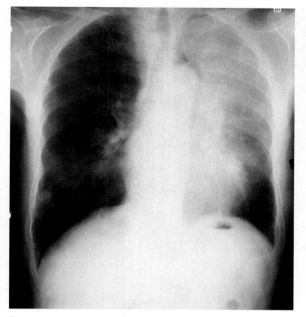
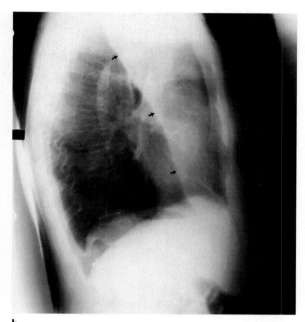

a   b

Figure 7.16 *Left upper lobe collapse.*
(a) PA film. Note:
* *decreased volume of left lung*
* *increased opacification of the left upper zone*
* *loss of definition of left cardiac border and of left hilum.*
(b) Lateral film. Note:
* *large anterior opacity due to left upper lobe which has collapsed upwards and anteriorly*
* *well-defined posterior margin (arrows) due to oblique fissure.*

(iv)   Elevation of left hilum.
(v)   Tracheal deviation to the left.
(vi)   Lateral film: increased opacity anteriorly, which has a well-defined posterior margin due to the oblique fissure.

* Left lower lobe – collapses downwards and posteriorly (*Fig. 7.17*):
(i)   Decreased volume of left lung.
(ii)   Triangular opacity behind the left heart.
(iii) Loss of definition of the left hemidiaphragm.
(iv)   Left heart border not obscured.
(v)   Elevation of left hemidiaphragm.
(vi)   Depression of left hilum.
(vii) Non-visualization of left lower lobe artery.
(viii) Lateral film: increased apparent density of lower thoracic vertebral bodies.

Pulmonary vascular patterns

The normal lung vascular pattern has the following features:

* Arteries branching vertically to upper and lower lobes.

* Veins running roughly horizontally towards the lower hila.

* Upper lobe vessels smaller than lower lobe vessels on erect CXR.

* Vessels difficult to see in the peripheral thirds of the lungs.

Pulmonary venous hypertension (*Fig. 7.18*)

* Vessels in upper lobe larger than vessels in lower lobe on erect CXR.

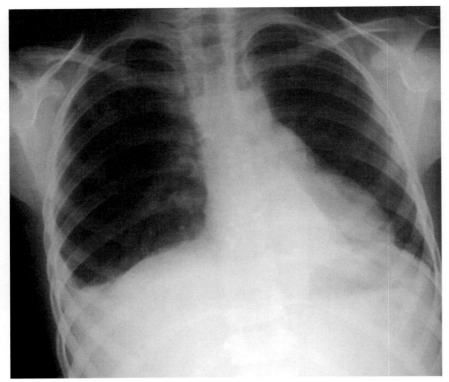

Figure 7.17 *Left lower lobe collapse.*
Note the following features:
- *loss of volume of the left lung*
- *triangular opacity behind the heart*
- *loss of definition of the left diaphragm medially*
- *depression of left hilum*
- *non-visualization of the left lower lobe artery.*

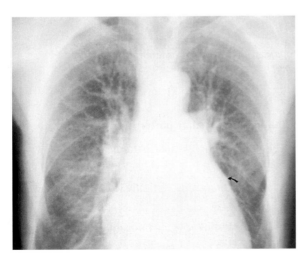

Figure 7.18 *Pulmonary venous hypertension – mitral valve disease.*
Upper lobe vessels are larger than those in the lobes, i.e. reversal of the normal pattern seen in the erect chest radiograph. Note:
- *cardiomegaly*
- *prominent left auricle indicating left atrial enlargement (arrow)*
- *Kerley B lines.*

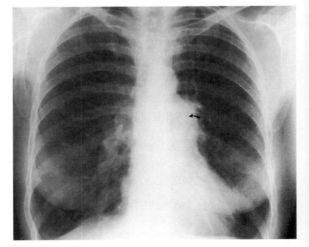

Figure 7.19 *Pulmonary arterial hypertension.*
Note:
- *prominent enlarged main pulmonary artery (arrow)*
- *rapid tapering in the calibre of more peripheral branches of the pulmonary artery.*

- Associated with cardiac failure and mitral valve disease.

- Associated with pulmonary oedema and pleural effusion.

Pulmonary arterial hypertension (*Fig. 7.19*)

- Pulmonary artery and its main left and right branches enlarged giving bilateral hilar enlargement.

- Rapid decrease in calibre of peripheral vessels ('pruning').

- Associated with long-standing pulmonary disease, e.g. emphysema, multiple recurrent pulmonary emboli, left to right shunts (VSD, ASD, PDA).

Pulmonary plethora

- Increased size and number of pulmonary vessels.

- Vessels seen in peripheral third of lung fields.

- Associated with left to right shunts (VSD, ASD, PDA).

Pulmonary oligaemia

- Decreased size and number of pulmonary vessels.

- Small main pulmonary arteries.

- General lucency (blackness) of lung fields. Associated with pulmonary stenosis/atresia, Fallot tetralogy, tricuspid atresia, Ebstein anomaly and severe emphysema.

Solitary pulmonary nodule

Factors to assess

- Size: greater than 4 cm diameter highly suspicious of malignancy.

- Margin: ill-defined margin suggests malignancy.

- Cavitation: malignancy or infection.

- Calcification: rare in malignancy.

- Comparison with previous CXR to assess growth.

Differential diagnosis

- Bronchial carcinoma:

- Evidence of rapid growth on serial CXR examinations.

    (i)   Ill-defined margin.
    (ii) Size greater than 4 cm.
    (iii) *No* calcification.
    (iv) For further notes see below.

- Solitary metastasis

- Tuberculoma:

    (i)   Calcification common.
    (ii) Well-defined margin.
    (iii) Usually 0.3–1.0 cm diameter.
    (iv) Unchanged on serial CXR examinations.

- Bronchial adenoma:
    (i)   Usually a carcinoid tumour.
    (ii) Around 2 cm diameter.
    (iii) Calcification in one-third.
    (iv) Hilar lymphadenopathy in 25%.

- Hamartoma:
    (i)   Well-defined, lobulated margin.
    (ii) Usually less than 4 cm diameter.
    (iii) Calcification more common in larger lesions.

- Arteriovenous malformations:
    (i)   Feeding arteries and draining veins may be seen.

Multiple pulmonary nodules (*Fig. 7.20*)

Metastases

- Usually well defined.

- Nodules of varying size.

- More common peripherally and in the lower lobes.

- Cavitation seen in squamous cell carcinomas, sarcomas and metastases from colonic primaries.

Abscesses

- Cavitation: thick, irregular wall.

- Usually *Staphylococcus aureus*.

Hydatid cysts

- Often quite large, i.e. 10 cm or more.

Rheumatoid nodules

Wegener's granulomatosis

- Cavitation common.

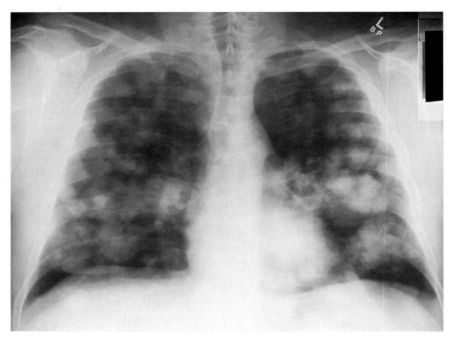

Figure 7.20 *Pulmonary metastases.*
Note multiple, well-defined masses throughout both lungs. Metastases tend to be more numerous peripherally due to haematogenous dissemination.

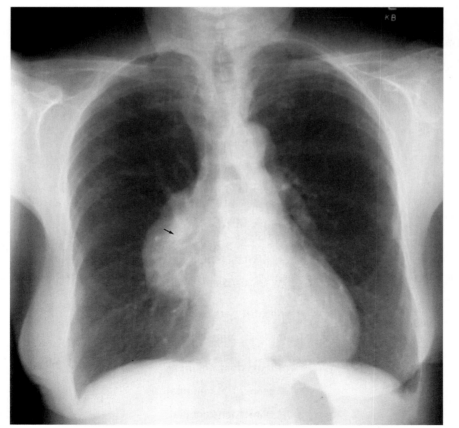

Figure 7.21 *Anterior mediastinal mass – Hodgkin's disease.*
Note:
- *right-sided mediastinal mass*
- *right hilar structures can still be seen (arrow) indicating that the mass is either anterior or posterior*
- *loss of definition of the upper right cardiac border indicates that the mass is anterior.*

- Associated paranasal sinus disease.

Multiple arteriovenous malformations

Mediastinal masses

Signs of a mediastinal versus a pulmonary lesion:

- Sharp margin.
- Convex margin.
- Absence of air bronchograms.

Logical classification and differential diagnosis of mediastinal masses is based on localization to the anterior, middle or posterior mediastinum. In this regard, the silhouette sign and the lateral film are of most use.

CXR signs of an anterior mediastinal mass (*Fig. 7.21*)

- Merge with cardiac border.
- Hila can be seen through the mass.
- Masses passing upwards into the neck merge radiologically with the soft tissues of the neck and so are not seen above the clavicles (cervico-thoracic sign); a lesion seen above the clavicles must lie adjacent to aerated lung apices, i.e. posterior and within the thorax.

Differential diagnosis of an anterior mediastinal mass

- Retrosternal goitre:
  (i) Cervico-thoracic sign, as above, i.e. mass not seen above the clavicles.
  (ii) Displaced trachea.
- Thymic tumour:
  (i) May be associated with myasthenia gravis.
- Thymic cyst.
- Lymphadenopathy:
  (i) Hodgkin disease
  (ii) Metastases.
- Aneurysm of ascending aorta.

CXR signs of a middle mediastinal mass

- Merge with hila and cardiac borders.

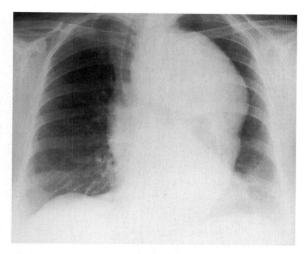

Figure 7.22 *Middle mediastinal mass – aortic aneurysm.*
There is a large aneurysm of the thoracic aorta causing displacement of the trachea.

Differential diagnosis of an anterior mediastinal mass

- Lymphadenopathy:
  (i) Mediastinal/hilar.
  (ii) Bronchial carcinoma, less commonly other tumours.
  (iii) Lymphoma.
- Bronchogenic cyst
- Aortic aneurysm (*Fig. 7.22*)

CXR signs of a posterior mediastinal mass

- Cardiac borders and hila clearly seen.
- Posterior descending aorta obscured.
- May be underlying vertebral changes.

Differential diagnosis of a posterior mediastinal mass

- Hiatus hernia:
  (i) Located behind the heart.
  (ii) May contain a fluid level.
- Neurogenic tumour:
  (i) Well-defined mass in the paravertebral region.
  (ii) Erosion or destruction of vertebral bodies/posterior ribs.

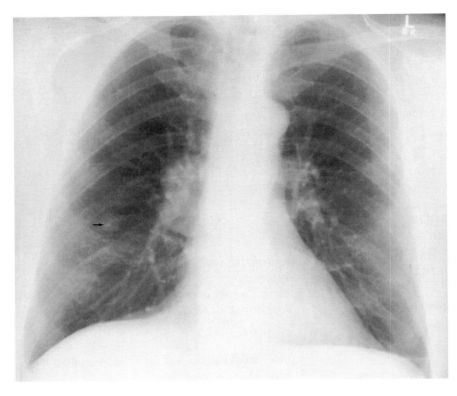

Figure 7.23 *Unilateral hilar enlargement – lymphadenopathy.*
Note:
- *enlarged right hilar lymph nodes*
- *small primary carcinoma in the right lower lobe (arrow).*

- Anterior thoracic meningocele:
  (i) Associated with neurofibromatosis.
- Neurenteric cyst:
  (i) Associated with vertebral abnormalities.
- Oesophageal duplication cyst.
- Paravertebral lymphadenopathy.

Hilar disorders

Each hilar complex as seen on the PA and lateral chest radiographs comprises the proximal pulmonary arteries, bronchus, pulmonary veins and lymph nodes. The lymph nodes are not visualized unless enlarged. In assessing hilar enlargement, be it bilateral or unilateral, one must decide whether it is due to enlargement of the pulmonary arteries or some other cause like lymphadenopathy or a mass. If the branching pulmonary arteries are seen to converge towards an apparent mass, this is a good sign of enlarged main pulmonary artery (hilum convergence sign).

Causes of unilateral hilar enlargement

- Bronchial carcinoma (*Fig. 7.23*).

- Infective causes:
  (i) TB.
  (ii) Mycoplasma.
- Perihilar pneumonia:
  (i) An area of pneumonia lying anterior or posterior to the hilum causing apparent enlargement on the PA film.
  (ii) Usually obvious on the lateral film.
- Other causes of lymphadenopathy (more commonly bilateral):
  (i) Lymphoma.
  (ii) Sarcoidosis.
- Causes of enlargement of a single pulmonary artery:
  (i) Post-stenotic dilatation on the left side due to pulmonary stenosis.
  (ii) Massive unilateral pulmonary embolus.
  (iii) Pulmonary artery aneurysm (often calcified).

Causes of bilateral hilar enlargement

- Sarcoidosis (*Fig. 7.24*):
  (i) Symmetrical.

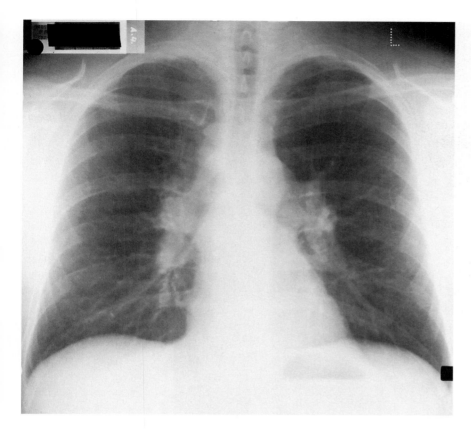

Figure 7.24 *Bilateral hilar enlargement – sarcoidosis. There is increased size and density of both hila.*

(ii) Lobulated.

(iii) Often associated with right paratracheal lymphadenopathy.

- Lymphoma:
  (i) Often asymmetrical.

- Metastatic malignancy:
  (i) Pulmonary primary.
  (ii) Non-pulmonary primary, e.g. testis, breast.

Pleural disorders

Pleural effusion

The X-ray appearances of pleural effusion are *not* related to the nature of the fluid, which may include:

- Transudate.

- Exudate.

- Blood.

- Pus.

- Lymph.

Classical appearance of pleural effusion (*Fig. 7.25*).

- Homogeneous dense opacity.

- Concave upper surface.

- Meniscus, i.e. higher laterally than medially.

- Large pleural effusions displace the mediastinum towards the contralateral side.

Variants

- Loculations that may look like pleural masses.

- Fluid in fissures.

- Subpulmonic effusion: fluid trapped beneath the lung produces opacity parallel to the diaphragm with a convex upper margin.

Causes of pleural effusion

- Cardiac failure:
  (i) Bilateral.
  (ii) Right larger than left.

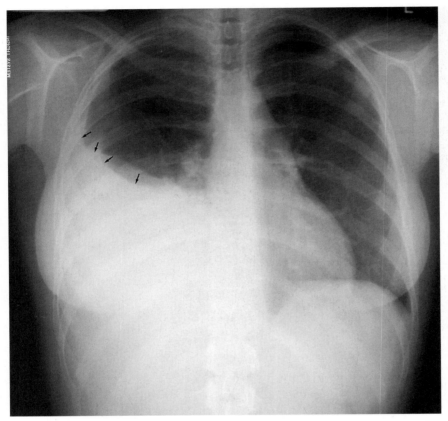

Figure 7.25 *Pleural effusion.*
Note:
- *non-visualization of right hemidiaphragm and costophrenic angle*
- *meniscus-shaped upper surface (arrows).*

- Malignancy:
  - (i) Bronchogenic carcinoma.
  - (ii) Metastatic.
  - (iii) Mesothelioma.

- Infection:
  - (i) Bacterial pneumonia.
  - (ii) TB.
  - (iii) Mycoplasma.
  - (iv) Empyema.
  - (i\v) Subphrenic abscess.

- Pulmonary embolus with infarct.

- Pancreatitis: effusion is usually left-sided.

- Trauma: associated with rib fractures.

- Connective tissue disorders:
  - (i) Rheumatoid arthritis.
  - (ii) SLE.

- Liver failure.

- Renal failure.

- Meig's syndrome:
  - (i) Associated with ovarian fibroma.

Pneumothorax

Pneumothorax is usually well seen on a normal inspiratory PA film. The diagnosis of small pneumothorax may be easier on an expiratory film. This is due to reduced volume of the lung in expiration, which makes the pneumothorax look relatively larger. Whether the film is performed in inspiration or expiration, the sign to look for is the lung edge outlined by air in the pleural space (*Fig. 7.26*).

CXR signs of tension pneumothorax

- Marked collapse and distortion of the lung.

- Increased volume of hemithorax with displacement of the mediastinum, depressed diaphragm and increased space between the ribs (*Fig. 7.27*).

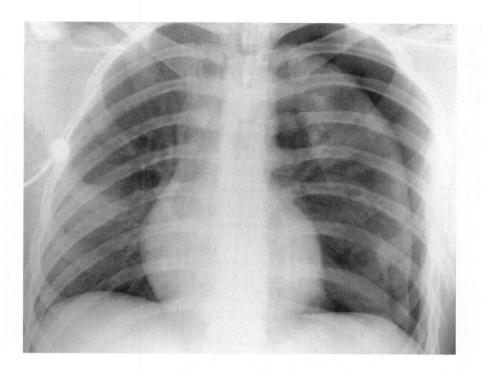

Figure 7.26
Pneumothorax.
The edge of the collapsed lung is well outlined by pleural air. Note multiple left rib fractures.

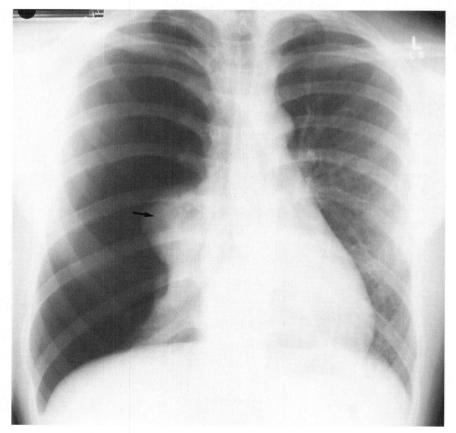

Figure 7.27 *Tension pneumothorax.*
Signs of tension pneumothorax as demonstrated in this case are as follows:

- *total collapse of right lung (arrow)*
- *increased size of right hemithorax*
- *increased space between right ribs*
- *shift of the mediastinum to the left.*

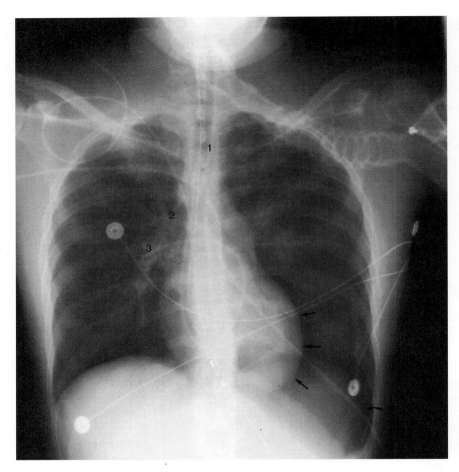

Figure 7.28 *Pneumothorax in a supine patient.*
Note:
* *deep left costophrenic angle due to air beneath the lung (curved arrow)*
* *sharp definition of the left cardiac border due to air located anteriorly (straight arrows)*
* *endotracheal tube (1), with tip just above the carina*
* *central venous catheter tip in SVC (2)*
* *Swann Ganz catheter tip in right pulmonary artery (3).*

Pneumothorax in the supine patient (Fig. 7.28)

Supine antero-posterior (AP) CXR may have to be performed in ICU patients or following severe trauma. Pleural air lies anteromedially and beneath the lung so that the usual appearance as described for an erect PA film is not seen. Signs of pneumothorax on a supine CXR include:

* Mediastinal structures are sharply outlined by adjacent free pleural air: heart border, inferior vena cava (IVC), SVC

* Upper abdomen appears lucent due to overlying air.

* Deep lateral costophrenic angle.

* Decubitus film with abnormal side up may be helpful.

Causes of pneumothorax

* Spontaneous:
  (i)   Tall, thin males.
  (ii) Smokers.

* Iatrogenic:
  (i)   Following percutaneous lung biopsy.
  (ii) Ventilation.
  (iii) CVP line insertion.

* Trauma:
  (i)   Associated with rib fractures.

* Emphysema.

* Malignancy:
  (i)   High incidence in osteogenic sarcoma metastases.

* Honeycomb lung.

- Cystic fibrosis.

Pleural thickening

- Secondary to trauma:
  (i)   Associated with healed rib fractures.
  (ii) Dense layer of soft tissue, often calcified.

- Following empyema:
  (i)   More common over the lung bases.
  (ii) Often calcified.

- TB.

- Asbestos exposure:
  (i)   Irregular pleural thickening and pleural plaques.
  (ii) Calcification common, especially of diaphragmatic surface of pleura.
  (iii) Note that pleural disease is not asbestosis; the term asbestosis refers to the interstitial lung disease secondary to asbestos exposure.

- Mesothelioma:
  (i)   Diffuse or localized pleural mass.
  (ii) Rib destruction uncommon.
  (iii) Large pleural effusions common.
  (iv) Pleural plaques elsewhere in 50%.

- Pancoast tumour:
  (i)   Primary apical lung neoplasm.
  (ii) Rib destruction with irregular pleural thickening.

- Pleural metastases:
  (i)   Often obscured by associated pleural effusion.

Assessment of the heart

See Chapter 8.

Other imaging investigations of the respiratory system

Virtually all symptoms and clinical situations related to the respiratory system will be investigated primarily by CXR. Interpretation of CXRs has been outlined above. Here I briefly outline the roles of the main imaging modalities in respiratory disease in general, before discussing the imaging findings in the more common respiratory conditions.

CT

CT is the investigation of choice for the following:

Mediastinal mass (*Fig. 7.29*)

- Accurate localization.

- Characterization of internal contents of mass, e.g. fat, air, fluid and calcification.

- Displacement/invasion of adjacent structures such as aorta, heart, trachea, oesophagus, vertebral column, chest wall.

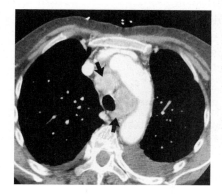

Figure 7.29 *Mediastinal lymphadenopathy – CT. This patient has widely disseminated breast carcinoma. Contrast enhancement of the aorta and SVC differientiates these structures from enlarged mediastinal lymph nodes (arrows).*

Hilar mass

- Greater sensitivity than plain films for the presence of hilar lymphadenopathy.

- Greater specificity in differentiating lymphadenopathy or hilar mass from enlarged pulmonary arteries.

Staging of bronchogenic carcinoma, lymphoma and other malignancies

- Greater sensitivity than plain films for the presence of mediastinal or hilar lymphadenopathy.

- Greater sensitivity for complications such as chest wall or mediastinal invasion, and cavitation.

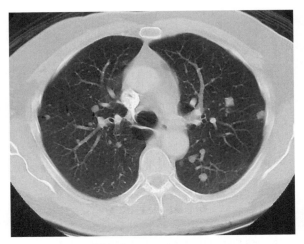

Figure 7.30 *Pulmonary metastases – CT.*
Multiple soft tissue masses throughout both lungs. Note that these masses are of variable size; this is a typical feature of metastases (arrows).

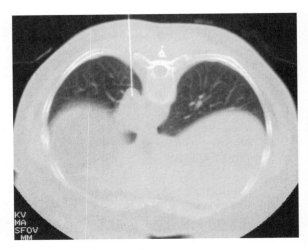

Figure 7.31 *CT-guided biopsy.*
Note placement of a biopsy needle into a mass in the left lower lobe. Cytology showed a squamous cell carcinoma.

Detection of pulmonary metastases (*Fig. 7.30*)

- CT has greater sensitivity than plain films for the detection of small pulmonary lesions, including metastases.

- This is particularly so in areas of the lung seen poorly on CXR including the apices, posterior segments of the lower lobes, and medial areas that are obscured by the hila.

Characterization of a pulmonary mass seen on CXR

- More accurate than plain films for the presence of calcification.

- Other factors also well assessed by CT include cavitation and relation of a mass to the chest wall or mediastinum.

- iv contrast material may help to identify aberrant vessels and arteriovenous malformations.

Demonstration of mediastinal vasculature

- Thoracic aortic aneurysm.

- Aortic dissection.

- SVC compression/invasion by tumour.

- Vascular anomalies, which may cause odd shadows on CXR, e.g. azygos continuation of IVC, partial anomalous pulmonary venous drainage.

Trauma

- Exclusion of mediastinal haematoma in a haemo-dynamically-stable patient with a widened mediastinum on CXR following chest trauma (see below).

Characterization of pleural disease

- CT gives excellent delineation of pleural abnormalities, which may produce confusing appearances on CXR.

- Pleural masses, fluid collections, calcifications and tumours such as mesothelioma are well shown, as are complications such as rib destruction, mediastinal invasion and lymphadenopathy.

Guidance of percutaneous biopsy and drainage procedures (*Fig. 7.31*)

- Especially useful for peripheral lesions not amenable to bronchoscopic biopsy.

High-resolution CT (HRCT)

HRCT is a technique used in the assessment of disorders of the lungs. Conventional CT of the chest uses sections 5–10 mm in thickness spaced 10 mm apart. The high-resolution technique uses much thinner

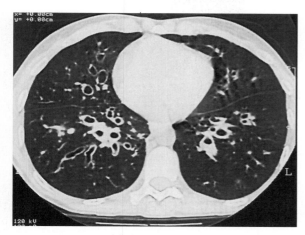

Figure 7.32 *Bronchiectasis – HRCT.*
There are dilated bronchi with thickened walls in the
right middle lobe and both lower lobes.

sections of around 1 mm thickness, spaced 10–15 mm apart. The thinner sections show much greater lung detail. Intravenous contrast material is not used and the mediastinal and chest wall structures are less well seen than with conventional chest CT. HRCT is useful in the following.

Bronchiectasis (*Fig. 7.32*)

- HRCT has replaced bronchography in the assessment of bronchiectasis.

- As well as showing dilated bronchi, HRCT accurately shows the anatomical distribution of changes, in addition to complications such as scarring, collapse, consolidation and mucous plugging.

Interstitial lung disease

- HRCT is more sensitive and specific than plain films in the diagnosis of many interstitial lung diseases.

- Sarcoidosis, interstitial pneumonia (fibrosing alveolitis), lymphangitis carcinomatosa and histiocytosis-X are examples of disorders that have specific appearances on HRCT, often obviating the need for biopsy in these patients.

- Where biopsy is felt necessary, HRCT may aid in guiding the operator to the most favourable biopsy site.

Atypical infections

- HRCT provides diagnosis of many atypical infections earlier and with greater specificity than plain CXR.

- Examples include: *Pneumocystis carinii*, aspergillosis and *Mycobacterium avium intracellulare*, infections which occur in immunocompromised patients, including those with AIDS.

- As well as diagnosis, HRCT may be useful for monitoring disease progress and response to therapy.

Normal CXR in symptomatic patients

- HRCT has a definite role in the assessment of patients with an apparently normal CXR, despite the clinical indications of respiratory disease, including dyspnoea, chest pain, haemoptysis and abnormal pulmonary function tests.

CT pulmonary angiography (CTPA: see Chapter 8)

Scintigraphy

A number of examples exist of the use of scintigraphy in the assessment of disorders of the respiratory system.

Pulmonary embolism

- Ventilation/perfusion lung scan (see Chapter 8).

Early infection

- Gallium-67 (^{67}Ga).

- The most common example in clinical use would be in the detection of early *Pneumocystis carinii* infection in AIDS patients: increased lung uptake of ^{67}Ga may be seen prior to the appearance of CXR changes (*Fig. 7.33*).

PET with FDG

- Characterization of a solitary pulmonary nodule: increased uptake in neoplastic masses.

- Differentiation of recurrent bronchogenic carcinoma from postoperative or postradiation changes. Such differentiation may be difficult or impossible with CXR and CT.

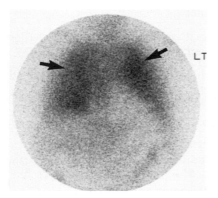

Figure 7.33 Pneumocystis carinii *pneumonia (PCP): gallium scan. Note diffuse uptake of gallium throughout both lungs in an HIV-positive patient (arrows). This pattern is typical of PCP.*

Ultrasound (US)

Echocardiography (see Chapter 8)

The commonest application for US in the chest is in echocardiography. Visualization of the heart may be difficult in emphysematous patients where the heart is covered by overexpanded lung. This difficulty is overcome with the use of transoesophageal probes.

Pleural fluid

- US is useful for the confirmation of pleural effusion suspected on CXR.

- US is also very useful for guidance of drainage of small pleural fluid collections.

Summary of CXR appearances in some common disorders

Emphysema (Fig. 7.34)

Emphysema refers to enlarged airspaces secondary to destruction of the alveolar walls. Centrilobular emphysema is the most common form. It occurs in smokers

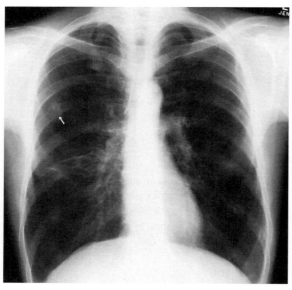

a

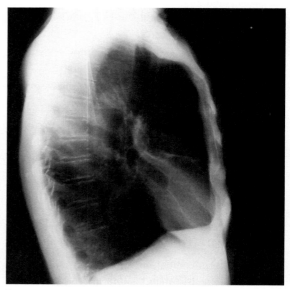

b

Figure 7.34 *Emphysema.*
(a) PA film. Note:
- *overexpanded lungs*
- *narrow mediastinum*
- *healed fracture of right 7th rib: incidental finding (arrow)*

(b) Lateral film. Note:
- *flattened diaphragms*
- *enlarged retrosternal space.*

and predominantly affects the upper lobes. Panlobular emphysema is seen in association with alpha-1 antitrypsin deficiency. It tends to predominantly affect the lower lobes.

CXR signs of emphysema include:

- Overexpanded lungs.
- Flat diaphragms lying below the 6th rib anteriorly.
- Increased retrosternal airspace on lateral film.
- Decreased vascular markings in lung fields.
- Increased antero-posterior diameter of the chest, with in some cases kyphosis and anterior bowing of the sternum.
- Bulla formation: bullae are seen as thin-walled air-containing cavities.
- Pulmonary arterial hypertension: prominent main pulmonary arteries.

Lung volume reduction surgery is being increasingly used in the treatment of emphysema. HRCT may be used prior to surgery for the following:

- Accurately assess the severity and distribution of disease.
- Quantitate the percentage of residual healthy lung.
- Identify conditions that would exclude surgical treatment such as bronchogenic carcinoma.

Asthma

Baseline changes

Between acute attacks, the CXR of an asthma sufferer is often normal. Changes that may be seen include:

- Overexpanded lungs.
- Thickening of bronchial walls most marked in the parahilar regions.
- Focal scarring from previous infections.

Complications

During acute exacerbations, the lungs are overinflated due to air trapping. Lobar or segmental atelectasis due to mucous plugging is common. It is important to differentiate atelectasis from consolidation to avoid

unnecessary use of antibiotics. Other complications include:

- Pneumonia.
- Pneumomediastinum and pneumothorax.
- Secondary aspergillosis.

Pneumonia

Organisms that commonly cause pneumonia include *Streptococcus pneumoniae*, *Haemophilus influenzae*, *Klebsiella pneumoniae* and *Mycoplasma pneumoniae*. Early subtle areas of alveolar shadowing progress to dense lobar consolidation. See above for notes on patterns of lobar consolidation.

Expansion of a lobe with bulging pulmonary fissures may be seen with klebsiella. Necrosis and cavitation may complicate severe cases of lobar pneumonia. Small pleural effusions commonly accompany pneumonia.

More aggressive organisms such as *Staphylococcus aureus* and *Pseudomonas* may cause more extensive consolidation. This may involve multiple lobes, with cavitation leading to abscess formation. Other complications include empyema and bronchopleural fistula.

For further information on pulmonary infections in children, see Chapter 16.

Tuberculosis (TB)

Primary TB

- Usually asymptomatic.
- Healed pulmonary lesion may be seen: small peripheral nodule, often calcified; calcified hilar lymph node (*Fig. 7.35*).

Post-primary pulmonary TB (reactivation TB)

- Predilection for apical and posterior segments of the upper lobes, plus the apical segments of the lower lobes.
- Variable appearances.
- Ill-defined areas of alveolar consolidation.
- Cavitation: thick-walled, irregular cavities (*Fig. 7.36*).

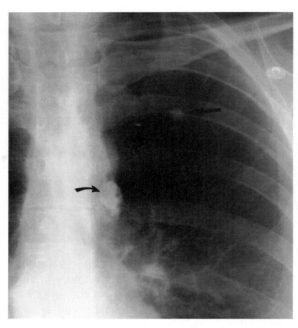

Figure 7.35 *TB: Ghon complex.*
There is a calcified granuloma in the left upper lobe (straight arrow), with a calcified lymph node in the mediastinum (curved arrow).

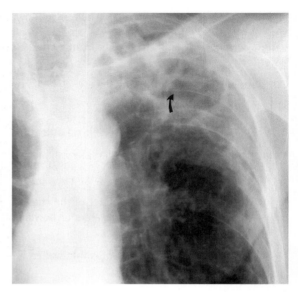

Figure 7.36 *Post-primary TB.*
An elderly patient with known emphysema presents with a cough, haemoptysis and shortness of breath. There is an area of consolidation in the left upper lobe with cavitation (curved arrow).

- Haemoptysis, aspergilloma, tuberculous empyema and broncho-pleural fistula may complicate cavitation.

- Fibrosis causing volume loss in the upper lobe.

- Calcification may occur with fibrosis.

- Fibrosis and calcification usually indicate disease inactivity and healing, but one should never diagnose inactive TB on a single CXR: serial films are essential to prove inactivity.

Miliary TB

- Haematogenous dissemination which may occur at any time following primary infection.

- Tiny foci of approximately 2 mm diameter spread evenly through both lungs.

Bronchogenic carcinoma

Bronchogenic carcinoma may produce a wide range of appearances depending on the stage of disease at the time of diagnosis. Usually, bronchogenic carcinoma is seen as a pulmonary mass (*Fig. 7.37*). This may be quite small, and may be an incidental finding on a CXR performed for other reasons, such as pre-anaesthetic or as part of a routine medical check-up. In this situation, characterization of a solitary pulmonary nodule is often a diagnostic challenge. Features that tend to indicate malignancy include:

- Mass greater than 4.0 cm diameter.

- Cavitation (may also be seen with infection).

- Ill-defined margin.

- Calcification is rare in malignancy.

Further assessment of the solitary pulmonary nodule could include the following:

- Comparison with previous X-rays, or obtain a follow-up X-ray:
  (i)   Lack of growth of a nodule over 2 years has been accepted as indicating a benign aetiology.
  (ii)   Recent research, however, has indicated that this is unreliable.

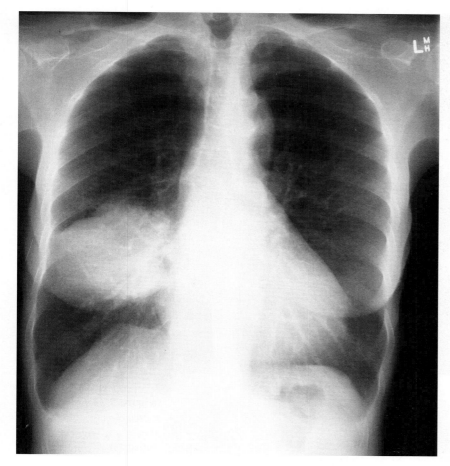

Figure 7.37 *Bronchogenic carcinoma.*
An elderly patient presents with cough and haemoptysis. CXR shows a large mass in the right middle lobe. Biopsy via bronchoscope revealed a bronchogenic carcinoma. The absence of air bronchograms indicates a mass, rather than a focus of alveolar consolidation.

- CT:
  (i)   Detection of even small amounts of calcification (granuloma) or fat (hamartoma) on CT virtually excludes bronchogenic carcinoma.
  (ii) Contrast enhancement tends to indicate malignancy rather than granuloma.
- PET:
  (i)   PET with FDG is based on increased glucose metabolism in neoplastic masses.
  (ii) PET may be useful to characterize solitary pulmonary nodules where other imaging is unhelpful.
  (iii) Neoplastic masses show increased uptake of FDG.

- Biopsy:
  (i)   Via bronchoscopy.
  (ii) Percutaneous with CT guidance.
  (iii) Open surgical biopsy and resection.

Complications of bronchogenic carcinoma that may be seen on CXR include:

- Invasion of adjacent structures: mediastinum, chest wall (*Fig. 7.38*).

- Segmental/lobar collapse (*Fig. 7.39*).

- Persistent areas of consolidation.

- Hilar lymphadenopathy.

- Mediastinal lymphadenopathy.

- Pleural effusion.

- Metastases: lungs, bones.

CT is used for the staging of bronchogenic carcinoma. It is more accurate than CXR for staging of bronchogenic carcinoma, especially for the following:

- Mediastinal lymphadenopathy.

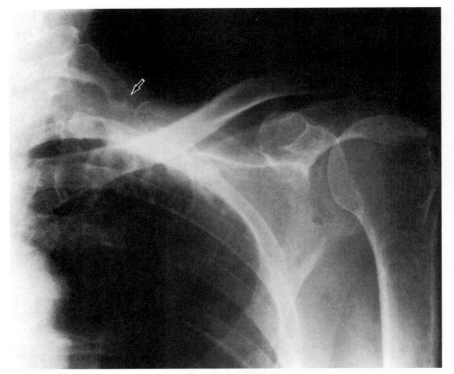

Figure 7.38 *Pancoast tumour*
Localized view showing a soft tissue mass at the apex of the left lung with destruction of the underlying 1st and 2nd ribs (arrow).

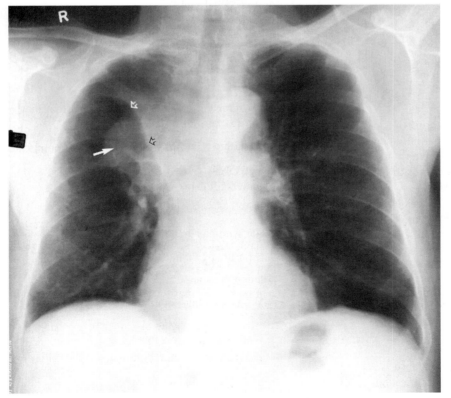

Figure 7.39 *Bronchogenic carcinoma.*
There is a large white hilar mass (white arrow) associated with collapse of the right lower lobe. Note signs of right upper lobe collapse:
- *decreased volume of right lung*
- *elevation of right hilum*
- *elevation of horizontal fissure (open arrows)*
- *non-visualization of right upper mediastinal margin.*

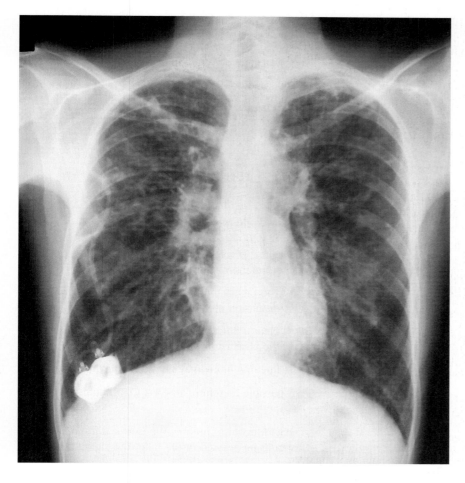

Figure 7.40 *Cystic fibrosis.*
Note:
- *overexpanded lungs*
- *extensive linear densities and bronchial wall thickening*
- *central venous catheter.*

- Hilar lymphadenopathy.

- Mediastinal invasion.

- Chest wall invasion.

CT may also be used for primary diagnosis where the CXR is negative and the presence of a tumour is suspected on clinical grounds, e.g. haemoptysis, positive sputum cytology or paraneoplastic syndrome.

Sarcoidosis (see *Figs 7.7, 7.10 & 7.24*)

Sarcoidosis is a disease of unknown aetiology characterized by the widespread formation of non-caseating granulomas. The chest is the commonest site with hilar and mediastinal lymphadenopathy and lung changes. Lymphadenopathy alone occurs in 50% of cases, lymphadenopathy plus lung changes in 25% of cases and lung changes alone in 15% of cases.

- Hilar lymphadenopathy:
  (i) Usually symmetrical and lobulated, associated with right paratracheal lymphadenopathy.

- Interstitial lung disease:
  (i) Multiple small nodules 2–5 mm diameter spread through both lungs.
  (ii) Predominantly in midzones.

- Rarely alveolar consolidation.

- Healing may lead to bilateral upperzone fibrosis.

- CXR normal in 10% of cases.

Other sites of involvement with sarcoidosis include:

- Liver and spleen.

- Peripheral lymph nodes.

- CNS: granulomatous meningitis.

- Eyes: uveitis.

- Bone.

- Salivary glands: bilateral parotid gland enlargement.

- Skin: erythema nodosum.

Cystic fibrosis (mucoviscidosis) (Fig. 7.40)

Cystic fibrosis is an autosomal recessive condition with dysfunction of exocrine glands and reduced mucociliary function. Pancreatic insufficiency leads to steatorrhoea and malabsorption. Meconium ileus may be seen in infants (see Chapter 16), with recurrent pancreatitis and meconium ileus equivalent occurring in older patients. Pulmonary symptoms include recurrent infections and chronic cough.
CXR changes include:

- Bronchiectasis: thickening of bronchial walls; dilated bronchi.

- Overinflated lungs.

- Localized areas of collapse.

- Mucoid impaction in dilated bronchi: finger-like opacities.

- High incidence of pneumonia.

- Pulmonary arterial hypertension: large pulmonary arteries.

Idiopathic pulmonary fibrosis

Idiopathic pulmonary fibrosis is a chronic lung disorder characterized by diffuse interstitial inflammation and fibrosis. Other names for this condition include chronic interstitial pneumonitis, fibrosing alveolitis, usual interstitial pneumonia (UIP) and Hamman–Rich syndrome. Peak incidence is 50–60 years of age.
CXR signs include:

- May see alveolar shadowing in the early stages of the disease.

- Interstitial linear and/or nodular pattern, predominantly at lung bases.

- Irregular 'shaggy' heart border.

- Progressive loss of lung volume, particularly lower zones.

- Later honeycomb lung.

This condition is indistinguishable radiologically from pulmonary fibrosis associated with systemic sclerosis (scleroderma), or complicating drug therapies such as bleomycin, cyclophosphamide and busulphan.

Chest trauma

Severely traumatized patients are unable to stand. For this reason, the CXR in the setting of acute trauma is often performed with the patient in the supine position. This leads to a number of problems with interpretation:

- The mediastinum appears widened due to normal distension of venous structures.

- Pleural fluid may be more difficult to diagnose in the absence of a fluid level.

- Pneumothorax may be more difficult to diagnose.

If possible therefore, an erect CXR should be performed.

Regardless of technique, the CXR of a trauma patient should be perused in the following logical fashion:

- Thoracic cage.

- Diaphragm.

- Pleura.

- Lungs.

- Mediastinum and airways.

Findings to look for include pneumothorax, haemothorax, haemopneumothorax, pulmonary contusion, mediastinal haematoma, ruptured diaphragm, and skeletal injuries including fractures of ribs, sternum and scapula.

Rib fractures

Extensive views looking for subtle rib fractures are not advised in the acute situation. Associated soft tissue injuries and complications are more important. Fractures of the upper three ribs indicate a high level of trauma, though there is no proven increase in the incidence of great vessel damage. Fractures of the

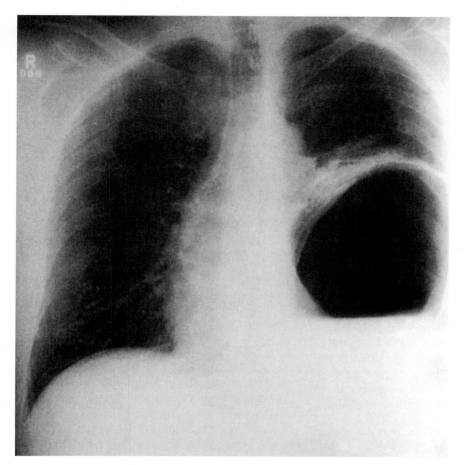

Figure 7.41 *Ruptured left diaphragm.*
The stomach has entered the left thoracic cavity and is dilated. Note:
- *collapse at the base of the left lung*
- *displacement of the heart to the right.*

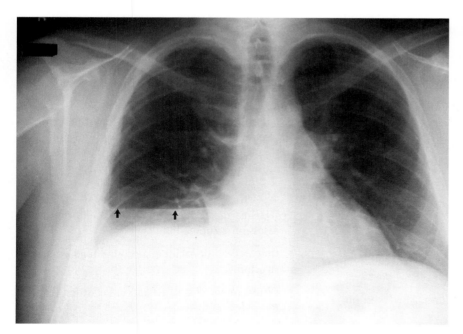

Figure 7.42
Haemopneumothorax.
Note the straight air – fluid level (arrows) in the right pleural space with no lateral meniscus.

lower three ribs have an association with upper abdominal injury (liver, spleen and kidney).

A flail segment refers to segmental fractures of three or more ribs. This produces paradoxical movement of a segment of the chest wall with respiration. This is often very difficult to appreciate clinically and as such flail segment is usually a radiological diagnosis. Flail segment has a high incidence of associated injuries such as pneumothorax, subcutaneous emphysema and haemothorax, and adequate pain management is crucial to prevent lobar collapse and pneumonia.

Other fractures

Sternal fractures usually involve the body of the sternum, rarely the manubrium. They are only seen on a lateral view. Sternal fracture has a high association with myocardial and pulmonary contusion and airway rupture. Dislocation of the sternoclavicular joint is an uncommon injury usually caused by a direct blow. This joint is notoriously difficult to see on plain films and CT is the investigation of choice where this injury is suspected. CT will show the medial end of the clavicle lying in an abnormally posterior position. Fractures of the clavicle, scapula and humerus may also be seen in association with chest trauma (thoracic spine; see Chapter 13).

Ruptured diaphragm (*Fig. 7.41*)

CXR signs of ruptured diaphragm include:

- Herniation of abdominal structures into the chest.
- Contralateral mediastinal shift.
- May occur months to years after trauma.

Pneumothorax (see *Figs 7.27, 7.28 & 7.29*)

- Tension pneumothorax indicated by depression of the diaphragm and contralateral mediastinal shift.
- Haemopneumothorax shows as a straight fluid level (*Fig. 7.42*).

Pulmonary contusion

- Solitary or multiple.
- Patchy consolidation which appears within hours of the trauma and usually clears after 4 days.
- Usually, though not always, associated with rib fractures.

Pneumomediastinum

- Vertical lucencies in the paratracheal tissues.
- Air may outline the mediastinal pleura, especially on the left.
- Associated with subcutaneous emphysema, especially in the neck.
- Often complicated by pneumothorax.

Ruptured major airway

- Severe pneumomediastinum.
- Pneumothorax.

Aortic rupture

Full thickness aortic rupture is usually fatal. Approximately 20% of aortic ruptures are not full thickness, i.e. the adventitia is intact. Untreated, there is a high mortality rate with delayed complete rupture occurring up to 4 months following trauma. Only around 5% of incomplete ruptures develop a false aneurysm associated with a normal life span. Note that incomplete aortic rupture implies an intact adventitia. Therefore mediastinal haematoma arises from other blood vessels, i.e. intercostal, internal mammary, etc. The mediastinal haematoma is associated with, not caused by, the aortic injury.

The CXR signs of aortic injury are due to the associated mediastinal haematoma. It is therefore important to recognize signs of mediastinal haematoma on CXR and CT. Twenty per cent of patients with mediastinal haematoma on CXR or CT will have an aortic injury. Absence of mediastinal haematoma is a reliable predictor of an intact aorta.

Incomplete rupture of the aorta is confirmed by aortogram or transoesophageal echocardiogram (TEE) with most tears occurring at the aortic isthmus, i.e. just distal to the left subclavian artery.

CXR signs of aortic rupture (*Fig. 7.43*):

- Widened mediastinum that may be difficult to assess on a supine film.
- Obscured aortic knuckle and other mediastinal structures.
- Displacement of trachea and nasogastric tube to the right.

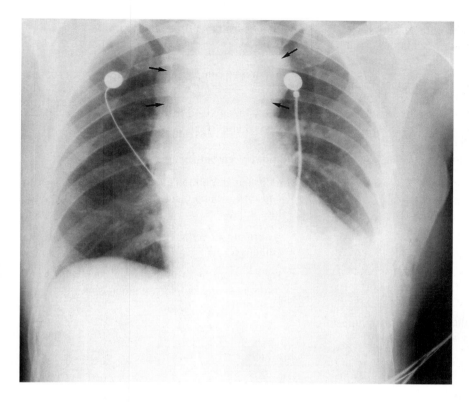

Figure 7.43 *Aortic rupture.*
Note:
- *mediastinal widening (arrows) with non-visualization of normal mediastinal structures due to haematoma*
- *non-visualization of the left hemidiaphragm due to haemothorax.*

- Depression of left main bronchus.

- Left haemothorax giving pleural opacification, including depression of the apex of the left lung.

Further investigations for aortic rupture:

- Where definite CXR signs of mediastinal haematoma are present, aortogram or TEE should be performed (*Fig. 7.44*).

- Where the CXR is equivocal, chest CT should be performed. Negative CT, i.e. no haematoma: no further investigations are required.

- Positive CT: perform aortogram or TEE.

CXR changes and complications following abdominal surgery

Atelectasis

- Caused by peripheral mucous plugs in small bronchi and by splinting from abdominal incisions.

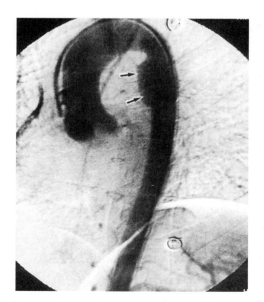

Figure 7.44 *Aortic rupture – aortogram.*
Disruption of the aorta at the isthmus (arrows), i.e. distal to the origin of the left subclavian artery. This is the most common site of a traumatic aortic rupture.

- Usually small to large areas of linear atelectasis seen as linear opacities with minimal loss of lung volume.

- In more severe cases may see lower lobe collapse.

Pleural fluid

- May be seen following upper abdominal surgery.

- Frequently accompanies lower lobe collapse.

- Signs of pleural fluid on supine CXR:
  (i)   Opacity over lung apex (pleural cap).
  (ii) Increased opacity of hemithorax.
  (iii) Blunting of costophrenic angle.

Pneumonia (see above)

Pneumothorax

- Usually due to pleural trauma complicating upper abdominal surgery, especially renal surgery.

Adult respiratory distress syndrome

- Bilateral widespread alveolar consolidation.

- Commonly complicated by left lower lobe collapse.

- Beware supine pneumothorax especially in ventilated patients and following insertion of central venous lines.

Pulmonary embolism

- CXR signs of pulmonary embolism are non-specific and may include pleural effusion, atelectasis and focal infiltrates.

- A normal CXR certainly does not exclude pulmonary embolism.

- For notes on the investigation of deep venous thrombosis and pulmonary embolism, see Chapter 8.

Methods of investigation of cardiac disease

Chest X-ray (CXR)

The most common use of plain films in cardiac disease is in the assessment of cardiac failure and its treatment. Plain films should also be perused for evidence of specific cardiac chamber enlargement, valve calcification, secondary changes to the pulmonary vascular pattern, and secondary signs such as rib notching.

Signs of specific chamber enlargement

On the PA view the right heart border is formed by the right atrium, outlined by the aerated right middle lobe. The left heart border is formed by the left ventricle, except where the right ventricle is enlarged. The left atrial appendage lies on the upper left cardiac border; it is not seen unless enlarged.

On the lateral view, the posterior cardiac border is formed by the left atrium superiorly and the left ventricle inferiorly. The anterior cardiac border is formed by the right ventricle. CXR signs of cardiac chamber enlargement may be seen as follows.

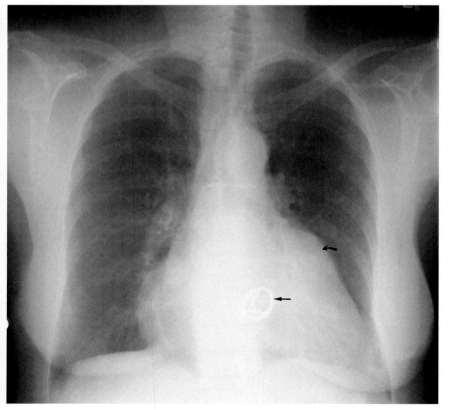

Figure 8.1 *Left atrial enlargement.*
Note:
- *'hump' on left upper cardiac border (curved arrow) due to prominence of the left auricle*
- *double edge to right cardiac border*
- *mistral valve prosthesis (straight arrow).*

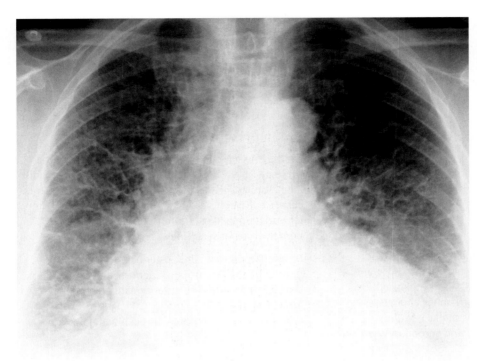

Figure 8.2 *Cardiac failure.*
Note the following signs:
- *cardiac enlargement*
- *interstitial markings and airspace shadowing bilaterally indicating pulmonary oedema*
- *bilateral pleural effusions.*

Right atrium

- Bulging right heart border.

Left atrium

- Prominent left atrial appendage on the left heart border (*Fig. 8.1*).
- Double outline of the right heart border.
- Splayed carina with elevation of the left main bronchus.
- Bulge of the upper posterior heart border on the lateral view.

Right ventricle

- Elevated cardiac apex.
- Bulging of anterior upper part of the heart border on the lateral view.

Left ventricle

- Bulging lower left cardiac border with depressed cardiac apex.

CXR signs of cardiac failure

Cardiac enlargement

- Cardiothoracic ratio is unreliable as a one-off measurement.
- Of more significance is an increase in heart size on serial CXRs, or a transverse diameter of greater than 15.5 cm in adult males or 14.5 cm in adult females.

Pulmonary venous hypertension

- Upper lobe blood vessels larger than those in the lower lobes (*see Fig. 7.18*).

Interstitial oedema

- Reticular (linear) pattern with Kerley B lines, i.e. thin lines predominantly in the lower lobes extending 1–2 cm horizontally inwards from the pleural surface of the lung (*see Fig. 7.9*).

Alveolar oedema

- Fluffy, ill-defined areas of consolidation in a perihilar or 'bat's wing' distribution (*Fig. 8.2*).

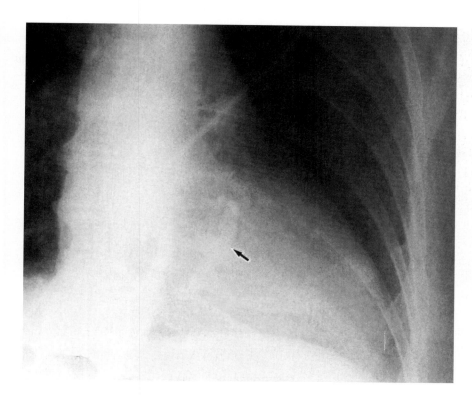

Figure 8.3 *Mitral valve annulus calcification. Dense calcification in the mitral valve (arrow).*

Pleural effusions

- Right larger than left.

Cardiac valve calcification

Mitral valve calcification

- Calcification of the mitral valve annulus is common in elderly patients. It may be associated with mitral regurgitation.
- Calcification of the mitral valve leaflets may occur in rheumatic heart disease or mitral valve prolapse.
- Mitral valve leaflet or annulus calcification is seen on the lateral view inferior to a line from the carina to the anterior costophrenic angle, and on the posterior to anterior (PA) view inferior to a line from the right cardiophrenic angle to the left hilum (*Fig. 8.3*)

Aortic valve calcification

- Usually associated with severe aortic stenosis.
- Aortic valve calcification is seen on the lateral view lying above and anterior to a line from the carina to the anterior costophrenic angle.

Changes of pulmonary vasculature

- Oligaemia, i.e. decreased pulmonary blood flow as occurs in pulmonary hypertension and in right outflow tract obstruction, e.g. Fallot tetralogy, Ebstein anomaly, pulmonary atresia, tricuspid atresia.
- Plethora, i.e. increased pulmonary blood flow as occurs with left to right shunts such as ASD, VSD, and PDA.

Rib notching

- Due to enlarged tortuous intercostal arteries associated with coarctation of the aorta (*Fig. 8.4*).

Echocardiography

Echocardiography has evolved from the early days of M-mode imaging into a highly sophisticated and accurate tool for investigation of a wide range of cardiac disorders. Direct visualization of cardiac anatomy is accompanied by Doppler analysis of flow rates through valves and septal defects. Colour

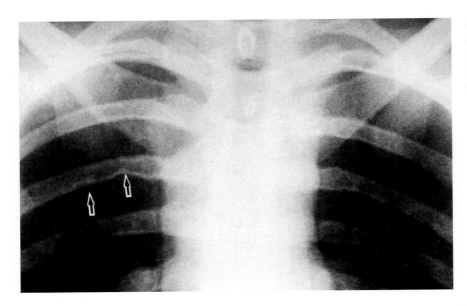

Figure 8.4 *Coarctation of the aorta.*
Rib notching (arrows) due to hypertrophy and tortuosity of the intercostal arteries.

Doppler helps in the identification of septal defects as well as high velocity jets through tightly stenosed valves.

A significant limitation of echocardiography has been the difficulty of imaging through the anterior chest wall. This is particularly true in large patients and in patients with emphysema in whom the heart may be largely obscured by overexpanded lung. These problems have been overcome with the use of transoesophageal probes giving transoesophageal echocardiography (TEE). The most useful applications of TEE include acute aortic dissection, endocarditis, congenital heart disease and paraprosthetic leaks.

In difficult cases, echocardiography may be further enhanced by the injection of ultrasound (US) contrast agents. Contrast agents currently under development may allow echocardiographic differentiation of viable from non-viable myocardium.

The following information may be obtained from echocardiography:

Cardiac anatomy

- Diagnosis and classification of congenital heart disease.
- Ventricular wall movement.
- Pericardial effusion.
- Cardiac masses.

- Postsurgical assessment (paravalvular/paraprosthetic leaks).

Measurements

- Chamber wall thickness.
- Chamber dimensions.
- Calculation of left ventricular ejection fraction and left ventricular fractional shortening.

Cardiac valves

- Valve anatomy, i.e. tricuspid or bicuspid.
- Thickness of valve leaflets.
- Measurement of valve dimensions.
- Detection of stenosis or regurgitation.
- Calculation of pressure gradients.

MRI

Advantages

- No radiation or iodinated contrast media.
- Good soft tissue differentiation.
- Multiplanar imaging.
- No interference from bone or air.

Applications

- Cardiac function: calculation of ejection traction, chamber volumes, stroke volumes and myocardial mass.

- Congenital heart disease: multiplanar imaging allows even very complex malformations to be imaged.

- Cardiomyopathies.

- Pericardial disease.

- Postsurgery: valve prosthesis assessment; bypass graft patency.

- Great vessel disease, e.g. aortic dissection, coarctation.

- Cardiac masses.

Scintigraphy

Multiple gated acquisition scan

- ^{99m}Tc-labelled red blood cells.

- Ejection fraction calculation.

- Regional wall motion analysis.

Most common indications include:

- Coronary artery disease.

- Drug-induced cardiomyopathy, most commonly doxorubicin (Adriamycin).

- Other cardiomyopathies.

- Chronic aortic regurgitation.

- Preoperative evaluation of patients with known coronary artery disease for whom major surgery is planned.

Myocardial perfusion scintigraphy

- Thallium-201 (^{201}Tl), ^{99m}Tc methoxyisobutylisonitrile (sestamibi).

- Areas of ischaemia or infarction show as areas of decreased or no uptake, i.e. 'cold' spots.

- Ischaemia: 'cold' spot on exercise; normal after 4 h (*Fig. 8.5*).

- Infarct: 'cold' spot on exercise and after 4 h of rest.

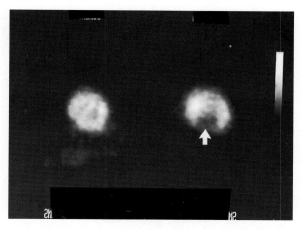

Figure 8.5 *Cardiac ischaemia – thallium scan. At rest (left) there is normal distribution of thallium. The exercise scan (right) shows a defect at the cardiac apex indicating an area of ischaemia (arrow).*

Indications include:

- Chest pain.

- Acute myocardial infarct.

- Coronary artery stenosis seen at angiography.

- Evaluation post-treatment of coronary artery disease, i.e. after angioplasty or coronary artery bypass graft (CABG).

- Evaluation of patients at high risk of coronary artery disease, especially preoperatively.

Helical CT

- Coronary artery graft patency.

- Great vessel disease, such as aortic dissection.

- Pericardial disease.

Ultrafast CT

- Not a widely used technique due to the high cost and limited availability of equipment.

- Where available, Ultrafast CT is used for quantification of cardiac function including ejection fraction, chamber volumes, stroke volumes and myocardial mass.

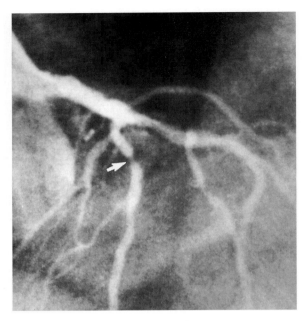

Figure 8.6 *Coronary artery stenosis.*
Left coronary angiogram shows a localized stenosis of the anterior descending branch (arrow).

Coronary angiography

- Still the investigation of choice for imaging coronary arteries (*Fig. 8.6*).

- Combined with angioplasty, stent placement or streptokinase infusion.

Indications for coronary artery angiography include:

- Angina, especially where risk factors such as cigarette smoking, positive family history or hypercholesterolaemia are present.

- Following cardiac arrest.

- Positive stress ECG or thallium scan.

- Occupation, e.g. airline pilot.

- Post CABG assessment.

Ischaemic heart disease/myocardial infarct

Myocardial infarct is obviously a medical emergency. Initial imaging assessment in the acute situation consists of a CXR to look for evidence of cardiac failure and to occasionally diagnose an unsuspected cause of chest pain such as pneumonia or pneumothorax. This will be followed by coronary angiography, as well as interventional procedures aimed at restoring coronary blood flow. These include coronary artery angioplasty and stent deployment.

Figure 8.7 *Left ventricular aneurysm.*
Note the marked convexity of the left cardiac border with elevation of the cardiac apex (arrow).

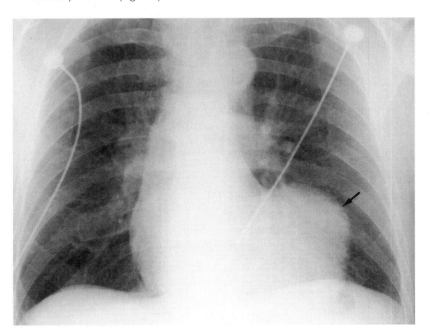

Further imaging consists of scintigraphy to assess the amount of viable versus non-viable myocardium, scintigraphy and echocardiography to quantitate cardiac function, and echocardiography to diagnose complications such as papillary muscle rupture, ventricular aneurysm and focal ventricular wall motion abnormalities.

CXR

- Normal in uncomplicated cases.

- Signs of cardiac failure (see above).

- Rarely, signs of left ventricular aneurysm may be seen, i.e. abnormal bulging contour of the left heart border associated with calcification (*Fig. 8.7*).

Coronary angiography *(see Fig. 8.6)*

To date, coronary angiography is the only imaging method available to accurately delineate the coronary arteries. It is commonly combined with intervention, i.e. angioplasty, stent placement or streptokinase infusion.

Scintigraphy

Thallium (^{201}Tl) exercise test (*see Fig. 8.5*)

The thallium exercise test is used to differentiate viable from non-viable myocardium and hence identify those patients who would benefit from coronary revascularization procedures such as angioplasty or bypass graft. Following injection with ^{201}Tl, imaging is performed immediately after exercise and then repeated 4 h later. Areas of infarct show as defects, i.e. 'cold' spots, on both series. Areas of ischaemia show as defects on the postexercise series which later fill in on the delayed series.

Infarct imaging

Infarct imaging is an uncommon test that uses ^{99m}Tc-labelled phosphates. An infarct shows as an area of increased uptake, i.e. a 'hot' spot.

Gated cardiac scan

Gated cardiac scan uses ^{99m}Tc-labelled red blood cells. It is used following myocardial infarction to provide the following information:

- Left ventricular ejection fraction, i.e. measurement of left ventricular function.

- Regional wall motion analysis.

- Left ventricular aneurysm.

Echocardiography

Echocardiography has largely replaced gated cardiac scan for the quantification of left ventricular ejection fraction. It will also provide a non-invasive diagnosis of complications such as:

- Papillary muscle rupture.

- Ventricular septal defect.

- Left ventricular aneurysm.

- Pericardial effusion.

Congenital heart disease

CXR

Plain-film assessment of suspected congenital heart disease is extremely difficult, as the changes are often non-specific. In addition, plain films are often normal or exhibit only subtle changes, despite the presence of a complex cardiac defect. Echocardiography is now widely available and is non-invasive. It is the investigation of choice for congenital heart disease. It is important, however, to be able to recognize relevant signs on CXR. The following approach would be recommended in the assessment of CXR for suspected congenital heart disease:

- Cardiac size.

- Specific chamber enlargement (see above).

- Cardiac situs.

- Situs of other structures, i.e. aortic arch and stomach.

- Pulmonary vascular patterns:
  (i)   Plethora: ASD, VSD and PDA.
  (ii) Oligaemia: Fallot's tetralogy, Ebstien's anomaly, pulmonary atresia, tricuspid atresia.

- Cardiac failure (see above).

- Skeletal changes:
  (i) Scoliosis.
  (ii) Rib notching as occurs in aortic coarctation.

Echocardiography

Echocardiography has largely replaced angiocardiography in the diagnosis and classification of congenital heart disease. It may provide non-invasive assessment of:

- Cardiac anatomy.

- Valvular function.

- Shunts, e.g. VSD, ASD.

- Anatomy of aortic root, aortic arch and main pulmonary arteries.

MRI

- MRI may supplement echocardiography in complex cases.

Hypertension

The great majority of hypertensive patients have essential hypertension. The clinical challenge is to identify the small percentage of patients with secondary hypertension and to delineate any treatable lesions. All hypertensive patients should have a CXR for the following reasons:

- Diagnosis of cardiovascular complications (e.g. cardiac enlargement, aortic valve calcification, cardiac failure).

- To establish a baseline for monitoring of future changes or complications such as aortic dissection.

Rarely, coarctation of the aorta may be detected. Signs of aortic coarctation on CXR are:

- Cardiac enlargement, especially left ventricle.

- Indentation of contour of aortic knuckle giving the configuration of a figure '3'.

- Bilateral rib notching involving the under surface of ribs 3–8 due to enlarged intercostal arteries (*see* Fig. 8.4).

Further imaging investigation is indicated in young patients, i.e. less than 40 years old, where hypertension is severe or malignant in nature; where antihypertensive medication fails to control hypertension; or in the presence of certain clinical signs such as a bruit heard over the renal arteries.

The more common causes of secondary hypertension are as follows:

- Renal:
  (i) Renal artery stenosis.
  (ii) Diseases leading to renal failure.

- Vascular:
  (i) Coarctation of the aorta.

- Endocrine:
  (i) Phaeochromocytoma.
  (ii) Conn syndrome, i.e. primary hyperaldosteronism.
  (iii) Cushing syndrome.

Initial investigations usually consist of:

- Biochemical testing of renal function.

- Endocrine studies.

- Screening tests for renal artery stenosis.

Renal artery stenosis

Screening tests for renal artery stenosis and renal disease are as follows:

US

- Measurement of renal size and assessment of renal morphology.

- Doppler examination of renal arteries: stenosis indicated by an increase in blood flow velocity.

A major limitation of US is the difficulty of imaging renal arteries due to:

- Overlying bowel gas.

- Obesity.

- Presence of multiple, aberrant arteries.

These problems may be overcome by direct Doppler examination of flow characteristics of small arteries within the kidneys.

Scintigraphy

^{99m}Tc-DTPA (diethylenetriamine pentaacetic acid). The use of intravenous captopril increases the accuracy of the study. Scintigraphy provides assessment of:

- Renal blood flow.
- Renal size and outline.
- Differential function.
- Drainage of collecting systems.

Note that this is a screening test only and renal artery morphology is not assessed.

Depending on the results of either or both of the above tests, more specific imaging for renal artery stenosis may be performed, as below:

Renal angiogram

First, an aortogram is performed to delineate the renal arteries including aberrant vessels. This is followed by selective injection of the renal arteries. Three types of arterial lesion may be found:

- Atheroma: localized narrowing of the renal artery origin.

- Atheroma of the renal artery distal to the origin.
- Fibromuscular hyperplasia: the renal artery has an irregular beaded appearance.

These three lesions may coexist in the same patient.

Renal vein renins

Via the femoral vein, catheters are positioned in the renal veins. Blood samples are taken from each renal vein to assess renin levels. Selective sampling from smaller branches may also be performed. A positive renal vein renin study indicates a favourable outcome from surgery or interventional radiology.

Renal artery percutaneous transluminal angioplasty (PTA) and stent insertion (*Fig. 8.8*)

Indications

- Renal artery stenosis.

- Three types of renal artery lesions are seen:
  (i)   Atheroma at the artery origin, i.e. ostial lesion.
  (ii) Distal atheroma.
  (iii) Fibromuscular hyperplasia.

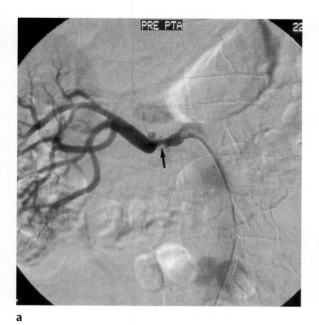

a

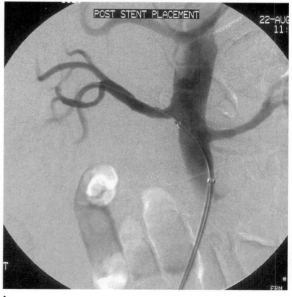

b

Figure 8.8 *Renal artery stent.*
(a) Angiogram shows a localized stenosis of the right renal artery (arrow). (b) Following stent deployment the stenosis is no longer seen.

Goals of treatment

- Normal blood pressure.

- Hypertension able to be controlled medically.

- Improved renal function.

Technique

Most lesions are initially treated with PTA though stents are now being more frequently used, especially in the following situations:

- Ostial lesion.

- Early or late restenosis following PTA.

- Complicated PTA, e.g. arterial dissection.

Advantages of stents

- Better technical results.

- Lower rate of restenosis, particularly in ostial and/ or severe disease.

Disadvantages of stents

- More invasive complex procedure with a large arterial sheath required.

- Stent positioning is critical.

- Higher cost.

Endocrine causes of hypertension

Endocrine causes, as indicated by clinical signs and symptoms as well as results of biochemical tests, may be outlined as follows:

Phaeochromocytoma

CT

- Concentrates initially on the adrenals with further studies of the remainder of the abdomen if no tumour is found.

Scintigraphy

- ^{99m}Tc-MIBG.

- MIBG (metaiodobenzylguanidine) is a noradrenaline analogue and is therefore taken up by cells of the adrenal medulla.

- Localization of phaeochromocytoma anywhere in the body.

Primary hyperaldosteronism

CT

- Use of fine sections and intravenous contrast gives optimal visualization of the adrenal glands.

Adrenal vein sampling

- Via the femoral veins, fine catheters may be placed within the adrenal veins for the purpose of selective venous sampling and hence diagnosis and localization of the source of hyperaldosteronism.

- Differentiate unilateral tumour, i.e. Conn tumour, from bilateral hyperplasia.

Cushing's disease

- CT of adrenal glands (see Chapter 11).

- MRI of pituitary fossa.

Aortic dissection

Depending on local availability and expertise, TEE and MRI are the investigations of choice for diagnosis and staging of aortic dissection. Where these modalities are not immediately available CT should be used.

Transoesophageal echocardiography (TEE)

- Where available TEE is the investigation of choice for diagnosis and staging of aortic dissection.

- Excellent spatial resolution makes TEE a highly sensitive technique.

- Potential errors include artefacts seen in the ascending aorta which may mimic dissection flaps; TEE must be performed and interpreted by experienced operators.

- As well as the dissection, TEE will diagnose complications such as aortic insufficiency and pericardial fluid.

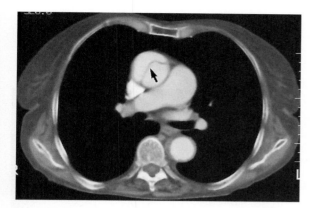

Figure 8.9 *Aortic dissection – CT.*
Note the intimal flap in the ascending aorta outlined by contrast in the true and false lumina (arrow).

MRI

Excellent contrast between flowing blood and soft tissue, plus the ability to image in sagittal as well as transverse planes, makes MRI an excellent modality for diagnosing and classifying aortic dissections. As MRI is very sensitive to flowing blood, the true and false

lumens can usually be distinguished, though certainly not in all cases. MRI is more specific, though slightly less sensitive, than TEE.

CT

Investigation of choice where TEE and MRI are unavailable or impractical (*Fig. 8.9*). Scans performed during the infusion of iv contrast may show the following:

- Visualization of the intimal flap.
- Differentiation of true and false lumen.
- Extent of dissection.
- Rupture.
- Involvement of branch vessels and infarction of organs.

Angiography

Angiography may be required for better definition prior to surgery, though less so with the advent of TEE and MRI.

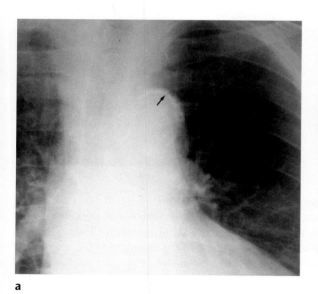

a

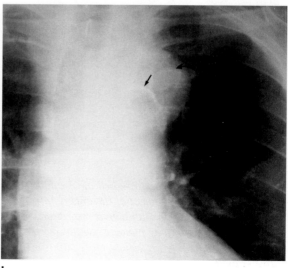

b

Figure 8.10 *Aortic dissection – CXR.*
(a) CXR performed a few months prior to presentation for other reasons. This shows calcification in the aortic arch (arrow). (b) CXR performed for acute chest pain. The aortic arch is now enlarged (curved arrow). The calcification is now separated from the outer wall of the aorta. Compare this appearance with (a).

CXR

CXR is unreliable in the diagnosis of aortic dissection. It is often normal, and positive findings are usually non-specific. Regardless of findings on CXR, more definitive imaging must be performed where a clinical suspicion of aortic dissection exists.

One may see any or all of the following signs:

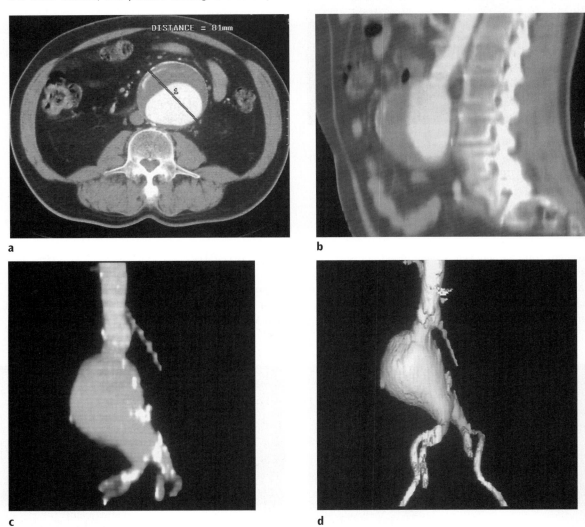

Figure 8.11 *Aortic aneurysm – helical CT and CT angiography.*
(a) Axial image. The diameter of the aneurysm is measured. Note the high attenuation lumen with thick lining thrombus anteriorly. (b) Multiplanar reconstruction (MPR). Following acquisition of data by helical CT reconstructions may be performed in any plane. A sagittal reconstruction shows the relationship of the aneurysm to the upper aorta. (c) Maximum intensity projection (MIP). MIP is a simple method of volume rendering which provides good differentiation of vascular structures and visualization of mural calcifications. Its principal disadvantage is lack of information on vessel depth; furthermore, extensive calcification may obscure the vessel lumen. (d) Shaded surface display (SSD). Also known as surface rendering. The outer surface of the contrast column is displayed as an opaque surface. The computer adds surface shading from an imaginary light source. This produces shades of grey on the surface and produces a striking 3D effect. Calcifications are not differentiated with SSD; overlapping vessels are better shown than with MIP. MIP and SSD should be regarded as complimentary 3D reconstruction techniques.

- Mediastinal widening.

- Pleural fluid.

- Separation of intimal calcification from the margin of the aortic outline (*Fig. 8.10*).

- Widening of the paravertebral stripe.

- Depression of the left main bronchus.

Abdominal aortic aneurysn (AAA)

CT

Investigation of first choice for measurement, definition of anatomy and diagnosis of complications such as leakage, hydronephrosis, etc.

Anatomy of aneurysm

- Shape.

- Size.

- Relationship to renal arteries and aortic bifurcation.

- Thrombus.

- Anatomical variants which may be important to know about preoperatively, e.g. horseshoe kidney, postaortic left renal vein.

Leakage

- Soft tissue surrounding the aneurysm.

- Active leakage may demonstrate extravasation of contrast material.

Complicated cases

- Inflammatory aneurysm.

- Retroperitoneal fibrosis.

Postoperative

- Assessment of grafts (infection, blockage, leakage); aortoduodenal fistula; retroperitoneal fibrosis.

Helical CT is particularly useful as the whole of the aorta may be scanned during peak contrast enhance-ment giving excellent definition. 2D and 3D reconstructions may be performed to further highlight the anatomy of the aneurysm. Three reconstruction techniques are commonly used (*Fig. 8.11*):

- Multiplanar reconstruction (MPR).

- Maximum intensity projection (MIP)

- Surface shading display (SSD).

US

- Used where CT is unavailable or for follow-up measurement of a known asymptomatic aneurysm.

- May be difficult owing to bowel gas or obesity.

- Anatomy of aneurysm, i.e. shape, size, relations to renal arteries and aortic bifurcation.

- Thrombus.

- Leakage: US is not as reliable as CT for detection of leakage.

Abdomen X-ray (AXR)

AAA may be seen as an incidental finding on AXR or X-ray of the lumbar spine. Plain-film signs of AAA may include:

- Soft tissue mass.

- Curvilinear calcification especially on the lateral view (*Fig. 8.12*).

- Loss of retroperitoneal planes (i.e. psoas margins and renal outlines), with leakage.

Angiography

Angiography is rarely required prior to surgery for AAA as CT and US usually provide adequate information.

Peripheral vascular disease

Clinical signs and symptoms of peripheral vascular disease include:

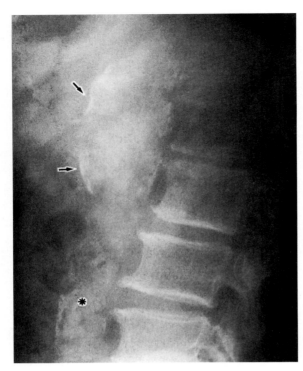

Figure 8.12 *Aortic aneurysm.*
Curvilinear calcification (arrows) marks the anterior wall of an aneurysm of the upper aorta. The lower aorta is calcified though not aneurismal (*).

- Intermittent claudication, i.e. muscle pain induced by exertion and relieved by rest.
- Rest pain.
- Tissue changes: ischaemic ulcers, gangrene.

Further assessment of limb ischaemia should combine physiological and anatomical information. The noninvasive vascular laboratory combines physiological tests with Doppler US imaging to define those patients requiring angiography and possible further treatment, either surgery or interventional radiology.

Physiological assessment

- Ankle-brachial index (ABI).
- Pulse volume recordings.
- Postexercise ABI and pulse volume recordings.

Doppler US

Signs of arterial stenosis:

- Narrowing of the vessel seen on 2D and colour images.
- Focal zone of increased flow velocity or turbulent flow.
- Altered arterial wave pattern distal to significant stenosis.

Doppler US is particularly useful to differentiate focal stenosis from diffuse disease and occlusion. Other arterial abnormalities such as aneurysm, pseudoaneurysm and arteriovenous malformation (AVM) are well seen. Doppler US is also useful for postoperative graft surveillance.

Magnetic resonance angiography (MRA)

MRA generally uses sequences which show flowing blood as high signal (bright white) and stationary tissues as low signal (dark). Increasingly for peripheral studies, contrast material (Gadolinium) is used to enhance blood vessels and reduce scanning times. Problems include long examination times and flow-related artefacts. These problems are being overcome and in centres where the technology is available, MRA has replaced diagnostic DSA in the assessment of patients with peripheral arterial disease.

Peripheral angiography; digital subtraction angiography (DSA)

See Chapter 1 for notes on the technique of DSA and Fig. 1.8.

Most peripheral angiography is done via a femoral artery puncture. Occasionally, if the femoral route cannot be used due to previous surgery or extreme tortuosity of the iliac arterias, the axillary or brachial arteries may be punctured. The method is that used for all angiography:

- The artery is punctured with a needle.
- A wire is threaded through the needle into the artery.

- The needle is removed leaving the wire in the artery.

- A catheter is inserted over the wire into the artery.

Contrast material is injected through the catheter and images are obtained to document the following:

- Site of stenosis.

- Length of stenosis.

- Status of distal run-off vessels.

With continued improvements in US and MRI techniques, less diagnostic angiography is now being performed. Angiography is increasingly being used in conjunction with interventional techniques as described below.

Venous insufficiency

For the patient with varicose veins for whom surgery is contemplated, US with Doppler is the imaging investigation of choice for assessment. The competence of a leg vein, deep or superficial, is determined with Doppler US using calf compression and release. A competent vein will show no or minor reflux (reversal of flow) on release of calf compression. Incompetence is defined as reflux of greater than 0.5 s in duration.

The following information may be obtained with Doppler US:

- Patency and competence of the deep venous system from the common femoral vein to the lower calf.

- Competence and diameter of saphenofemoral junction.

- Competence and diameter of long saphenous vein.

- Duplications, tributaries, varices arising from the long saphenous vein.

- Competence and diameter of the saphenopopliteal junction.

- Document location of saphenopopliteal junction.

- Anatomical variants of the saphenopopliteal junction.

- Course and connections of superficial varicose veins.

- Incompetent perforator veins connecting deep system with superficial system and their position in relation to anatomical landmarks such as groin crease, knee crease and medial malleolus.

To assist further with surgical planning marks may be placed on the skin over incompetent perforating veins pre-operatively. For clarity, a diagram of the venous system based on the US examination is usually provided.

Deep venous thrombosis (DVT)

Doppler US

In combination with colour Doppler imaging (CDI), US is the investigation of choice for DVT. It is non-invasive and painless, relatively inexpensive, and reliable for the femoral and popliteal veins.

With the use of colour Doppler, US can reliably image calf veins, and can also assess the pelvic veins and IVC. US will also detect conditions that may mimic DVT, e.g. ruptured Baker's cyst.

Signs of DVT on US examination include:

- Non-compressibility of the vein (*Fig. 8.13*).

- Failure of venous distension with Valsalva's manoeuvre.

- Lack of normal venous Doppler signal.

- Loss of flow on colour images.

- Acute blood clot may be anechoic and hence not visible.

- Chronic clot is usually hyperechoic and adherent to the vein wall.

The main disadvantage of Doppler US is operator dependence, and the above comments assume a skilled operator using high-quality equipment.

Venography

With the advent of Doppler US, venography is no longer the investigation of choice for DVT. Venography

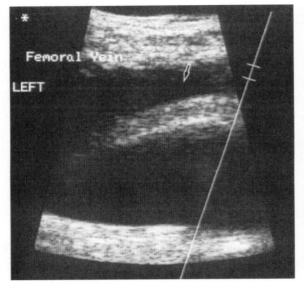

a

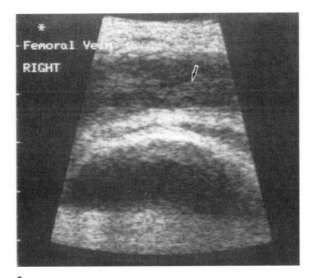

b

c

Figure 8.13 *Deep venous thrombosis (DVT).*
(a) Normal left femoral vein. The left femoral vein is seen in longitudinal section (arrow). (b) Compression. With only light pressure the normal femoral vein is easily compressed (arrow). (c) Thrombosed right femoral vein. The right femoral vein is distended and filled with echogenic thrombus (arrow). The vessel cannot be compressed.

may be performed where US is equivocal or unavailable. Signs of DVT on venogram include:

- Filling defects within contrast-filled vessels.
- Non-filling of occluded deep veins.
- Collateral flow via the superficial system or cross-pelvic collaterals with iliac vein thrombosis.

Pulmonary embolism (PE)

Pulmonary embolism (PE) is a common cause of morbidity and mortality in postoperative patients, as well as in patients with other risk factors such as prolonged bed rest, malignancy and cardiac failure.

Diagnosis of PE, however, remains problematical. Symptoms include: pleuritic chest pain, shortness of breath, cough and haemoptysis, though a large number of pulmonary emboli are clinically silent. Clinical signs such as hypotension, tachycardia, reduced oxygen saturation and ECG changes (S1 Q3 T3) are non-specific and often absent. Imaging studies are used to try to increase the accuracy of diagnosis. These include: CXR, ventilation/perfusion nuclear lung scan (V/Q scan), pulmonary angiography and, more recently, helical CT pulmonary angiography.

CXR

Signs of PE on CXR include:

- Pleural effusion.

- Localized area of consolidation contacting a pleural surface.

- Localized area of collapse.

These signs are non-specific and often absent; the CXR in a patient with PE is often normal.

Scintigraphy: V/Q SCAN

In V/Q scans, a ventilation phase is first performed with the patient breathing a radioactive tracer ^{99m}Tc-labelled aerosol. Six images are performed using anterior, posterior and oblique projections. This is followed by the perfusion phase in which images are obtained using an intravenous injection of ^{99m}Tc-labelled macroalbumen aggregates (MAA). These aggregates which have a mean diameter of 30–60 μm are trapped in the pulmonary microvasculature on first pass through the lungs. The same six projections are performed and the perfusion phase compared with the ventilation phase.

The diagnostic hallmark of PE is one or more regions of ventilation/perfusion mismatch, i.e. a region of lung where perfusion is reduced or absent and ventilation is preserved. After correlation with an accompanying CXR, lung scans are graded as low, intermediate or high probability of PE. Many studies have shown that a high probability scan is an accurate predictor of PE, whilst a low probability scan accurately excludes the diagnosis. Unfortunately, a large proportion of patients (up to 75% in some series) have an intermediate probability scan. The difficulty is compounded by

25–30% disagreement between experts in interpretation of low and intermediate probability scans.

Where the diagnosis is 'intermediate probability scan', either:

- Treat on clinical grounds.

- Investigate further with pulmonary angiogram or CTPA (see below).

Pulmonary angiography

Pulmonary angiography has long been considered the gold standard for imaging of PE. A catheter is introduced usually via the femoral vein and passed through the right atrium and right ventricle and into the pulmonary arteries. Thrombo-emboli are seen as filling defects in the arteries with secondary signs such as non-filling of peripheral vessels. As the performance of pulmonary angiography requires highly skilled operators, expensive angiography equipment and adequate patient monitoring, it is performed only in large multi-modality institutions and even then only rarely.

Pulmonary angiography is also performed for selective urokinase infusion where this is clinically indicated.

CT pulmonary angiography (CTPA)

The advent of helical CT has added a further dimension to the imaging of PE. Helical CT is much faster than conventional CT and allows imaging of the thorax in a single breath hold. This in turn allows imaging of the entire pulmonary vascular bed during optimum peak contrast enhancement. Pulmonary emboli are seen on CTPA as filling defects within contrast-filled blood vessels (*Fig. 8.14*).

Recent literature has shown that helical CT demonstrates thrombo-emboli in central pulmonary arteries, i.e. main, lobar and segmental arteries, with greater than 90% sensitivity and specificity. CTPA is less accurate is depicting PE confined to smaller subsegmental arteries. The clinical importance of such small subsegmental emboli is yet to be firmly established. If, as many believe, these are not clinically important, then CTPA may well be the imaging modality of choice for diagnosis of PE. However, if subsegmental PE is shown to be clinically important, either as an indicator of larger thrombo-emboli to come, or as a cause of death in patients with severe pre-existing cardiopulmonary disease, then CTPA alone may not be adequate.

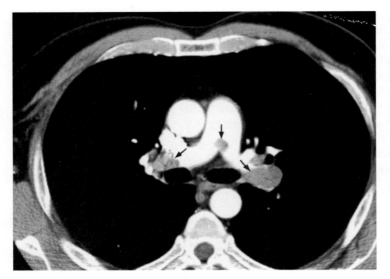

Figure 8.14 *Pulmonary embolism: CT pulmonary angiography (CTPA). Pulmonary emboli are seen as filling defects within the pulmonary arteries (arrows).*

Suggested protocol for imaging investigation of PE

Given the current state of knowledge and availability of technology, the following protocol for investigation of PE is suggested. Clinical suspicion of PE in a high-risk patient should be first investigated with CTPA. If this is positive, i.e. thrombus is shown in the first three divisions of the pulmonary artery, treatment is commenced. If negative, the patient may be observed or, where there is a persisting high level of clinical suspicion, perform a V/Q lung scan. If this is positive, treatment is commenced; if negative or equivocal, either the patient is observed or, in the occasional difficult case, go on to pulmonary angiography.

Interventional radiology of the peripheral vascular system

Percutaneous transluminal angioplasty (PTA)

Indications

- Short segment arterial stenosis with associated clinical evidence of limb ischaemia.

Technique

- Arterial puncture: femoral, brachial/axillary, popliteal.
- Wire passed across stenosis.
- Balloon catheter passed over wire and balloon positioned in the stenosis.
- Balloon dilated.
- Pressure readings proximal and distal to the stenosis pre- and postdilatation may be performed.
- Post-dilatation angiogram also performed (*Fig. 8.15*).

Postprocedure care

- Haemostasis and bed rest as for angiography.
- Low-dose aspirin.
- Heparin following complicated procedure.

Complications

- Complications of angiography.
- Arterial occlusion due to dissection.
- Arterial rupture and haemorrhage.
- Distal embolization.

Stent placement

Arterial stents are of two types:

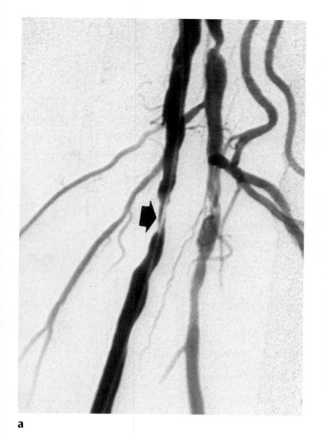

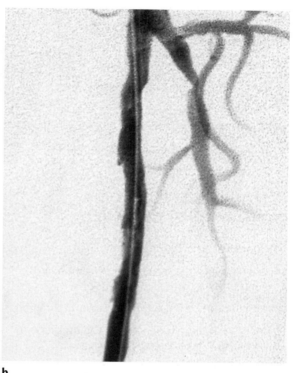

a

b

Figure 8.15 *Percutaneous transluminal angioplasty (PTA).*
(a) Pre-angioplasty. There is a localized stenosis of the left superficial femoral artery (arrow). Note that a wire has been passed across the stenosis. (b) Post-angioplasty. Following PTA there is good resolution of the stenosis with restoration of normal vessel calibre.

1. Balloon-expandable (Palmaz):

- Stent-balloon assembly passed to the stenosis over a guide wire and within a protected sheath.

- Sheath withdrawn and stent deployed by balloon inflation.

- Balloon catheter removed leaving stent in place.

2. Self-expanding (Wallstent):

- Delivered to stenosis on a catheter over a guide wire.

- When stent properly positioned, catheter withdrawn leaving stent in place.

- Stent consists of stainless steel spring filaments woven into a flexible self-expanding band.

Indications for stent placement

- Stents are being used more often by interventional radiologists in the management of stenotic and occlusive vessel disease.

- Severe or heavily calcified iliac artery stenosis/occlusion.

- Acute failure of PTA due to recoil of the vessel wall.

- PTA complicated by arterial dissection.

- Late failure of PTA due to restenosis.

Thrombolysis

Indications

- Acute, or acute on chronic arterial ischaemia.
- Arterial thrombosis postangioplasty.
- Graft thrombosis.
- Acute upper limb DVT.

Acute upper limb DVT may be caused by:

- Central venous catheters.
- Underlying venous stenosis.
- Mediastinal tumour/radiotherapy.

Technique

- Arterial puncture: may be performed under US control when the artery is occluded.
- Position catheter in or just proximal to thrombosis.
- Infusion of thrombolytic agent, e.g. urokinase by continuous or pulsed spray infusion.
- Regular follow-up angiograms to ensure dissolution of thrombus with repositioning of catheter as required.
- PTA/stent for any underlying stenosis.
- Anticoagulation following thrombolysis.

Contraindications

- Bleeding diathesis.
- Active/recent bleeding from any source.
- Anticoagulation therapy.
- Recent surgery, pregnancy, trauma.

Complications

- Complications of angiography, especially haematoma.
- Distal embolization of partly lysed thrombus.
- Systemic bleeding: gastrointestinal, cerebral, haematuria, epistaxis.

Inferior vena cava (IVC) filtration

Indications

- PE or DVT, where anticoagulation therapy is contraindicated.
- Recurrent PE despite anticoagulation.
- During surgery in high-risk patients.

Technique

- Inferior cavogram to check IVC patency, exclude anatomical anomalies, measure IVC diameter and document position of renal veins.
- Filter type depends upon approach to be used, i.e. via femoral or jugular vein.

Complications (rare)

- Femoral vein/IVC thrombosis.
- IVC perforation.
- Filter migration.

Embolization

Indications

Systemic arteriovenous malformation

- Definitive treatment.
- Preoperative.
- Palliative.

Trauma

- MVA, especially with pelvic/lower limb fracture/dislocation.
- Penetrating injuries, e.g. gunshot wounds.

Tumours

- Palliative: embolic agents labelled with cytotoxics, radioactive isotopes or monoclonal antibodies.
- Definitive treatment for tumours of vascular origin, e.g. aneurysmal bone cysts.
- Preoperative to decrease vascularity or deliver chemotherapy.

Complications

- Complications of angiography.
- Inadvertent embolization of normal structures.
- Pain.
- Postembolization syndrome, i.e. fever, malaise, leukocytosis 3–5 days postembolization.

9   Gastrointestinal system

Methods of imaging investigation of gastrointestinal diseases

Abdomen X-ray (AXR)

With the proliferation over the past two decades of imaging techniques, such as CT and ultrasound (US), and other modalities, such as endoscopy, the role of plain abdominal radiography has decreased. The AXR is still a quite useful primary investigation in the patient with acute abdomen, depending on the specific presentation as outlined below. It is no longer recommended as a first-line investigation of abdominal masses, haematemesis, malaena, urinary tract infection or vague abdominal pain. A number of less-common indications will be encountered such as swallowed (or inserted) foreign body.

The standard abdominal series

The standard plain-film abdominal series consists of three films as follows:

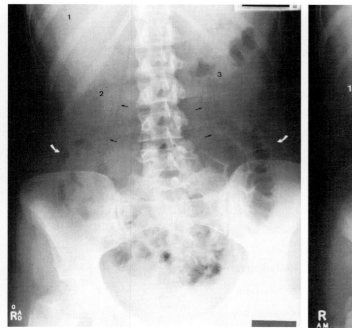
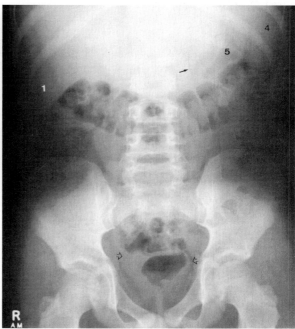

a   b

Figure 9.1 *(a) and (b) Normal abdomen.*
Identify the following features on the two radiographs: 1, liver;
2, right kidney; 3, left kidney; 4, spleen; 5, stomach. Black arrows: psoas margins; white arrows: properitoneal fat stripes; open arrows: bladder.

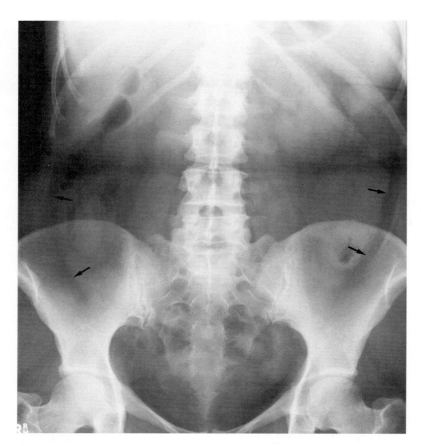

Figure 9.2 *Normal abdomen. The properitoneal fat stripes are well shown in this patient (arrows). These stripes are seen as low-density lines down each flank. They are caused by fat, which lies between the peritoneum and the muscles of the abdominal wall. Each fat stripe is therefore a radiographic marker of the lateral border of the peritoneum; they normally lie close to the outer wall of the bowel. Inflammatory processes such as appendicitis may obscure the properitonial fat stripe. Fluid or a mass in the paracolic gutter will cause separation of the bowel from the properitonial fat stripe.*

Supine antero-posterior (AP) abdomen

Erect AP abdomen

- Used to look for fluid levels and free gas.

- Therefore used for cases of possible intestinal obstruction or perforation.

- If the patient is too ill for the erect position, a decubitus film may be a useful substitute.

Erect chest

An erect chest X-ray (CXR) should be a part of a routine abdominal series for the following reasons:

- Free gas beneath the diaphragms.

- Chest complications of abdominal conditions such as pleural effusion in pancreatitis.

- Chest conditions presenting with abdominal pain such as lower lobe pneumonia.

Method of assessment of an AXR (*Fig. 9.1*)

Owing to a number of variable factors including body habitus, distribution of bowel gas and the size of individual organs, such as the liver, the 'normal' AXR may show a wide range of appearances. For this reason, a methodical approach is important and the following check-list ('things to look for') should be used.

Hollow organs

- Stomach.

- Small bowel: generally contains no visible gas, although a few non-dilated gas-filled loops may be seen in elderly patients as a normal finding.

- Large bowel.

- Bladder: seen as a round, soft tissue 'mass' arising from the pelvic floor.

Solid organs

- Liver.
- Spleen.
- Kidneys.
- Uterus.

Margins

- Diaphragm.
- Psoas muscle outline (*see Fig. 1.4*).
- Flank stripe, otherwise known as the properitoneal fat line (*Fig. 9.2*).

Bones

- Lower ribs.
- Spine.
- Pelvis, hips and sacro-iliac joints.

Calcifications

- Aorta.
- Other arteries: the splenic artery is often calcified in the elderly and is seen as tortuous calcification in the left upper abdomen.
- Phleboliths: small, round calcifications within pelvic veins; very common even in young patients and should not be confused with ureteric calculi.
- Lymph nodes: lymph node calcification may be due to previous infection and is common in the right iliac fossa and the pelvis.

Barium swallow: examination of the oesophagus

Indications

- Dysphagia.
- Swallowing disorders in the elderly, following stroke or CNS trauma.
- Suspected gastro-oesophageal reflux.
- Postoesophageal surgery.

Patient preparation

- Nil by mouth for a couple of hours.

Method

The patient is asked to swallow contrast material and films are taken. Barium is usually used, although for checking of surgical anastomoses, where leakage may be seen, a water-soluble material, such as Gastrografin, is preferable. Note that Gastrografin should not be used if pulmonary aspiration is suspected as it is highly osmolar and may induce pulmonary oedema if it enters the lungs. Images of the patient's oesophagus are recorded on cine-film, video or X-ray film. Video is particularly useful in the assessment of swallowing disorders and these studies are often undertaken with the help and co-operation of a speech or swallowing therapist.

Postprocedure care

- Physiotherapy and antibiotics if pulmonary aspiration has occurred.

Contraindications

- Known severe pulmonary aspiration.

Complications

- Pulmonary aspiration.

Barium meal: examination of the stomach and duodenum

Indications

- Dyspepsia.
- Suspected upper gastrointestinal tract (GIT) bleeding.
- Weight loss/anaemia of unknown cause.
- Assessment of anastomoses post-gastric surgery: use water-soluble contrast (e.g. Gastrografin).

Patient preparation

- Nil by mouth for 4–6 h.
- No smoking on the day of examination.

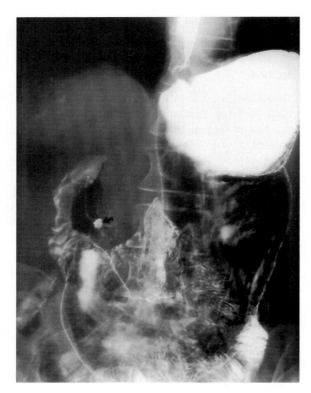

Figure 9.3 *Barium meal – duodenal ulcer.*
Double-contrast barium meal. Duodonal ulcer (arrow)
seen as a crater filled with barium. Note mucosal folds
radiating from the ulcer.

Method

A single contrast study is one where a hollow organ is
filled with contrast material such as barium. The
outline of the organ can be appreciated, although not
its mucosal surfaces. If gas is then used to dilate the
organ, the mucosal surfaces can be seen coated with
barium. This is 'double contrast' (*Fig. 9.3*). The great
majority of barium meals and enemas are performed
in double contrast as it provides much better mucosal
detail than single contrast. Single contrast studies
using barium only may be performed in children, and
occasionally in the very elderly.

In the case of a barium meal, the patient drinks a
small amount of barium followed by gas-forming
liquids and films are taken. An antispasmodic is
commonly used to temporarily halt peristalsis and
allow accurate imaging of the duodenum. Intravenous
hyoscine is used. It rapidly halts peristalsis for

15–20 min. The side-effects are rare and due to
anticholinergic effects such as blurred vision and dry
mouth. Hyoscine is contraindicated in patients with
cardiac ischaemia or glaucoma and intravenous
Glucagon may be used in these cases.

Postprocedure care

- Advise patient to drink plenty of water to aid the
  passage of barium from the bowel.

Contraindications

- Bowel obstruction.

Complications

- Pulmonary aspiration.

Barium follow-through: examination of the small bowel

This is a simple procedure used to demonstrate and
locate the site of a suspected partial small bowel
obstruction. The patient drinks a quantity of barium
and films are taken until the contrast either reaches
an obstruction or enters the large bowel. Gastrografin
should be used if there is any suspicion of a perforation.

Small bowel enema (enteroclysis)

Indications

- Ulcero-inflammatory disease, especially Crohn's
  disease.

- Malabsorption syndromes.

- Miscellaneous small bowel conditions, such as
  tumour and Meckel diverticulum.

Patient preparation

- Laxative on the evening before the examination.

- Nil by mouth on the day of examination.

Method

A nasogastric tube is passed into the stomach and
with the aid of a steering wire is then guided through

the duodenum to the duodeno-jejunal flexure. A mixture of barium with either water or methyl cellulose introduced rapidly through the tube into the small bowel gives a double-contrast effect.

Advantages of this technique over simple barium follow-through include:

- Better assessment of mucosal pattern.
- Much more rapid procedure.

The major disadvantage is the use of a nasogastric tube, which is unpleasant to the patient.

Postprocedure care

- The patient is warned of diarrhoea due to the large amount of fluid passed into the small bowel.

Contraindications

- Complete small bowel obstruction.

Complications

- Problems with the nasogastric tube.

Barium enema: examination of the large bowel

Indications

- Altered bowel habit.
- Lower GIT bleeding (*Fig. 9.4*).
- Weight loss/anaemia of unknown cause.

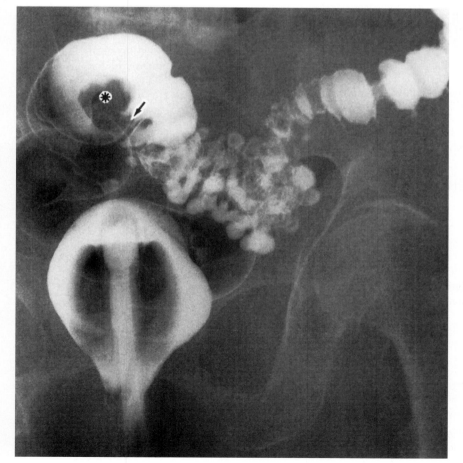

Figure 9.4 *Pedunculated polyp.*
Filling defect in the sigmoid colon (*). Note the stalk of the polyp (arrow).

- To outline and define a suspected obstruction (single contrast).

- Suspected perforation (Gastrografin).

- Check surgical anastomoses (Gastrografin).

Patient preparation

Various bowel preparation regimes have been described, e.g. low-residue diet for 2–3 days, plus laxatives, with a bowel wash-out performed on the day of examination.

Method

Barium is passed into the large bowel via a rectal cannula followed by air giving a double-contrast technique. Single-contrast technique may be used in the very elderly, or in children, or for suspected obstruction, as above.

Contraindications

- Toxic megacolon as may occur in ulcerative colitis.

Complications

- Bowel perforation.

- Rare cases of allergy to the balloon used on the rectal catheter have been reported.

- Transient bacteraemia: patients with artificial heart valves should receive antibiotic cover.

Coelic axis/mesenteric angiography

Indications

- GIT bleeding.

- GIT ischaemia.

- Preoperative demonstration of vascular supply of liver tumour (i.e. surgical 'road map').

See Chapter 1 for general notes on angiography.

Dysphagia

Barium swallow

Barium swallow is the simplest and cheapest screening test for the investigation of dysphagia. For many

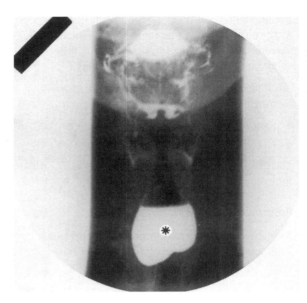

Figure 9.5 *Pharyngeal pouch – barium swallow. Large pharyngeal pouch (*) well outlined with barium.*

conditions, barium swallow is sufficient for diagnosis; for others it will guide further investigations. The more common conditions encountered on barium swallow are outlined below:

Pharyngeal pouch (Zenker's diverticulum) (*Fig. 9.5*)

- Projects posteriorly and to the left above cricopharyngeus through the inferior constrictor muscle.

- May be quite large with a fluid level seen on CXR.

Oesophageal diverticulum

- Most common from the level of the tracheal bifurcation to the diaphragm.

- Project anteriorly and laterally.

- Large diverticulae above the diaphragm may be associated with hiatus hernia.

Achalasia

- Dilated oesophagus that may also be elongated and tortuous.

- Poor peristalsis.

- Smoothly tapered lower end.

- CXR may show a mediastinal fluid level, absent

gastric air bubble, and evidence of aspiration pneumonia.

Sliding hiatus hernia

- Range in size from a small clinically insignificant hernia to the entire stomach lying in the thorax (i.e. thoracic stomach) which is at risk of volvulus.

- On CXR may show as an apparent mass behind the heart containing a fluid level.

Reflux oesophagitis

- Erosions give a granular appearance to the mucosa.

- Ulcers seen as larger mucosal defects.

- Chronic reflux may cause a peptic stricture that usually has smooth tapering edges.

Carcinoma of the oesophagus

- Appearances depend on pattern of tumour growth.

- Early lesions may show only an area of mucosal irregularity and ulceration.

- More advanced lesions present with irregular strictures with elevated margins (*Fig. 9.6*).

- May also present as an irregular intraluminal mass, ulceration or with sinus/fistula formation.

- Further staging of carcinoma of the oesophagus consists of CT to assess local invasion and mediastinal lymphadenopathy, as well as to exclude liver and pulmonary metastases.

Endoscopy and biopsy

All strictures seen on barium swallow should undergo endoscopic assessment and biopsy, as should areas of ulceration and mucosal irregularity.

Acute abdomen

In assessing the patient with an acute abdomen the surgeon may complement a full history and examination with other investigations, including laboratory tests (e.g. white cell count, ESR), laparoscopy and imaging studies. Plain abdominal films remain the first line of imaging investigation for most patients with an acute abdomen, and the most common findings are outlined below. A plain film of the supine abdomen may show the following:

- Abnormal gas patterns such as dilated bowel loops, free gas or gas in the biliary tree.

- Soft tissue masses.

- Foreign bodies.

- Abnormal calcifications such as renal calculi and pancreatic calcification.

A plain film of the erect chest may show free gas beneath and above the diaphragm, chest conditions which may present as acute abdomen such as basal pneumonia, or chest complications of abdominal conditions such as pleural effusion and basal atelectasis.

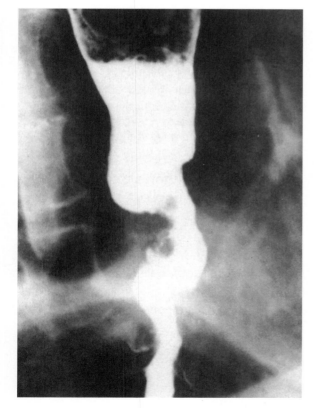

Figure 9.6 *Oesophageal carcinoma – barium swallow. There is a stricture of the lower oesophagus with prominent margins and an intraluminal mass.*

Plain films of the erect abdomen are less frequently used. These should be reserved for cases of suspected intestinal obstruction or suspected perforation.

Other imaging modalities, i.e. CT, US and contrast studies are used where appropriate. In particular, CT has found an increasing role in the diagnosis of bowel disorders. CT provides excellent delineation of bowel wall thickening, bowel masses, pericolonic inflammation, and sinus and fistula tracts. As is discussed in this and subsequent chapters, CT is useful in the investigation of small bowel obstruction, small bowel neoplasms, inflammatory bowel disease and lower abdominal pain.

Intestinal obstruction

Small bowel obstruction

Plain films remain the primary investigation of choice in suspected small bowel obstruction.

Plain-film signs of small bowel obstruction include:

- Dilated small bowel loops, which have the following features:
  (i)   Tend to be central.
  (ii)   Numerous.
  (iii) 2.5–5.0 cm diameter.
  (iv)   Have a small radius of curvature.
  (v)   Valvulae conniventes, which are thin, numerous, close together and extend right across the bowel.
  (vi)   Do not contain solid faeces.

- Multiple fluid levels on the erect film.

- 'String of beads' sign on the erect view due to small gas pockets trapped between valvulae conniventes.

- Absent or little air in the large bowel (*Fig. 9.7*).

Limitations of plain films include:

- Partial or early obstruction.

- Strangulation.

- Closed-loop obstruction.

CT is the investigation of choice when clinical and plain-film assessment are inconclusive. CT is highly accurate for establishing the diagnosis of small bowel obstruction, defining the location and cause of obstruction, and diagnosing associated strangulation.

CT signs of small bowel obstruction:

- Small bowel loops measuring >2.5 cm in diameter.

- Identifiable focal transition zone from prestenotic dilated bowel to post-stenotic collapsed bowel loops (*Fig. 9.8*).

Oral contrast studies (small bowel follow-through) using barium or water-soluble contrast are often misleading, i.e. unable to differentiate obstruction from paralytic ileus, and may in fact delay diagnosis. Enteroclysis (small bowel enema) remains the investigation of choice for grading severity and location of partial obstruction.

In summary, the majority of small bowel obstructions are diagnosed with clinical assessment and plain films. CT is the investigation of choice in doubtful cases, with enteroclysis occasionally useful in partial obstruction.

Large bowel obstruction

Plain-film signs of large bowel obstruction include:

- Dilated large bowel loops which have the following features:
  (i)   Tend to be peripheral.
  (ii)   Few in number.
  (iii) Large: above 5.0 cm diameter.
  (iv)   Wide radius of curvature.
  (v)   Haustra, which are thick and widely separated, and may or may not extend right across the bowel (compare these features with the valvulae conniventes found in the small bowel).
  (vi)   Contain solid faeces (*Fig. 9.9*).

- Caecum may be dilated.

- Small bowel may be dilated.

Contrast enema may be helpful for the following:

- To differentiate 'pseudo-obstruction', which occurs most commonly in elderly patients and may be indistinguishable on plain films from mechanical obstruction.

- To localize the point of obstruction.

- To diagnose the cause of obstruction, e.g. tumour, inflammatory mass.

Paralytic ileus

Localized ileus

Localized ileus refers to dilated loops of bowel ('sentinel loops'), usually small bowel, overlying a local

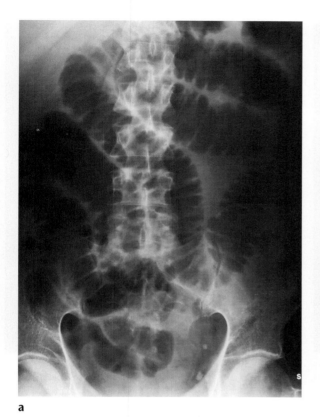

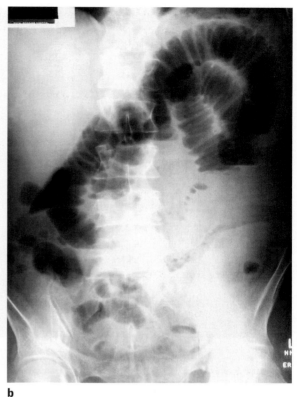

a   b

Figure 9.7 *Small bowel obstruction.*
(a) Supine film. Note that small bowel loops are mainly central in position; numerous; measure less than 5 cm in diameter; have a small radius of curvature; contain valvulae conniventes which pass across the bowel lumen and are thin and close together. (b) Erect film. Note:
* *features of small bowel loops, as above*
* *numerous air-filled levels.*

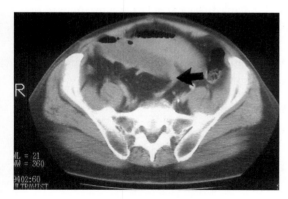

Figure 9.8 *Small bowel obstruction – CT.*
Typical case of small bowel obstruction due to adhesions. Note the dilated small bowel loops with a focal transition zone to distal collapsed bowel (arrow).

inflammation. Sentinel loops may be seen in the following sites:

* Right upper quadrant: acute cholecystitis.

* Left upper quadrant: acute pancreatitis (*Fig. 9.10*).

* Lower right abdomen: acute appendicitis.

Generalized ileus

Generalized ileus refers to non-specific dilatation of small and large bowel, which may occur post-operatively or with peritonitis. Scattered irregular fluid levels are seen on the erect X-ray.

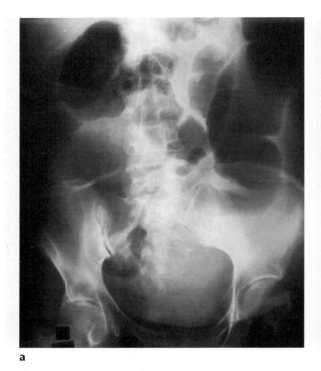
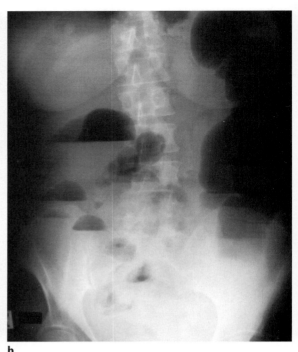

a

b

Figure 9.9 *(a) and (b) Large bowel obstruction.*
Note the features of large bowel loops:

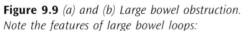

- *peripheral*
- *few in number*
- *wide radius of curvature*
- *greater than 5 cm in diameter*
- *contain haustra which are thick and widely separated.*

Specific causes of intestinal obstruction that may be diagnosed with plain films

Caecal volvulus (*Fig. 9.11*)

- Markedly dilated caecum containing one or two haustral markings.

- The dilated caecum may lie in right iliac fossa or left upper quadrant.

- Attached gas-filled appendix.

- Small bowel dilatation.

- Collapse of left half of colon.

Sigmoid volvulus (*Fig. 9.12*)

- Massively distended sigmoid loop in the shape of an inverted 'U', which can extend above T10 and overlap the lower border of the liver.

- Usually has no haustral markings.

- The outer walls and adjacent inner walls of the 'U' form three white lines that converge towards the left side of the pelvis.

- Overlap of the dilated descending colon, i.e. 'left flank overlap' sign.

Strangulated hernia

- Gas-containing soft tissue mass in the inguinal region.

- May have a fluid level on the erect view.

- Gas in the bowel wall in the presence of infarction.

Gallstone ileus (*Fig. 9.13*)

- Small bowel obstruction.

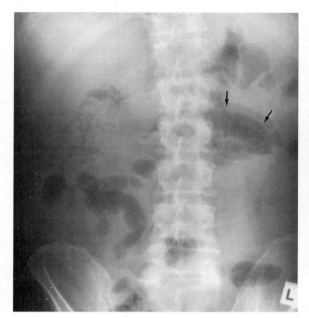

Figure 9.10 *Sentinel loops.*
Multiple dilated loops of small bowel (arrows) are grouped in the left upper abdomen in a patient with pancreatitis.

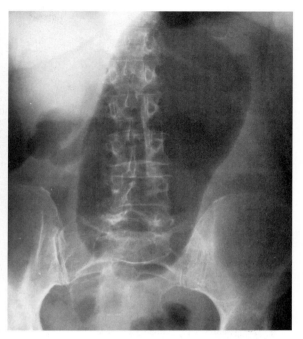

Figure 9.11 *Caecal volvulus.*
Massively dilated caecum in the central abdomen. Note that the distal large bowel is not dilated.

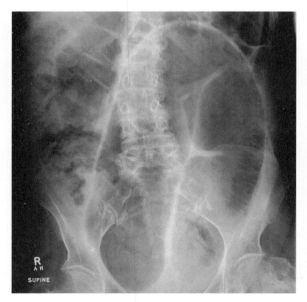

Figure 9.12 *Sigmoid volvulus.*
There is dilatation of the sigmoid colon. The dilated bowel loop forms an inverted 'U' arising from the pelvis. Note that the remainder of the large bowel is dilated. This helps to differentiate this condition from caecal volvulus.

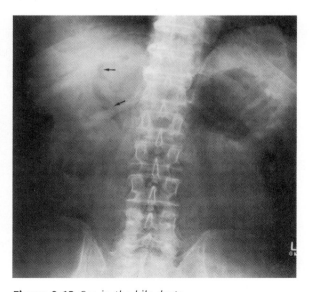

Figure 9.13 *Gas in the bile ducts.*
Gas in the bile ducts is seen as a low-density branching pattern in the right upper abdomen (arrows). This is separate to the colon, overlies the liver shadow, and conforms to the anatomy of the biliary tree.

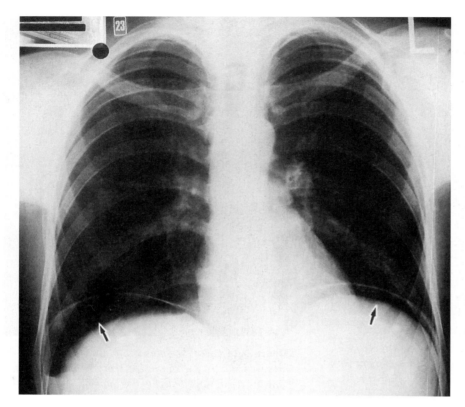

Figure 9.14 *Perforation of the colon.*
Excellent demonstration of free gas beneath the diaphragm (arrows).

- Gas in the biliary tree seen as a branching pattern of gas density in the right upper quadrant.

- Calcified gallstone lying in an abnormal position is occasionally seen.

Intussusception (see Chapter 16)

Perforation of the gastrointestinal tract (GIT)

Plain-film signs of free gas

- Erect CXR: gas beneath diaphragm (*Fig. 9.14*).

- Supine abdomen: gas outlines anatomical structures such as the liver, falciform ligament and spleen; bowel walls are seen as white lines outlined by gas on both sides, i.e. inside and outside the bowel lumen (*Fig. 9.15*).

- Free gas is also identified on erect abdomen film.

- If the patient is too ill to stand then either decubitus or shoot-through lateral films can be performed.

Contrast studies

Use water-soluble contrast (Gastrografin) as opposed to barium where perforation is suspected. Contrast meal is performed for suspected perforated duodenal or gastric ulcers, with contrast enema for suspected perforated colon. Contrast enema may also identify sinus and fistula tracts, e.g. colovesical fistula in diverticular disease.

Acute appendicitis

The plain-film diagnosis of acute appendicitis is unreliable and some, all, or indeed none of the following signs may be seen:

- Faecolith: calcified opacity usually in the right iliac fossa.

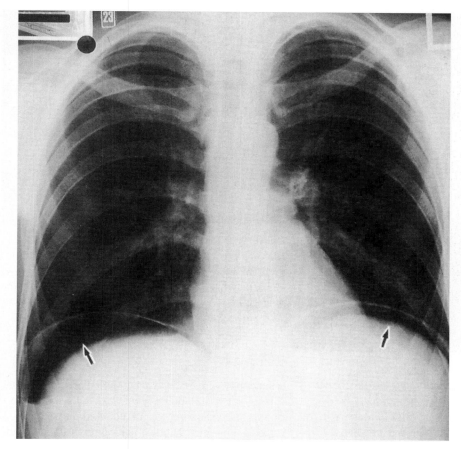

Figure 9.15
Pneumoperitonium-supine abdomen.
The bowel wall is outlined by gas within the lumen and by free gas outside the bowel within the peritoneal cavity (arrows).

- Distal small bowel obstruction or localized paralytic ileus.

- Blurred right psoas margin and right properitoneal fat stripe.

- Lumbar scoliosis convex to the left.

- Decreased abdominal gas due to vomiting and diarrhoea.

- Gas in the appendix.

- Appendix abscess: soft tissue mass in the right iliac fossa which may separate gas-filled ascending colon from properitoneal fat stripe.

US and CT have an increasing role in the assessment of right lower quadrant pain and are useful for the following:

- Diagnosis of appendicitis.

- Diagnosis of complications of appendicitis, e.g. abscess, mucocele.

- Diagnosis of alternate causes of right lower quadrant pain, e.g. pelvic inflammatory disease.

Choice of modality will depend to some extent on local expertise, though CT should be used in obese patients or in severely ill patients in whom complications such as peritonitis or abscess are suspected. US is highly accurate for appendicitis in children and thin patients, particularly where compression and colour Doppler imaging (CDI) are used, and where the examination is concentrated to the point of maximal tenderness as indicated by the patient (*Fig. 9.16*).

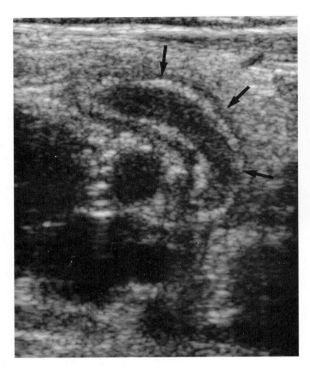

Figure 9.16 *Acute appendicitis – US.*
Ten-year-old male presenting with right iliac fossa pain. US shows an inflamed appendix as a sausage-shaped thick-walled mass in the right iliac fossa (arrows). The mass was non-compressible to probe pressure.

Acute cholecystitis

Ultrasound (US)

US is the investigation of choice for suspected acute cholecystitis.

US signs of acute cholecystitis include:

- Gallstones: hyperechoic lesions with acoustic shadowing which are mobile (*see Fig. 2.3*).

- Thickening of gallbladder wall to greater than 4 mm. (*Fig. 9.17*).

- Hypoechoic gallbladder wall due to oedema.

- Surrounding fluid or localized fluid collection.

- Distended gallbladder.

- Localized tenderness to direct probe pressure.

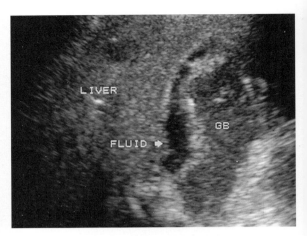

Figure 9.17 *Acute cholecystitis – US.*
The inflamed gallbladder (GB) in this case has a thick irregular wall. The bile within the gallbladder is echogenic in keeping with inflammatory debris. Note the fluid between the gallbladder and the liver. A gangrenous gallbladder was found at surgery.

Scintigraphy

Scintigraphy with ^{99m}Tc-labelled iminodiacetic acid (IDA) compounds has a limited role in difficult cases where clinical assessment and US are doubtful. Acute cholecystitis is indicated by non-visualization of the gallbladder with good visualization of the common bile duct and duodenum 1 h after injection (*Fig. 9.18*). Visualization of the gallbladder excludes acute cholecystitis.

Plain films

Plain films are insensitive for acute cholecystitis.

Plain-film signs are also usually non-specific and include:

- Gallstones (only seen in 10%).

- Soft tissue mass in the right upper quadrant due to distended gallbladder.

- Paralytic ileus in the right upper quadrant.

Acute pancreatitis

CT

CT is the imaging investigation of choice for acute pancreatitis, and is particularly useful for the following:

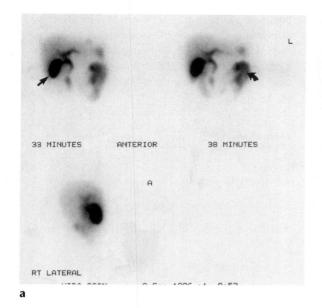
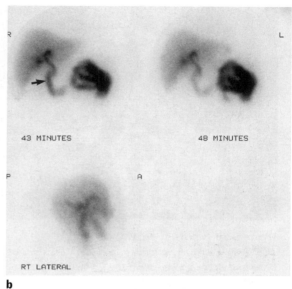

a   **b**

Figure 9.18 *Acute cholecystitis – HIDA scan.*
(a) Normal HIDA scan. Following normal hepatic uptake there is good filling of the bile ducts and the gallbladder (straight arrow). Note also normal activity in the duodenum and jejunum (curved arrow). (b) Acute cholecystitis. There is normal hepatic uptake of tracer. The bile duct is outlined (arrow) and tracer has entered the bowel. The gallbladder is not seen due to acute cholecystitis. Compare this appearance with (a).

- Confirmation of the diagnosis.

- Identification of necrotic gland tissue.

- Diagnosis of complications.

- Guidance of interventional procedures.

CT signs of acute pancreatitis include:

- Diffuse or focal pancreatic enlargement with decreased density and indistinct gland margins.

- Fine sections during infusion of contrast (i.e. dynamic scans) can differentiate necrotic non-enhancing tissue from viable enhancing tissue.

- Thickening of surrounding fascial planes, e.g. left paranephric fascia (*Fig. 9.19*).

- Acute fluid collections, most commonly related to the pancreas though also in the lesser sac and in the left pararenal space.

- Phlegmon appears as an irregular mass spreading along fascial planes and can be quite extensive.

- Abscess.

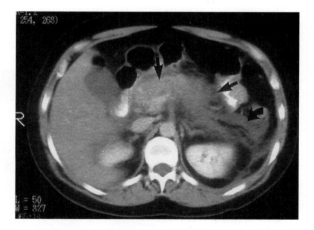

Figure 9.19 *Acute pancreatitis – CT.*
The pancreas is swollen and has indistinct margins due to inflammation of surrounding fat (straight arrows). There is thickening of the left pararenal fascia (curved arrow).

- Pseudocyst (*Fig. 9.20*).

CT can be used to guide aspiration procedures and placement of drains in abscesses and pseudocysts, and

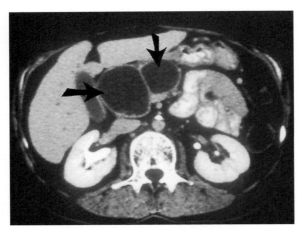

Figure 9.20 *Pancreatic pseudocysts – CT.*
Two well-defined low-attenuation cysts in the pancreatic head and neck (arrows). Note the following features:
- *thin wall*
- *homogeneous low-attenuation fluid contents.*

for follow-up either postoperatively or in conservative management.

US

US examination may be difficult in the acute situation owing to overlying dilated bowel loops. The acutely inflamed pancreas appears enlarged with decreased echogenicity and blurred irregular margins. Fluid collections are seen as hypoechoic areas anatomically localized as described above. As with CT, US can be used to guide aspiration and drainage procedures, and for follow-up.

Plain films

Unreliable: no significant plain-film findings in up to two-thirds of patients with acute pancreatitis.

Plain-film signs may include:

- Paralytic ileus in the left upper quadrant (*see Fig. 9.10*).
- Generalized ileus.
- Loss of left psoas outline.
- Separation of greater curve of stomach from transverse colon.
- Pancreatic calcification with chronic pancreatitis.

CXR signs that may be seen include:

- Left pleural effusion.
- Atelectasis of left lower lobe.
- Elevated left hemidiaphragm.

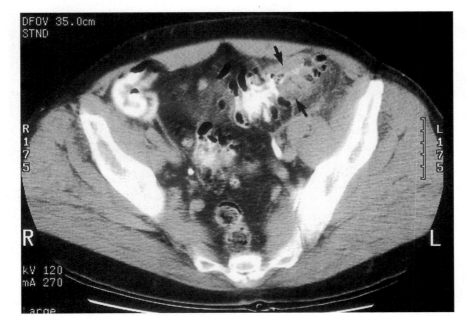

Figure 9.21 *Acute diverticulitis – CT. The wall of the sigmoid colon is thickened with intramural abscess formation (arrows). Note also inflammatory stranding in the pericolonic fat.*

Acute diverticulitis

Diverticulitis refers to diverticular perforation with intramural, pericolonic or peritoneal inflammation, abscess formation and sinus/fistula formation. Plain films are usually unhelpful. In the past, barium enema has been used to study patients with diverticulitis. Limitations of barium enema include:

- Inability to diagnose pericolonic and peritoneal inflammation.

- Low sensitivity for intramural inflammation.

- Low sensitivity for alternative diagnoses.

CT is now the investigation of choice for assessment of acute left lower quadrant pain. CT is highly accurate for the diagnosis of diverticulitis. It is able to visualize intramural and pericolonic inflammation, and where diverticulitis is not present it may suggest alternative diagnoses such as small bowel obstruction, pelvic inflammatory disease, pancreatitis, pyelonephritis, etc.

CT signs of diverticulitis (*Fig. 9.21*):

- Localized wall thickening >5 mm.

- Pericolonic inflammation: soft tissue stranding or haziness in pericolonic fat.

- Abscess/phlegmon: soft tissue mass containing fluid and/or gas.

- Sinus/fistula tracts: linear tracts filled with contrast/gas.

- Contrast/gas in bladder, vagina or abdominal wall.

Abdominal abscess

Plain films

Although the following signs may be seen, plain films are unreliable for the diagnosis of abdominal abscess, and US or CT are usually required.

CXR signs associated with subphrenic abscess:

- Raised hemidiaphragm.

- Pleural fluid.

- Lower lobe collapse.

- Subdiaphragmatic fluid level.

Signs that may be seen on AXR include:

- Mass, perhaps containing gas or even a fluid level on the erect view.

- Displaced bowel loops.

- Localized or generalized ileus.

- Loss of outline of adjacent structures, e.g. psoas muscle.

US

US should be the primary investigation of choice for suspected intra-abdominal abscess. Advantages of US include:

- Portability.

- Localized fluid collections are well shown and usually easily differentiated from dilated bowel loops.

- Guide needle aspiration and drainage.

- Especially sensitive for subdiaphragmatic, subhepatic and pelvic collections (*Fig. 9.22*).

The principal disadvantage of US is that it is less sensitive for central abdominal collections due to overlying intestinal gas. US may also be difficult to perform where surgical dressings and drains are present.

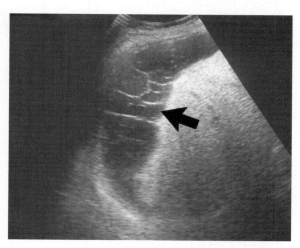

Figure 9.22 *Subphrenic abscess – US.*
A complex fluid collection (arrow) is seen between the right diaphragm and the liver.

CT

CT is an excellent modality for the diagnosis of abdominal abscess, especially where US is unhelpful. Complete bowel opacification with oral and rectal contrast is mandatory as non-opacified bowel loops may mimic fluid collections. CT may also be used for guidance of needle aspiration and drain placement. CT signs of abscess include:

- Low attenuation mass.
- Irregular enhancing wall.
- May contain gas and fluid levels.

Scintigraphy

Scintigraphy is used to sort out difficult cases where clinical suspicion of an abscess is high, but CT and US are negative.

Labelled white cells studies using Indium or ^{99m}Tc-HMPAO (hexamethylpropyleneamineoxime) may be performed. ^{99m}Tc-HMPAO provides better image resolution, lower radiation dose and easier handling compared with Indium. An abscess (or other inflammatory process) shows as an area of focal increased activity.

Gallium scanning is also extremely sensitive in detecting sites of inflammation. Gallium scans may be difficult to interpret due to normal gallium uptake in bowel, liver and spleen.

Acute mesenteric ischaemia (AMI)

AMI is caused by abrupt disruption of blood flow to the bowel. The goal of diagnosis and therapy is prevention or limitation of bowel infarction. Plain-films are insensitive for AMI. Plain-films signs when present usually indicate bowel infarction and include:

- Bowel wall thickening.
- Bowel dilatation.
- Gas in the bowel wall (*Fig. 9.23*).
- Portal vein gas.

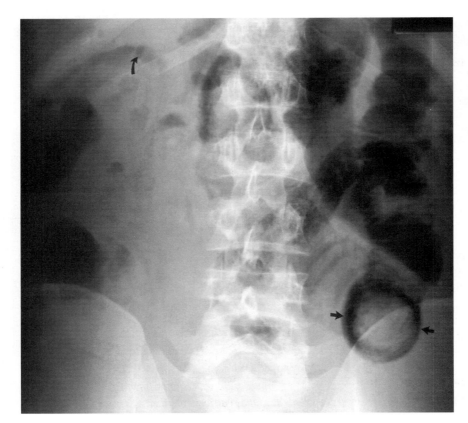

Figure 9.23 *Small bowel infarction.*
There is a large amount of gas in the wall of the small bowel indicating infarction (straight arrows). Note gas in the portal vein (curved arrow).

Early diagnosis requires a high index of suspicion and early angiography in patients with clinical evidence of AMI, i.e. sudden onset of severe abdominal pain and bloody diarrhoea. The most common causes of AMI are superior mesenteric artery (SMA) embolus, SMA thrombosis and non-occlusive SMA vasospasm. Depending on the cause and clinical situation, particularly the presence or absence of peritoneal signs, treatment will be immediate surgery or interventional radiology.

SMA embolus

The patient may have a history of cardiac disease, previous embolic event or simultaneous peripheral artery embolus. Angiography shows occlusion of SMA usually several centimetres from its origin. SMA embolus is usually treated with immediate surgery.

SMA thrombosis

SMA thrombosis is usually associated with an underlying stenotic atherosclerotic lesion in the SMA. The onset of pain may be less acute than in SMA embolus. Angiography shows occlusion of the SMA within 1–2 cm of its origin with collateral vessels to the more distal SMA. Interventional radiology consists of thrombolytic therapy via a selective catheter, which may be followed by angioplasty of any underlying stenosis.

Non-occlusive SMA vasospasm

Mesenteric vasospasm may persist after an episode of severe systemic hypotension. Angiography shows diffuse arterial narrowing due to vasospasm, poor filling of distal branches, low arterial flow rate and delayed filling of veins. Interventional radiology consists of papaverine bolus and infusion via a catheter placed in the SMA.

Inflammatory bowel disease

Plain films

Plain films are relatively insensitive and non-specific for the diagnosis of inflammatory bowel disease. They may be useful in acute colitis, where barium studies are contraindicated and endoscopy may be difficult and painful.

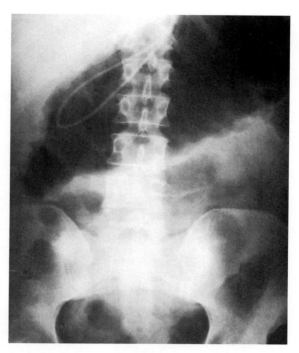

Figure 9.24 *Toxic megacolon.*
Grossly dilated transverse colon. There is also a nasogastric tube lying curled in the stomach.

X-ray signs of acute colitis:

- Affected bowel shows wall thickening, blurred mucosal margins, absent haustral markings.
- Gasless colon strongly suggests severe disease.

X-ray signs of toxic megacolon:

- Marked large bowel dilatation, most often of the transverse colon, often greater than 8 cm diameter (*Fig. 9.24*).
- May be complicated by perforation and peritonitis.

CT

CT is the investigation of choice in the acute situation particularly where barium studies and endoscopy may be difficult or contraindicated. CT is used in inflammatory bowel disease to define:

- Extent and site of bowel involvement.
- Extracolonic inflammation and abscess formation.
- Sinus/fistula formation.

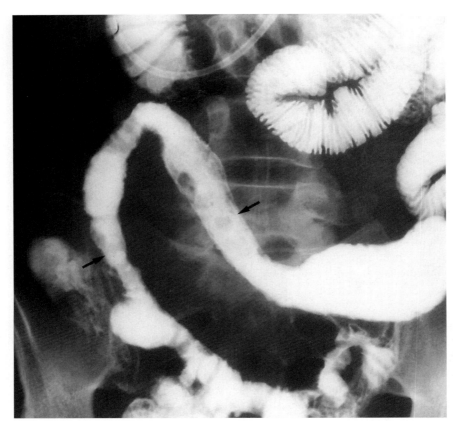

Figure 9.25 *Crohn's disease – enteroclysis.*
The diseased small bowel loop (arrows) shows the following features:

- *thickened bowel wall with loss of normal mucosal pattern*
- *ulceration*
- *'cobblestoning'*
- *separation from adjacent bowel loops due to mesenteric inflammation*
- *note the normal small bowel loops proximal and distal to the diseased segment.*

Barium studies for Crohn's disease

- Small bowel study: best images obtained by enteroclysis (small bowel enema).
- Barium enema for large bowel involvement.

Signs of Crohn's disease on barium studies are numerous and include:

- 'Skip' lesions (i.e. diseased segments separated by segments of normal bowel).
- Ulcers.
- Strictures.
- 'Cobblestoning' due to fissures separating islands of intact mucosa.
- Thickened bowel wall.
- Fistulae and sinuses.
- Separation of bowel loops due to mesenteric infiltration or abscesses (*Fig. 9.25*).

Barium studies for ulcerative colitis

Barium enema is absolutely contraindicated in toxic megacolon.

Signs of ulcerative colitis on barium enema:

- Rectum involved.
- Retrograde involvement of large bowel with no skip lesions.
- Early there is fine ulceration that later becomes more florid.
- Pseudopolyp formation due to postinflammatory granulation tissue and fibrosis.
- Loss of haustral markings (*Fig. 9.26*).
- Shortening and narrowing of large bowel.
- Involvement of distal ileum in total colitis with fine ulceration giving a granular mucosal pattern.

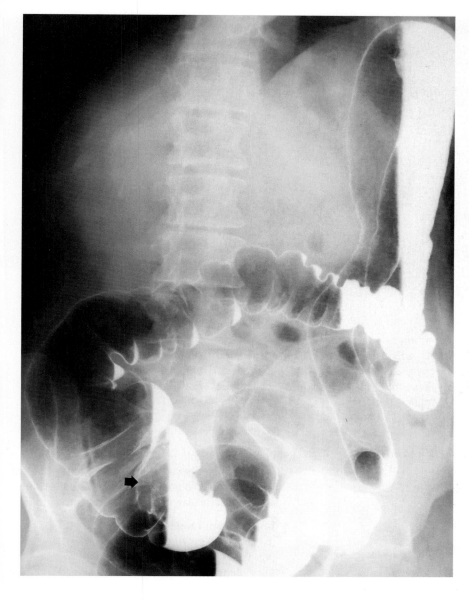

Figure 9.26 *Ulcerative colitis – barium enema. Note:*
- *loss of normal haustra in the left colon*
- *pattern of fine mucosal ulceration giving the bowel a 'shaggy' outline*
- *this case is complicated by a carcinoma, seen as a mass in the caecum (arrow).*

Scintigraphy

Scintigraphy for assessment of inflammatory bowel disease is performed with a variety of techniques, e.g. ^{99m}Tc-HMPAO and ^{99m}Tc-labelled sucralfate. Affected bowel segments show as areas of increased tracer uptake, i.e. 'hot' areas. Scintigraphy may be useful in defining anatomical location of disease, to a lesser extent in assessing disease severity, to diagnose relapse in patients with known inflammatory bowel disease,

and in acutely ill patients in whom barium studies are contraindicated.

Gastrointestinal bleeding

Endoscopy is the primary investigation of choice for acute upper and lower GIT bleeding. In a significant proportion of patients, however, endoscopy will either

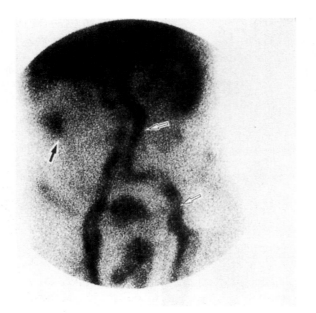 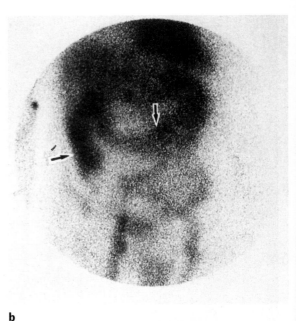

a   b

Figure 9.27 *Gastrointestinal haemorrhage – scintigraphy.*
(a) ^{99m}Tc-labelled red blood cells. An early scan shows a 'hot' area (solid arrow) on the right side of the abdomen indicating haemorrhage into the upper ascending colon. Note that the aorta and iliac vessels are well outlined (hollow arrows). (b) A later scan shows tracer filling much of the bowel (solid arrows) indicating extensive haemorrhage. (Courtesy of Dr F. Smith, Aberdeen.)

fail to find a bleeding point, or fail to achieve haemostasis, and it is in these cases that radiological techniques have an important role.

The goals of diagnosis and treatment of the patient with acute GIT bleeding are:

- Haemodynamic resuscitation.

- Localization of the source of bleeding.

- Control of blood loss either by surgery, interventional radiology, or a combination of both.

An upper GIT source for GIT bleeding is excluded by:

- Nasogastric aspirate.

- Upper GIT endoscopy.

Lower GIT bleeding is first investigated by sigmoidoscopy. If this is negative, scintigraphy and angiography are used to further assess the patient.

Causes of acute lower GIT bleeding include:

- Angiodysplasia.

- Colonic diverticulum:
  (i)   Although diverticular disease is most prevalent in the sigmoid colon, up to 50% of bleeding from colonic diverticulae occurs in the ascending colon.

- Less common causes:
  (i)   Inflammatory bowel disease.
  (ii) Colonic carcinoma.
  (iii) Solitary rectal ulcer.
  (iv) Postpolypectomy.

RBC scintigraphy with ^{99m}Tc-labelled red blood cells (RBCs)

A bleeding point shows as an area of increased uptake outside normal areas of activity. These normal areas of activity include the aorta, inferior vena cava (IVC), portal vein, renal veins, kidneys and bladder (*Fig. 9.27*). Scintigraphy is more sensitive than angiography, i.e. a lower rate of haemorrhage is required (0.1–0.2 mL/min) to produce a positive result.

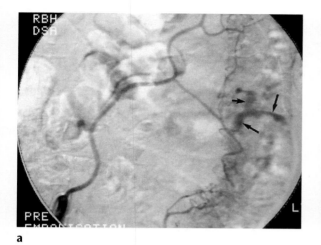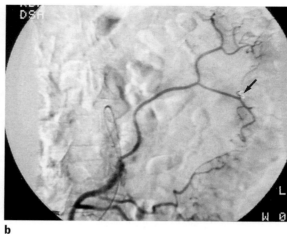

a   b

Figure 9.28 *Bleeding diverticulum – angiogram.*
(a) Inferior mesenteric angiogram. Selective catheterization of the inferior mesenteric artery. Acute haemorrhage is seen as a blush of contrast in the bowel arising from a branch of the left colic artery (arrows). (b) Embolization. Following superselective catheterization a steel coil is used to occlude the bleeding artery (arrow). Note that leakage of contrast is no longer seen indicating successful embolization.

Scintigraphy is less anatomically specific than angiography. For this reason surgery based on RBC scintigraphy alone is not recommended. Rather, RBC scintigraphy should be seen as a screening test that will increase the accuracy of subsequent angiography.

RBC scintigraphy is therefore usually used in a complementary role to establish whether or not acute haemorrhage is occurring prior to angiography. A patient with clinical evidence of bleeding and negative scintigraphy should be investigated with elective colonoscopy and barium studies.

Angiography

Angiography is performed for two reasons:

- To locate a bleeding point.

- To achieve haemostasis by infusion of vasoconstrictors, or embolization (*Fig. 9.28*).

Active haemorrhage is seen as extravasation of contrast material into the bowel if bleeding of 0.5–1.0 mL/min^{-1} is occurring at the time of injection. Angiodysplasia is seen as a small nest of irregular vessels with early and persistent filling of a draining vein.

Interventional radiology

Interventional radiology is most useful where surgery is thought to be too risky, or for stabilization prior to surgery. Options for the patient with GIT bleeding include:

- Selective infusion of vasoconstrictors such as vasopressin.

- Embolization of small distal arterial branches following superselective catheterization.

Barium studies

In centres where endoscopy services are limited, or where colonoscopy is technically impossible, barium studies of upper and lower GIT have a role in chronic and intermittent bleeding. These studies are especially useful for making certain specific diagnoses such as peptic ulceration, to exclude malignancy of either upper or lower GIT in chronic blood loss, and in the diagnosis of other lesions such as polyps (*see Fig. 9.4*), diverticular disease and inflammatory bowel disease.

Barium studies have no role in the patient with acute bleeding.

Carcinoma of the stomach

Endoscopy and biopsy

Endoscopy is now widely performed in the assessment of symptoms suspicious for gastric carcinoma, including dyspepsia, upper abdominal pain, anaemia and weight loss. It is highly accurate, may be combined with biopsy, and has largely replaced barium meal in the diagnosis of gastric disorders.

Barium meal

Barium meal is occasionally performed where endoscopy is not freely available. See above for technique. The appearance of a gastric tumour on barium meal depends on the pattern of growth. The following may be seen:

- Gastric mass producing an irregular filling defect.
- Ulcer, usually with elevated margins (*Fig. 9.29*).
- Mucosal infiltration with gastric fold thickening, mucosal irregularity and distorted gastric outline.

- 'Linitis plastica': small non-distensible stomach (*Fig. 9.30*).

Staging

Further imaging for staging of gastric carcinoma includes CT for liver metastases and lymphadenopathy, chest CT and CXR for pulmonary metastases, plus scintigraphy where bone metastases are suspected.

Small bowel neoplasms

Small bowel neoplasms may present in a variety of ways and are often very difficult to diagnose. The patient may present with a quite specific clinical picture such as carcinoid syndrome or intussusception, or with less specific signs such as anaemia, weight loss or frank bleeding. The two principal imaging investigations are barium studies and CT. These studies are complementary in that barium studies show intraluminal and mucosal tumours whilst CT will image intramural tumours and extra-intestinal spread.

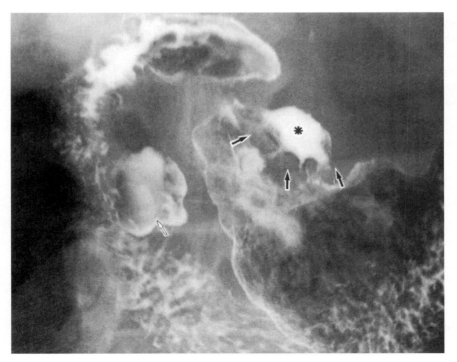

Figure 9.29 *Gastric carcinoma – barium meal. Tumour of the gastric antrum shown as heaped-up folds of soft tissue (black arrows) surrounding a large central ulcer crater (*). A diverticulum of the second part of the duodenum is also shown (white arrow).*

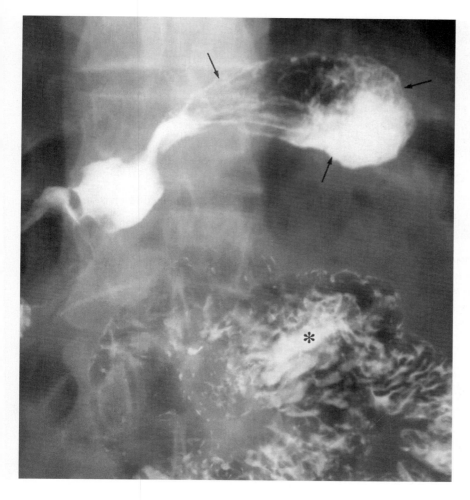

Figure 9.30 *Linitis plastica – barium meal. Small, contracted stomach which fails to distend despite double-contrast technique (arrows). There is rapid passage of contrast and gas into the small bowel (*).*

CT will also show lymphadenopathy, liver metastases and tumour complications such as invasion of adjacent structures, fistula formation and intussusception.

The primary sign of a small bowel neoplasm on CT is asymmetric thickening of the bowel wall, usually >1.5 cm. This is compared with bowel wall thickening in benign processes such as Crohn's disease or ischaemia; such thickening is usually concentric, symmetrical and may show the 'target' sign.

CT is highly accurate for presence, site and size of tumour, as well as the presence of metastases. CT is less accurate at predicting histology. The exception is lipoma where the fat content is well seen; carcinoid tumour may also have a fairly specific appearance.

Benign tumours commonly present as the lead point in an intussusception. Intussusception appears on CT as a soft tissue mass containing multiple layers giving a target-like appearance.

Carcinoid tumour

- Majority occurs in the ileum.

- Often involves the mesentery inciting a desmoplastic reaction.

- CT: soft tissue mass that may be heavily calcified.

- Mesenteric infiltration seen as strands of soft tissue radiating from the mass; adjacent small bowel loops tend to be separated and may be kinked and angular in appearance (*Fig. 9.31*).

- Patients with clinical evidence of carcinoid syndrome will usually also have hepatic metastases.

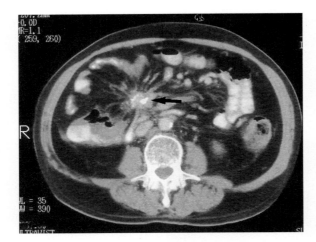

Figure 9.31 *Carcinoid tumour – CT.*
A calcified mesenteric mass (arrow) is surrounded by radiating soft tissue strands due to desmoplastic reaction.

Adenocarcinoma

- Localized mass or focal area of asymmetric bowel wall thickening.

Non-Hodgkin lymphoma

- Tends to involve a longer segment of bowel than adenocarcinoma.

- Usually a well-defined mass with concentric bowel wall thickening.

- Most commonly involves the ileocaecal region.

- With involvement of mesenteric lymph nodes may see large masses, which encase the mesenteric vessels and displace bowel loops.

- In children, may present as a lead point in intus-susception.

- May also see other CT signs such as lymphadenopathy and splenomegaly.

Small bowel metastases

- Most common primary sites are melanoma, lung, breast and ovary.

- Direct invasion of the small bowel may also occur from the large bowel and pancreas.

Colorectal carcinoma (CRC)

Probably the most widely used classification of CRC is Kirklin's modification of Dukes' original system as below:

- Stage A: Tumour confined to mucosa.

- Stage B1: Tumour extension into, but not through, muscularis propria.

- Stage B2: Tumour extension through muscularis propria but confined to bowel wall.

- Stage C: Stage B1 or B2 with lymph node metastases.

- Stage D: Distant metastases.

As can be seen, the two most critical factors influencing survival data are depth of invasion of the bowel wall and presence or absence of lymph node metastases. Unfortunately, two major limitations of imaging of CRC are assessment of depth of wall invasion and detection of microscopic metastases in non-enlarged lymph nodes. Whilst accurate pretreatment staging of CRC is probably useful for planning of surgery, radiotherapy and chemotherapy, it remains controversial due to the limitations of imaging plus the fact that most patients with CRC will have surgery for either cure or palliation.

Colonoscopy/barium enema

Both of these investigations are most useful for initial detection of CRC and adenomatous polyps and in localization, characterization and diagnosis of multiple lesions. Colonoscopy is more accurate than barium enema for detection of small and sessile polyps and has the added advantages of biopsy and polyp removal at the time of examination. Barium enema remains a highly accurate and relatively non-invasive technique. It is particularly useful for assessment of an elongated, tortuous colon where redundant loops may not be amenable to negotiation with a colonoscope (*Fig. 9.32*).

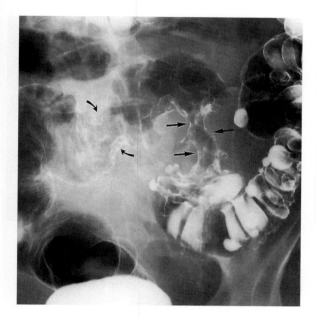

Figure 9.32 *Double-contrast barium enema –*
carcinoma.
Note:
- *'apple-core' stricture (straight arrows)*
- *mucosal irregularity in the more distal colon*
  indicating extensive involvement with carcinoma
  (curved arrows)
- *diverticular disease of the more proximal colon.*

CT

CRC may be seen on CT as a mass or thickening of the bowel wall. Invasion beyond the bowel wall and invasion of adjacent structures are usually well demonstrated by CT. CT is unable to assess the depth of wall invasion and to detect small metastases in non-enlarged lymph nodes. Therefore, CT is accurate for advanced disease though less so for earlier non-invasive disease.

Transrectal ultrasound (TRUS)

The layers of rectal wall are well seen and therefore TRUS is able to evaluate the depth of wall invasion. TRUS may also be used for guided biopsy of perirectal lymph nodes. Limitations of TRUS include overstaging due to peritumoral inflammation mimicking invasion beyond the muscularis propria, as well as understag-

ing due to microscopic tumour invasion too small to be seen with TRUS.

Distant spread

- Liver metastases: CT.
- Lung metastases: CXR/CT.
- Bone metastases: scintigraphy/plain films.

Abdominal trauma

As with the acute abdomen discussed above, the patient with abdominal trauma can be assessed by many aids that supplement the clinical history and examination. These aids to diagnosis include peritoneal lavage, laparoscopy, 'mini-lap' and laparotomy.

Imaging plays an important role and the more common findings in each of the modalities are outlined below. It should be emphasized that haemodynamically unstable patients should undergo immediate surgery. Contrast enhanced CT is the investigation of choice for suspected abdominal injuries in haemodynamically stable patients. US is used in some centres, particularly in children; it is less sensitive than CT. With CT now widely available, plain films are performed less often in the setting of trauma. They are, however, used to assess spinal and pelvic fractures and it is therefore important to also recognize plain-film signs of abdominal trauma.

CT

CT for the assessment of abdominal trauma is usually performed with iv and oral contrast material; oral contrast material may need to be administered by nasogastric tube. CT provides excellent anatomical definition of intra-abdominal fluid collections and solid organ damage. Intraperitoneal and retroperitoneal gas is also seen, and CT may show haematoma in the wall of traumatized gut. Blood appears as hypodense material in more dependent parts of the peritoneal cavity, i.e. pelvis (*Fig. 9.33*), hepatorenal pouch and paracolic gutters.

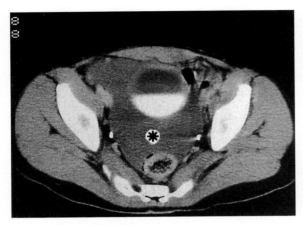

Figure 9.33 *Peritoneal blood – CT.*
Blood in the peritoneal cavity due to traumatic splenic rupture. Blood is seen as low-attenuation material (*) separating the bladder from the rectum.

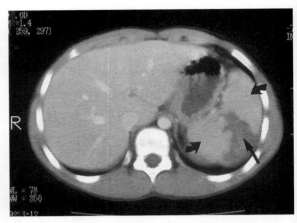

Figure 9.34 *Splenic rupture – CT.*
A large laceration of the spleen is seen as an irregular low-attenuation area (straight arrow) separating high-attenuation splenic fragments (curved arrows).

Splenic trauma

Splenic lacerations appear as hypodense lines separating more dense splenic fragments (*Fig. 9.34*).

Hepatic trauma

CT provides accurate localization of hepatic haematoma, intrahepatic or subcapsular. Intrahepatic haematoma may be of increased or decreased attenuation. Lacerations appear as hypodense lines in the liver substance.

Pancreatic trauma

Laceration through the pancreas is seen as a low attenuation cleft.

Bowel trauma

Pneumoperitoneum occurs in only 60% of cases of traumatic bowel perforation. Free retroperitoneal gas may be seen with duodenal rupture. Free fluid may be seen lying between bowel loops; fluid may be of high attenuation if it contains leaked oral contrast material. Intramural haematoma is seen as localized bowel wall thickening or intramural mass. Associated injuries such as solid organ damage or Chance fracture occur in over 50% of cases.

Other CT signs in abdominal trauma:

- Sentinel clot sign: high attenuation blood immediately adjacent to the site of injury.
- Collapsed IVC and renal veins indicate severe shock.

US

US examination may be difficult in the traumatized patient owing to distended bowel loops, dressings, chest tubes, etc. US is most useful for the diagnosis of free intraperitoneal blood. Blood in the peritoneum appears as anechoic fluid, sometimes with septations, separating bowel loops and surrounding solid organs. US is less sensitive than CT for the diagnosis of solid organ injury or bowel injury.

Plain films: AXR

Signs to look for on the AXR of a traumatized patient include:

- Free gas.
- Free fluid.
- Fractures:
  (i) Fractured lower ribs: high association with liver/spleen injury.

(ii)   Spinal fractures including fractured transverse processes and Chance fracture: see Chapter 13.

(ii)   Pelvic fractures: see Chapter 13.

• Foreign material, e.g. pieces of glass, etc.

CXR changes associated with abdominal trauma:

• Pleural effusion.

• Lower lobe collapse.

• Ruptured diaphragm.

• Rib fractures.

Angiography

Angiography has a limited role in abdominal trauma. It is used to localize bleeding where other imaging techniques have failed to do so, often as a precursor to embolization.

For notes on 'Trauma to kidneys and ureters' and 'Trauma to bladder and urethra', see Chapter 11.

10 Liver, gallbladder and pancreas

Investigation of liver masses

Helical CT of the liver

The ability to visualize a mass in the liver on CT, i.e. lesion conspicuity, is due to the difference in density between the lesion and the surrounding liver. Lesions that are of low attenuation such as liver cysts are well seen on plain, non-contrast CT. Lesions containing calcification such as mucin-producing metastases and hydatid cysts are also well seen. Unfortunately, a large percentage of liver malignancies are of equal or similar attenuation to liver tissue and are therefore difficult, if not impossible, to see on an unenhanced CT. Intravenous contrast material is used to improve lesion conspicuity.

The liver receives a dual blood supply. The hepatic artery supplies 20% whilst the portal vein supplies 80% of hepatic blood flow. Following intravenous injection of a bolus of contrast material there are three phases of contrast enhancement. An early arterial phase begins at around 25 s following commencement of injection. After blood has circulated through the mesentery, intestine and spleen there is a later portal venous phase of enhancement beginning at around 70 s following commencement of injection. Given that 80% of the liver's blood supply is from the portal vein it follows that maximum enhancement of liver tissue will occur in the later portal venous phase. After several minutes there is redistribution of contrast material to the extracellular space giving the third or equilibrium phase of contrast enhancement.

Most liver tumours are supplied by the hepatic artery. Furthermore, most tumours are hypovascular, i.e. they receive less blood supply than surrounding liver. It follows then that maximum lesion conspicuity for most liver tumours including metastases will occur in the portal venous phase of contrast enhancement. Please note that this is due to liver enhancement, not enhancement of the lesion. These hypovascular lesions are seen as low-attenuation masses well visualized against high-attenuation enhancing liver (*Fig. 10.1*).

A few liver tumours are hypervascular, i.e. they receive more blood supply than surrounding liver. For these tumours maximum lesion conspicuity will occur in the arterial phase of contrast enhancement. This is due to enhancement of the lesion, not the liver. These lesions are seen as high-attenuation masses compared with the relatively low-attenuation liver tissue (*Fig. 10.2*).

Examples of hypervascular lesions best seen in the arterial phase are:

- Small hepatocellular carcinomas.

- Focal nodular hyperplasia.

- Hypervascular metastases.

The speed of helical CT allows imaging of the entire liver in around 20 s, i.e. during a single breathhold.

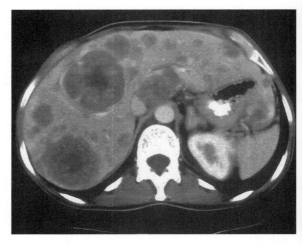

Figure 10.1 *Liver metastases – CT. Contrast-enhanced helical CT, portal venous phase. Liver tissue shows dense enhancement. The hypovascular metastases which are supplied by the hepatic artery are well seen as low-attenuation masses in the portal-venous phase of contrast enhancement.*

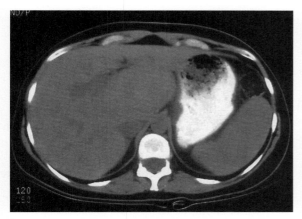

a

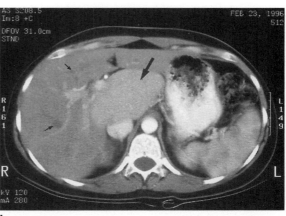

b

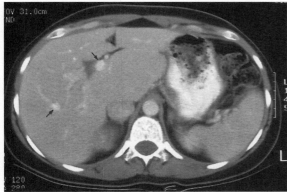

c

Figure 10.2 *Focal nodular hyperplasia – CT.*
Focal nodular hyperplasia is a good example of a hypervascular mass supplied by the hepatic artery and therefore best seen in the arterial phase of contrast enhancement. (a) Non-contrast CT. The mass is of equal density to surrounding liver and could easily be missed. (b) Contrast CT – arterial phase. The mass is well seen (large arrow) due to dense enhancement compared with relatively unenhanced surrounding liver tissue. Note other normal features of the arterial phase:
* *patchy enhancement of the spleen*
* *unenhanced hepatic veins (small arrows) not to be confused with metastases.*
(c) Portal-venous space. The mass is once again of equal density to surrounding liver tissue. Note that the spleen now shows homogeneous enhancement and that the hepatic and portal veins are now filled with contrast (arrows).

This means that the entire liver may be scanned during the separate phases of contrast enhancement. This technique is termed 'dual phase' liver CT. Overlapping reconstruction implies that all of the liver is accurately imaged so that even small lesions of the order of 1 cm should be seen.

Helical CT is now the imaging investigation of choice for assessment of liver masses. It is the most sensitive technique for the presence of a mass. It is also useful for the following:

* Good anatomical localization.

* Definition of tumour margins.

* Characterization of contents: fluid, necrosis, fat, calcification, gas, etc.

* Diagnosis of complications: invasion of the portal vein, arteriovenous shunting.

* Biopsy guidance.

Ultrasound (US)

US is often the first investigation performed for a suspected liver mass as it is non-invasive and relatively cheap (*Fig. 10.3*). As with CT it gives good anatomical

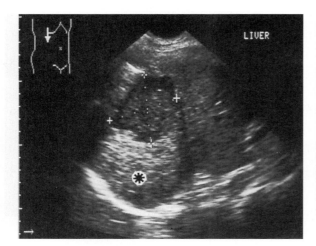

Figure 10.3 *Liver abscess – US.*
Abscess seen as an area of reduced echogenicity in the liver. Note the following features:
- *irregular wall*
- *echogenic contents due to inflammatory debris*
- *acoustic enhancement.*

localization. It is highly sensitive for fluid-filled lesions such as cysts and abscesses though less accurate than CT for characterization of solid lesions. Being non-invasive, US is particularly useful for masses requiring follow-up:

- Haemangioma, to confirm lack of growth.

- Metastases and other tumours receiving chemotherapy.

- Abscess, following drainage/antibiotic therapy.

Intraoperative US is now widely used in the diagnosis and management of metastases.

Scintigraphy

Liver scintigraphy uses ^{99m}Tc-labelled sulphur colloid compounds, which are taken up by Kupffer cells in the liver (not hepatocytes), as well as by the spleen and, to a lesser extent, the bone marrow. Liver lesions larger than 1 cm can be seen. Scintigraphy is especially useful for the diaphragmatic surface which may be difficult to image with other techniques. It generally complements CT and US, and may occasionally find metastases missed by other modalities. Most liver masses appear as filling defects except for focal

nodular hyperplasia, which usually contains Kupffer cells and therefore shows tracer uptake.

Plain films

Plain films are not useful as a primary investigation for suspected liver mass. Various secondary signs such as elevation of the right diaphragm or displacement of the hepatic flexure may infer the presence of a liver mass on an abdominal X-ray (AXR). Occasionally, more specific signs may be seen such as gas in an abscess, or calcification in hydatid cyst.

Angiography

Angiography is used more often for liver masses than for masses in other organs, not so much for diagnostic purposes but as a surgical 'road map'. This includes outlining the arterial supply, portal vein (hepatocellular carcinoma and some metastases may invade the portal vein), and occasionally the inferior vena cava (IVC). Angiography may also be used for selective infusion of chemotherapy or embolization.

Imaging investigation of jaundice

US is the first imaging investigation of choice for the jaundiced patient. If the bile ducts are not dilated, a diffuse hepatic disease is considered. If this cannot be diagnosed by imaging and biochemical analysis, then liver biopsy may be required.

If the bile ducts are dilated on US without an obvious cause seen, endoscopic retrograde cholangiopancreatography (ERCP) or percutaneous transhepatic cholangiography (PTC) is then performed. In some centres CT may also be performed, as this has a higher rate of diagnosis of the cause of biliary obstruction than US. Newer, less invasive techniques for imaging the biliary system are also now available, i.e. 3D CT cholangiography and magnetic resonance cholangiopancreatography (MRCP).

HIDA scans have a limited role.

Table 10.1 *Imaging findings of the more common liver masses*

Mass	Ultrasound (US)	CT	Other imaging
Metastases	Multiple masses of variable echotexture	Most are seen as low attenuation lesions on contrast enhanced scans	Intraoperative US is a highly accurate technique used at surgery for carcinoma of the colon, or to localize metastases prior to partial hepatic resection
HCC	3 patterns may be seen: single mass, multiple masses, diffuse infiltration	Small HCC tends to be hypervascular and best seen as enhancing mass on arterial phase of contrast enhancement. Larger tumours seen as low-attenuation masses. Complications: portal vein invasion, arterio-venous shunting.	
Simple cyst	Well defined, anechoic, acoustic enhancement	Well defined, low attenuation, homogeneous	
Pyogenic abscess	Poorly defined, irregular margin; hypoechoic contents	Low-attenuation lesion with an irregular enhancing wall	
Hydatid cyst	Simple cyst or multiloculated cyst	Low-attenuation cyst or multiloculated cyst. Calcifications well shown on CT	
Amoebic abscess	Usually sited peripherally in the right lobe. Well-defined margin with homogeneous low-attenuation contents	Well-defined margin. Homogeneous low-attenuation contents	
Haemangioma*	Homogeneous hyperechoic mass	Peripheral globular enhancement on arterial phase scans; central enhancement on delayed scans	MRI: intense high signal on T2-weighted scans Scintigraphy with ^{99m}Tc-labelled red blood cells shows a focal area of increased activity
Focal nodular hyperplasia	Well-defined mass. Central scar seen in 50%	Equal attenuation to liver on portal venous phase of contrast enhancement. Dense enhancement on arterial phase	Scintigraphy with ^{99m}Tc-sulphur colloid: no filling defect (see above)
Hepatic adenoma	Most common in young women taking oral contraceptives. Well-defined mass with hyperechoic areas due to haemorrhage	Well-defined margin. Heterogeneous texture due to haemorrhage	

*Haemangioma is the most common benign hepatic mass. It is usually asymptomatic though large lesions may bleed. Multiple masses are seen in up to 20% of cases. The greatest significance in clinical practice is to differentiate haemangioma from a more sinister liver mass, especially in a patient with a primary tumour elsewhere. In these patients haemangioma is often seen as an incidental finding. If seen initially on US it is suggested that CT be performed to define the enhancement pattern. If this is typical of haemangioma then this is usually adequate (*see Fig. 3.3*). Doubtful lesions may be followed up with a further US or CT in a few months time to confirm lack of growth. MRI and/or scintigraphy may occasionally be used where immediate clarification is required.
HCC, hepatocellular carcinoma.

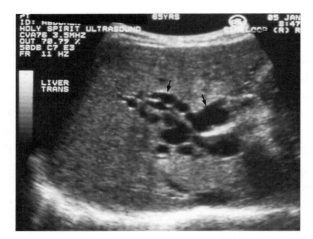

Figure 10.4 *Dilated bile ducts – US.*
Dilated intrahepatic bile ducts seen as branching fluid-filled structures in the liver (arrows).

US

US is the initial investigation of choice to differentiate obstructive from non-obstructive jaundice, i.e. to distinguish dilated from non-dilated bile ducts. Common bile duct measurements may be as follows:

* Normal <6 mm.

* Equivocal 6–8 mm.

* Dilated >8 mm.

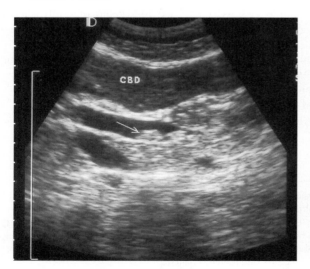

Figure 10.5 *Common bile duct stones – US.*
The common bile duct is dilated. Stones are seen as hyperechoic foci in the lower common bile duct (arrow).

Dilated intrahepatic bile ducts show a stellate branching pattern radiating from the porta, often best seen in the left hepatic lobe (*Fig. 10.4*). The site and cause of obstruction are defined in only 25% of cases as overlying duodenal gas often obscures the lower end of the common bile duct (*Fig. 10.5*). Associated dilatation of the main pancreatic duct suggests obstruction at the level of the pancreatic head/ampulla of Vater.

In the absence of ductal dilatation, diffuse or focal liver diseases such as metastases, fatty infiltration or cirrhosis may be seen. US is also useful for biopsy guidance. Studies have shown that the use of US guidance both to localize the liver accurately and to avoid large vascular structures will increase the safety of liver biopsy.

Endoscopic retrograde cholangiopancreatography (ERCP)

Indications

* Obstructive jaundice: to define the site and cause of biliary dilatation (*Fig. 10.6*).

* Other biliary disorders, e.g. sclerosing cholangitis.

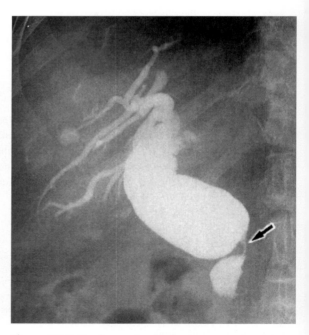

Figure 10.6 *Carcinoma head of pancreas.*
Mass encircling and compressing the lower common bile duct (arrow). The duct above is grossly dilated.

- Pancreatic disease, e.g. chronic pancreatitis.

Patient preparation

- Nil by mouth for 4–6 h.
- Mild sedation as for endoscopy.
- Antibiotic cover.

Method

The ampulla of Vater is identified and a small cannula passed into it under direct endoscopic visualization. Contrast is then injected into the biliary and/or pancreatic ducts and films taken. Sphincterotomy, basket retrieval of stones and stent placement may be performed at the time of ERCP.

Postprocedure care

- Standard observations postsedation.

Contraindications

- Acute pancreatitis.

Complications

- Acute pancreatitis.

Percutaneous transhepatic cholangiography (PTC)

Indications

- High biliary obstruction, i.e. at level of porta (*Fig. 10.7*).
- Biliary obstruction not able to be outlined by ERCP.
- Precursor to stent placement for relief of biliary obstruction.

Patient preparation

- Clotting studies.
- Sedation.
- Antibiotic cover.
- Nil by mouth 4–6 h.

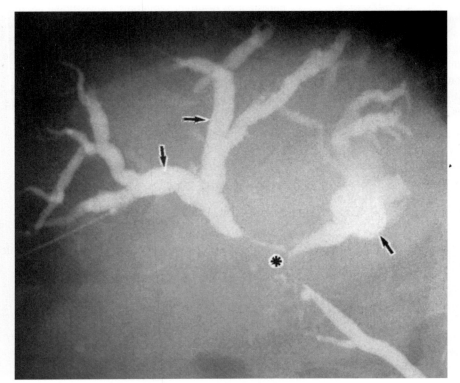

Figure 10.7 *Hepatocellular carcinoma – PTC.*
The tumour is causing compression of the bile ducts at the porta (*). The proximal ducts are dilated (arrows).*

Method

A needle is passed into the liver and then slowly withdrawn as small amounts of contrast are injected. Once a bile duct is entered, contrast is more rapidly injected to outline the biliary system.

Postprocedure care

- Standard observations of blood pressure, pulse rate and temperature.

Contraindications

- Bleeding tendency.
- Biliary infection.

Complications

- Haemorrhage.
- Septicaemia.
- Bile leak leading to biliary peritonitis.

CT

Parameters of bile duct dilatation are as for ultrasound, i.e. common bile duct >8 mm is dilated. Dilated intrahepatic ducts show a low-attenuation branching pattern radiating from the porta. As with US, main pancreatic duct dilatation localizes the obstruction to the lower common bile duct. The site and cause of bile duct obstruction may be suggested on CT in up to 90% of cases.

In the absence of bile duct dilatation, CT can assess the liver for other diseases causing jaundice. These include diffuse processes such as fatty infiltration, cirrhosis and metastases, or focal lesions such as hepatocellular carcinoma. CT may be used for biopsy guidance, particularly in the biopsy of focal masses.

Cholescintigraphy: HIDA scan

Scintigraphy of the biliary system (cholescintigraphy) is performed with ^{99m}Tc-labelled iminodiacetic acid (IDA) compounds. These compounds are taken up by liver cells and rapidly excreted in bile and are therefore used to delineate the biliary system and gallbladder. HIDA scans have a limited role in jaundice owing to impaired excretion and poor visualization of the bile ducts in the presence of elevated bilirubin.

Abnormal findings on HIDA scans for jaundice may be as follows:

- Failure of liver uptake indicates severe liver dysfunction.
- Liver uptake with non-visualization of bile ducts indicates cholestasis or a high obstruction.
- Visualization of bile ducts but not duodenum indicates low obstruction.

Newer methods of imaging the bile ducts

Visualization of the biliary system prior to surgery is required for two reasons:

- Presence of bile duct stones.
- Diagnosis of bile duct variants that may complicate surgery.

Bile duct visualization following surgery is required to exclude or detect bile duct stones in patients with persistent or recurrent symptoms. Conventional US and CT techniques have a relatively low sensitivity for detection of bile duct calculi, especially where the bile ducts are not dilated. Furthermore, anatomical variants of the biliary system may be difficult to appreciate. ERCP has been the 'gold standard' for opacification of the biliary system. It has the advantage of therapeutic applications such as sphincterotomy. It is, however, invasive, highly operator-dependent, and not always possible technically. Two relatively non-invasive techniques are now available for reliable delineation of the biliary system:

- 3D helical CT cholangiography.
- MRCP.

These techniques are gaining wide acceptance for assessment of the bile ducts, pre- and postlaparoscopic cholecystectomy.

Indications

- Prelaparoscopic cholecystectomy.
  (i) Outline variants of the biliary system that may increase the risk of bile duct injury.
  (ii) Diagnose bile duct stones.

- Postlaparoscopic cholecystectomy.
  (i)   Diagnose missed stones in patients with recurrent symptoms.
- Pancreatitis where ERCP is not suitable.

3D helical CT cholangiography

3D helical CT cholangiography involves a slow infusion of cholangiographic agent to opacify the bile ducts. Helical CT scans and 3D reconstructions are performed. Limitations include poor bile duct opacification in jaundiced patients, poor opacification of the cystic duct when obstructed by a calculus and difficulty of visualization of some calculi, depending on their composition. Risk of allergy to contrast material is also a factor.

MRCP

Heavily T2-weighted images are obtained. These show stationary fluids such as bile as high signal with moving fluids and solids as low signal. The bile ducts and gallbladder are therefore seen as bright structures

on a dark background (*Fig. 10.8*). 3D or multiplanar reconstructions may also be performed.

Indications

- Prelaparoscopic cholecystectomy to diagnose bile duct calculi and bile duct variants, and to avoid intraoperative exploration of the common bile duct.
- Failed ERCP.

Depending on availability of the technique and cost considerations, MRCP may in the future replace diagnostic ERCP in the assessment of jaundiced patients with dilated bile ducts on US.

Advantages of MRCP over other techniques for showing the bile ducts include:

- Less expensive than ERCP.
- Non-invasive.
- No radiation.
- No iv contrast material required.

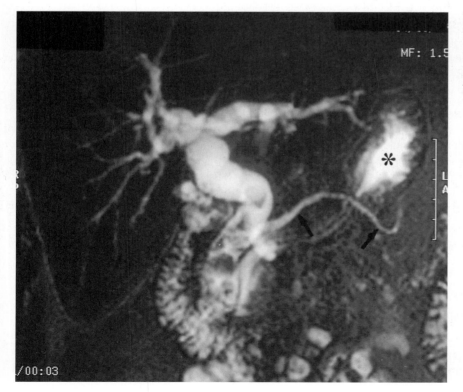

Figure 10.8 *MRCP – biliary calculi.*
Post-cholecystectomy patient. Note the following findings:
- *dilated bile ducts with several large calculi in the common bile duct*
- *pancreatic duct (arrows)*
- *stomach (*), duodenum and small bowel loops are also seen.*

Table 10.2 *Imaging findings in common surgical causes of jaundice*

Cause of jaundice	Ultrasound	CT	ERCP or PTC
Bile duct calculus	Hyperechoic focus in bile duct +/- acoustic shadow (*Fig. 10.5*)	Appearance varies depending on composition. Calcium: high attenuation; cholesterol: low attenuation; mixed: may be very difficult to see on CT	Filling defect in bile duct. May be single/ multiple, round/ faceted, mobile/ impacted
Carcinoma of the head of pancreas (*Fig. 10.11*)	Dilated bile ducts. Dilated pancreatic duct. Distended gallbladder. Hypoechoic mass in pancreatic head	Dilated bile ducts. Dilated pancreatic duct. Distended gallbladder. Mass in pancreatic head. Complications such as vascular encasement, liver metastases and lymphadenopathy	Smooth tapering stricture at the lower end of the common bile duct (*Fig. 10.6*)
Carcinoma of the ampulla of Vater	Dilated bile ducts. Dilated pancreatic duct. Distended gallbladder.	Dilated bile ducts. Dilated pancreatic duct. Distended gallbladder. No soft tissue mass. Abrupt termination of a dilated lower common bile duct without an obvious mass or calculus visible is highly suggestive of a small carcinoma of either the ampulla of Vater or the pancreatic head	Abrupt termination of the common bile duct at its lower end. May see small soft tissue filling defect
Cholangiocarcinoma	Dilated bile ducts that terminate at a soft tissue mass in and around the duct	Abrupt transition from dilated to absent bile duct. Soft tissue mass	Biliary stricture or filling defect
Carcinoma of the gallbladder	Irregular thickening of gallbladder wall. Soft tissue mass replacing gallbladder and invading liver	Irregular soft tissue mass replacing gallbladder. Liver invasion. Liver metastases	Extrinsic bile duct compression or irregular duct narrowing due to invasion
Extrinsic biliary compression due to a mass	Dilated bile ducts above a liver mass. For ultrasound features of common liver masses see *Table 10.1*	Dilated bile ducts above a liver mass. For CT features of common liver masses see *Table 10.1*	Extrinsic bile duct compression or irregular duct narrowing due to invasion (*Fig. 10.7*)

- Simultaneous imaging of ducts proximal and distal to obstruction.
- Unaffected by bilirubin levels.

Disadvantages include:

- Relative unavailability of MRI in some areas.
- Patients unsuitable for MRI, e.g. cardiac pacemakers, claustrophobia.
- Limited spatial resolution, therefore difficulty visualizing stones <3 mm, tight biliary stenosis, small peripheral bile ducts and small side branches of the pancreatic duct.
- No therapeutic applications, i.e. unable to perform sphincterotomy, insert stents, etc.

Imaging in portal hypertension

Imaging is performed in suspected and known portal

hypertension and cirrhosis to document and outline complications such as varices and ascites, to diagnose small hepatocellular carcinomas (see above), and to assist in various interventional procedures as described below.

US

US signs of liver cirrhosis are:

- Increased echogenicity of liver parenchyma (due to associated fatty infiltration).

- Irregular liver surface.

- Loss of normal liver architecture, i.e. loss of visibility of hepatic blood vessels.

- Enlarged spleen.

- Enlarged portal vein >13 mm.

- Decreased or reversed portal vein flow on Doppler studies.

- Varices may be seen in the splenic hilum and around the head of the pancreas, and the recanalized umbilical vein may be seen in the falciform ligament.

- Ascites.

CT

CT signs of liver cirrhosis include:

- Irregular contour.

- Decreased density with fatty change or increased density with haemochromatosis.

- Enlarged caudate lobe.

- Enlarged spleen.

- Varices: discrete round or tubular structures that enhance with contrast.

- Ascites (*Fig. 10.9*).

Angiography

- To demonstrate anatomy and flow pattern of the portal vein and its feeding branches.

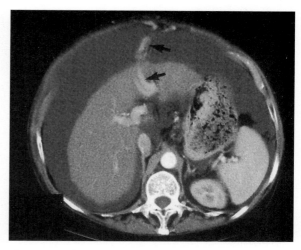

Figure 10.9 *Portal hypertension – CT.*
There is a large amount of ascites seen as low-attenuation fluid surrounding the liver, stomach and spleen. Note the recanalized umbilical vein (arrows) secondary to portal hypertension.

- Aim to outline portal system and measure pressures and flow rates.

- Complemented, and often superseded, by Doppler studies.

- Angiography may also be used postportosystemic stent shunt to demonstrate shunt patency.

Transjugular intrahepatic portosystemic stent shunting (TIPSS)

- Performed for portal hypertension with chronic, recurrent variceal haemorrhage not amenable to sclerotherapy.

- Patient imaged with Doppler US prior to procedure to exclude malignancy and confirm patency of portal vein.

- Technique:
  (i) Jugular vein puncture, often under US control.
  (ii) Wire passed into IVC and hepatic vein catheterized.
  (iii) Puncture device passed through catheter.
  (iv) Using US to select the most direct route, the portal vein is punctured and a wire passed.
  (v) Tract from hepatic vein to portal vein dilated.

a

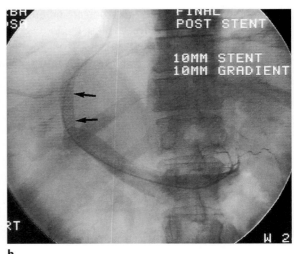

b

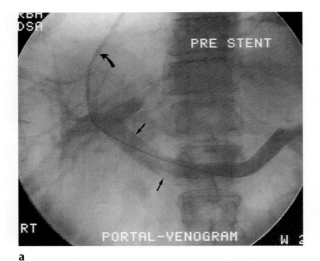

c

Figure 10.10 *TIPPS procedure.*
(a) Pre-stent. A guiding catheter is inserted via the right internal jugular vein. Its tip lies in the right hepatic vein (curved arrow). A puncture into the portal vein is then performed via the guiding catheter establishing communication between the portal and systemic venous systems. A fine catheter is passed through the puncture; its tip lies in the splenic vein. Contrast is injected with good opacification of the portal vein (straight arrows). (b) Post-stent. A self-expanding stent is deployed to maintain communication between the portal and systemic venous systems (arrows). (c) Post-stent. A subtraction film shows contrast outlining the portal vein (straight arrow), the shunt (open arrow) and the right hepatic vein (curved arrow).

(vi)   Stent inserted, usually a metallic prosthesis expanded by balloon (*Fig. 10.10*).

Imaging of pancreatic masses

CT is the investigation of choice for imaging of pancreatic masses. Helical CT using a dual phase technique is preferable, i.e. fine sections through the pancreas during the arterial phase of contrast enhancement followed by scans of the liver and pancreas during the portal venous phase. Most large pancreatic tumours will be seen on US examination. However, smaller masses (<2 cm) are frequently missed on US due to overlying intestinal gas or obesity. This particularly applies to small carcinomas of the pancreatic head and islet cell tumours. MRI has been widely described in the assessment of pancreatic tumours and it may occasionally be useful in difficult cases.

Imaging, particularly CT, may be used to guide biopsy of pancreatic masses or percutaneous aspiration of fluid collections such as pseudocysts.

Table 10.3 *Imaging features of pancreatic masses*

Mass	Clinical features	Location	CT	Ultrasound
Adenocarcinoma of the pancreas (*Fig. 10.11*)	Commonest pancreatic neoplasm. Those located in the head tend to present earlier due to biliary obstruction	Head: 60% Body: 25% Tail: 15%	See also *Table 10.2* Soft tissue mass Complications: local invasion, encasement of mesenteric artery and vein, metastases	See also *Table 10.2* Hypoechoic mass
Pseudocyst (*see Fig. 9.20*)	Complication of acute/ chronic pancreatitis and pancreatic trauma	Most within pancreas. Also lesser sac, mesentery, rarely mediastinum	Well-defined cyst with low-attenuation contents	Well-defined cyst with anechoic contents
Serous microcystic neoplasm	Benign neoplasm with multiple cysts of up to 2 cm diameter	Most common in the head	Complex mass with multiple low-attenuation cysts	Hyperechoic mass
Mucinous macrocystic neoplasm	Cystadenoma: benign cystadenocarcinoma: malignant.	Most common in the tail	Multilocular cystic mass. Local invasion	Multilocular cystic mass
Islet cell tumours	Endocrine syndrome depending on tumour type: insulinoma, gastrinoma, glucagonoma, somatostatinoma, VIPoma Non-functioning tumours present as a mass	Anywhere in the pancreas Occasionally extrapancreatic, especially gastrinoma	Enhancing mass. Insulinoma tends to be small (1–2 cm) Gastrinoma tends to be larger, up to 15 cm	Hypoechoic masses Intraoperative and endoscopic US highly accurate for diagnosis and localization

Summary of interventional procedures of the liver and biliary tree

Liver biopsy

Liver biopsy may be performed under CT or US guidance. Core biopsy is often required as fine-needle aspiration may not provide sufficient material for diagnosis. Two basic indications for guided liver biopsy:

- Localized mass/masses: imaging guidance to confirm position of needle in mass.

- Diffuse liver disease: imaging guidance not strictly required though may increase safety and diagnostic yield.

Imaging is also required prior to biopsy to exclude a vascular mass such as haemangioma or arteriovenous malformation (AVM).

Non-surgical management of bile duct stones

ERCP

- Sphincterotomy.

- Basket removal.

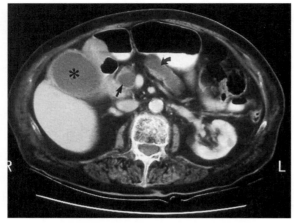

a

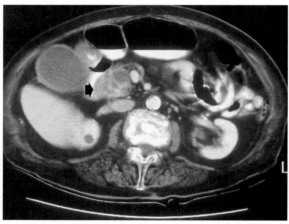

b

Figure 10.11 *Carcinoma head of pancreas – CT.*
(a) Note the following features:
- *dilated common bile duct (straight arrow)*
- *dilated pancreatic duct (curved arrow)*
- *distended gallbladder (*).*
(b) Enlarged irregular head of pancreas (arrow).

Basket removal through T-tube tract

- T-tube should be *in situ* for at least 4 weeks postsurgery to ensure a 'mature' tract able to accept wires and catheters.

- T-tube cholangiogram to assess position and number of stones.

- Wire through T-tube; T-tube removed.

- Steerable catheter and wire manipulated to stone; basket sheath over guide wire.

- Stone engaged in basket and removed.

- Rare complications include pancreatitis, cholangitis and bile leak.

Flexible choledochoscope through T-tube tract

- May be accompanied by intracorporeal lithotripsy.

Chemical dissolution

- Not widely practised or accepted.

Non-surgical management of malignant biliary obstruction

This section briefly describes a range of palliative procedures used to assist in the management of biliary obstruction caused by malignancies arising from the liver, bile ducts, pancreas and gallbladder. Indications are as follows:

- Performed for symptomatic relief, i.e. relief of pruritis, pain, cholangitis.

- Non-resectable tumour of bile ducts, head of pancreas, or liver.

- Medical risk factors which make surgery impossible.

Methods vary with the type of tumour, its location, and local expertise and preferences. Various methods include:

- Endoscopic, i.e. 'from below' for mid to low biliary obstruction.

- Percutaneous, i.e. 'from above', or combined percutaneous–endoscopic for high obstruction or where the second part of duodenum is inaccessible due to tumour or prior surgery.

Regardless of approach the basic technique is the same:

- Opacify ducts by ERCP or PTC.

- Pass wire across obstruction.

- Insert stent or internal–external drain.

Occasionally in severe obstruction a two-stage procedure is required. This involves placement of a drainage tube above the obstruction for a few days. After decompression of the biliary system, a wire is passed across the obstruction and a stent inserted.

Internal biliary stents are made of plastic or self-expanding metal and are better accepted by patients as they avoid the potential problems of external biliary drains such as skin irritation, pain, bile leaks and risk of dislodgement.

Percutaneous cholecystostomy (gallbladder drainage)

Indications

- Acute cholecystitis where the surgical risks are unacceptable.

Technique

- US guidance.
- Transhepatic approach preferable due to reduced risk of bile leak.
- Puncture gallbladder, wire through needle, drainage catheter over wire.

Postprocedure care

- Non-resolution of pyrexia within 48 h may indicate gangrene of the gallbladder requiring surgery.
- Cholecystogram once acute illness has settled: stones causing cystic duct obstruction may require surgery; otherwise the catheter is removed.

Liver embolization

Embolization of various liver lesions may be performed via catheter selectively placed in the hepatic artery or its branches.

Indications

- Metastases for selective delivery of chemotherapy and occasionally to reduce bulk and therefore relieve mass effect of large lesions.
- Non-resectable hepatocellular carcinoma for palliation of symptoms.
- AVM or false aneurysm.
- Haemostasis in bleeding adenoma or haemangioma.

11 Urinary tract

Radiological procedures

Intravenous pyelogram (IVP)

Indications

- Renal colic.

- Haematuria.

For other conditions, such as prostatism, urinary tract infection and renal cell carcinoma, other imaging techniques, especially ultrasound (US), CT and scintigraphy, have replaced IVP. At the time of writing, CT is rapidly replacing IVP in the assessment of renal colic and haematuria. It may well be that in the near future IVP will only rarely be performed for very specific reasons, such as sorting out complex congenital anomalies or for follow-up following surgical repair or reconstruction of the ureters.

Patient preparation

Some sort of bowel preparation is usually recommended; however, I feel that this has limited usefulness. Dehydration of the patient is no longer recommended. For patients at risk of contrast-medium reaction oral steroid may be given prior to IVP (see Chapter 6).

Method

Preliminary films are taken mainly to identify the kidneys and diagnose any area of renal tract calcification. This is particularly important in renal colic where a ureteric stone is being sought. Intravenous contrast is then injected. Films are taken to show the kidneys, the collecting systems, ureters and bladder. When overlying bowel gas obscures the kidneys, tomography and/or oblique projections are used to outline the collecting system. This is especially important in patients with haematuria where a small transitional cell carcinoma (TCC) of the collecting system may be the cause. A postmicturition film confirms drainage of both ureters and emptying of the bladder.

Postprocedure care

- Nil.

Contraindications and complications

- See Chapter 6 on contrast medium.

Retrograde pyelogram

Indications

- To better delineate lesions of the upper renal tract identifed by other imaging studies such as IVP.

- Haematuria, where other imaging studies are normal or equivocal.

Patient preparation

- Standard preoperative preparation.

Method

This procedure is usually performed in conjunction with formal cystoscopy. The ureteric orifice is identified and a catheter passed into the ureter. Contrast is then injected via this catheter to outline the collecting system and ureter. In my experience better images are attained by performing the contrast injection in the X-ray department after the patient has left the recovery ward, rather than obtaining mobile films in theatre.

Postprocedure care

- Standard postoperative care and observations.

Contraindications

- Urinary tract infection.

Complications

- Rupture of ureter and collecting systems.

Ascending urethrogram

Indications

- Prior to urethral catheterization in any patient with an anterior pelvic fracture/dislocation, or with blood at the urethral meatus following trauma.

- Pre- and postoperative assessment of urethral stricture.

- Outline urethral anomalies (e.g. hypospadias).

Patient preparation

- Nil.

Method

A small catheter is passed into the distal urethra and contrast-injected. Films are obtained in the oblique projection. The posterior urethra is usually not opacified via the ascending method. Should this area need to be examined, a micturating cysto-urethrogram will be required.

Postprocedure care

- Nil.

Contraindications

- Urinary tract infection.

- Recent urethral instrumentation.

Complications

- Urethral trauma (rare).

Micturating cysto-urethrogram (MCU)

Indications

- Urinary tract infection in children, i.e. for assessment of vesico-ureteric reflux (see Chapter 16).

- Suspected posterior urethral valves in male children.

- Posterior urethral problems in male adults.

- Stress incontinence in female adults.

- Postprostatic surgery, i.e. to check anastomoses and the integrity of the bladder base.

Patient preparation

- Antibiotic cover is often used.

Method

The bladder is filled with contrast via a urethral catheter. The catheter is withdrawn and films are taken during micturition. The particular indication will dictate the type and number of films performed.

Postprocedure care

- Nil.

Contraindications

- Acute urinary tract infection should not be present at the time of examination.

Complications

- Urinary tract infection.

- Trauma due to catheterization.

Investigation of a renal mass

The goals of imaging a suspected renal mass include:

- Confirmation of presence and site of mass.

- Differentiation of benign from malignant.

- Accurate characterization of features.

- Diagnose metastases, including lung, liver and bone metastases, as well as lymphadenopathy.

- Assess the other kidney.

US provides a cheap, safe and reliable screening test for a renal mass suspected clinically or found on IVP during investigation of haematuria/renal colic. It is the initial investigation of choice for assessment of a renal mass, followed by CT.

US

US will accurately differentiate a simple cyst from either a complicated cyst or a solid mass. If a simple cyst is found then no further imaging is required. If a

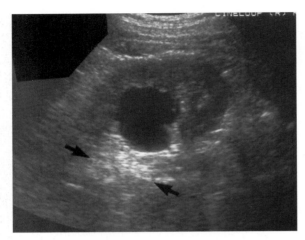

Figure 11.1 *Simple renal cyst – US.*
Note the following features of a simple cyst on US:
- *anechoic (black) contents*
- *well-defined posterior wall*
- *acoustic enhancement (arrows).*

complicated cyst or solid mass are found, further assessment will be needed.

US features of a simple cyst:

- Well-defined thin wall.

- Anechoic.

- Acoustic enhancement (*Fig. 11.1*).

Any lesion not fitting the above parameters of a simple cyst requires further assessment.

The term 'complicated cyst' refers to a cyst with:

- Internal echoes which may be due to haemorrhage or infection.

- Soft tissue septa.

- Associated soft tissue mass.

Causes of a complicated cyst include benign and malignant processes as follows:

- A simple cyst complicated by haemorrhage or infection.

- Tumour which has undergone necrosis.

- Cystic tumour.

The diagnosis of complicated cyst on US therefore usually implies that further assessment is required. This could take the form of further imaging with CT, follow-up US to exclude a growing lesion, biopsy or even surgical exploration.

A solid lesion on ultrasound may show areas of increased echogenicity due to calcification or fat, or areas of decreased echogenicity due to necrosis (*Fig. 11.2*). Where renal cell carcinoma is suspected, US is also used to look for complications such as:

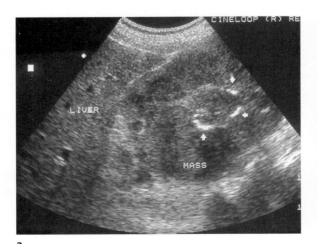

a

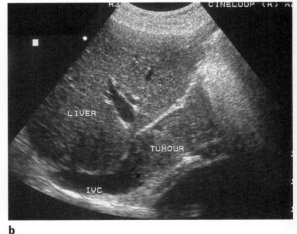

b

Figure 11.2 *Renal cell carcinoma – US.*
(a) Carcinoma of the right kidney. US shows a large heterogeneous tumour beneath the liver. Note hyperechoic areas due to calcification (arrows). (b) US shows tumour invading the IVC. The distal extent of tumour invasion is well seen (arrows). Note that the upper IVC is clear.

- Invasion of renal vein and inferior vena cava (IVC) (*Fig. 11.2*).

- Lymphadenopathy.

- Metastases in the liver and contralateral kidney.

US may be used as a guide for:

- Biopsy of solid lesions or complicated cysts.

- Cyst aspiration for diagnostic and therapeutic purposes.

- Cyst ablation by injection of ethanol.

CT

Contrast-enhanced CT is used for further characterization of a solid lesion or complicated cyst. CT is more accurate than US for characterization of internal contents of a mass, as well as for staging of renal cell carcinoma. It will accurately show areas of calcification, fat, necrosis, or marked enhancement with a vascular lesion.

For renal cell carcinoma, CT is also used to assess complications such as:

- Invasion of local structures seen as tumour tissue extending into perirenal and pararenal fat and into surrounding muscles and organs.

- Vascular invasion seen as increased calibre and decreased density of renal vein or IVC with failure to enhance with contrast.

- Lymphadenopathy.

- Metastases in liver.

- Tumour in the other kidney (*Fig. 11.3*).

CT can be used to guide biopsy of masses, or cyst aspiration and ablation.

The majority of renal masses will be adequately characterized and staged with US and/or CT. Other imaging investigations are only occasionally performed.

MRI

MRI gives similar information to CT. Its potential advantages are:

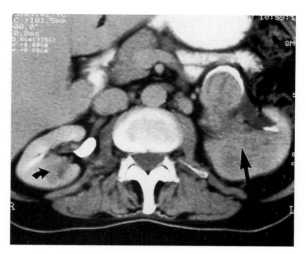

Figure 11.3 *Renal cell carcinoma – CT.*
Note:
- *irregular mass arising from the left kidney (straight arrow)*
- *small contralateral tumour in the right kidney (curved arrow).*

- Accurate for assessing vascular invasion.

- Iodinated contrast material is not required.

- Multiplanar imaging gives more accuracy in assessing the renal pole and for showing invasion of surrounding structures.

Angiography

Angiography is performed rarely for renal cell carcinoma in the following situations:

- Prior to tumour embolization.

- To provide a surgical 'road map'.

- Where results of the above imaging modalities are equivocal with respect to vascular invasion.

Biopsy and the indeterminate renal mass

Occasionally, a renal mass will be encountered which cannot be definitively classified with imaging. A common example is a cyst complicated by haemorrhage or infection. This will appear as a well-defined

Table 11.1 *US and CT features of the more common renal masses*

Mass	Clinical	Ultrasound	CT
Renal cell carcinoma (*Figs. 11.2 & 11.3*)	Imaging for primary diagnosis, as well as diagnosis of complications as above	Heterogeneous mass with areas of haemorrhage, necrosis and calcification	Heterogeneous mass. Less enhancement than normal kidney. Complications: local invasion, lymphadenopathy, venous invasion and metastases
Angiomyolipoma	Benign fat containing tumours with two types seen: • Sporadic: solitary, in females 40–60 years • Associated with tuberous sclerosis: multiple and bilateral	Heterogeneous mass Hyperechoic due to fat content. Common incidental finding	Fat content well shown on CT as low-attenuation areas. The presence of fat in a renal mass virtually excludes malignancy (*Fig. 11.4*)
Oncocytoma	Benign uncommon renal tumour seen in adults. May be difficult to differentiate from renal cell carcinoma on imaging and even on biopsy	Well-defined hypoechoic mass	Low-attenuation mass with well-defined pseudocapsule. Central stellate scar seen in 30%
Lymphoma	Three patterns of renal lymphoma are seen: • Diffuse infiltration • Discrete masses • Direct invasion form perirenal disease	Diffusely enlarged hypoechoic kidney Multiple hypoechoic masses	Diffusely enlarged low-attenuation kidney Multiple low-attenuation masses Other evidence of lymphoma: lymphadenopathy, splenomegaly
Multilocular cystic nephroma	Rare benign neoplasm of male children aged 3 months to 4 years, and adult females aged 50–60 years. Occasional malignancy in both age groups	Anechoic mass with multiple echogenic soft tissue septae	Low-attenuation mass with multiple higher-attenuation septae
Nephronia	Refers to acute focal bacterial nephritis; if untreated leads to abscess formation	Poorly defined hypoechoic mass	Poorly defined low-attenuation mass
Metastases	Commonest primary sites are lung, breast and stomach	Multiple heterogeneous masses	Multiple heterogeneous masses

hypoechoic lesion on US and as a high to intermediate attenuation lesion on CT, and as such may be difficult to differentiate from a solid mass. Biopsy of renal masses is usually not indicated for the following reasons:

• Histological interpretation is often difficult.

• Biopsy may alter radiological parameters for further follow-up, e.g. haemorrhage into a cyst.

Biopsy of a solitary renal mass may be indicated in the following uncommon situations:

• High suspicion for lymphoma.

• Known or previous primary carcinoma elsewhere, especially lungs, breast or stomach.

• Where a positive biopsy result would indicate a non-operative approach.

Generally, a decision will be made to either remove or observe an indeterminate renal mass. A suggested imaging protocol for observation would be:

• Repeat imaging in 6 months.

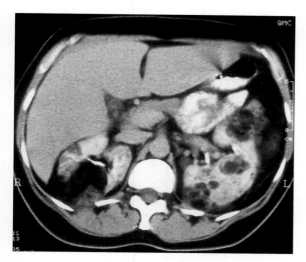

Figure 11.4 *Tuberous sclerosis – CT.*
Multiple angiomyolipomas are seen in both kidneys. The low-attenuation fat content of these tumours is well seen on CT.

- If increased in size then remove.

- If unchanged go to annual follow-up.

Painless haematuria

Haematuria may be seen in association with urinary tract infection and ureteral stones. In these situations, other clinical symptoms and signs such as acute flank pain and fever are usually present.

The common causes of painless haematuria are as follows:

- Tumour:
  (i)   Renal cell carcinoma.
  (ii) Transitional cell carcinoma of kidney, ureter or bladder.

- Prostatomegaly.

- Papillary necrosis.

- Medical renal disease, e.g. acute glomerulonephritis.

- Anticoagulant therapy.

- Coagulopathy.

It follows from the above list that imaging assessment of painless haematuria requires visualization of the renal parenchyma to exclude a renal mass, plus visualization of the urothelium. This includes imaging of the collecting system, renal pelvis, ureters and bladder.

The most commonly used initial tests are IVP plus cystoscopy. If these are negative, US or CT to diagnose a small renal mass are performed. If these are negative, a medical renal cause is considered for which renal biopsy is required.

Increasingly, CT is replacing IVP as the initial screening test for the patient with haematuria.

IVP

In combination with cystoscopy, IVP remains the best initial screening test for painless haematuria. It provides visualization of the calyces, renal pelvis and ureter with an anatomical resolution not possible with other imaging modalities. For example, a small transitional cell carcinoma (TCC) will not be seen on US or CT unless the pelvicalyceal system is dilated. Such a lesion should be seen on IVP as a filling defect in the pelvicalyceal system, whether it is dilated or not.

Signs of a TCC on IVP are as follows:

- Lucent filling defect (differential diagnosis includes blood clot, sloughed papilla, uric acid or xanthine calculus) (*Fig. 11.5*).

- Dilatation of the urinary tract above the tumour.

- Obstructed kidney may show delayed opacification.

- Often multiple so the whole urinary tract must be closely examined.

Fine section non-contrast CT is sometimes useful to further delineate a lucent filling defect. All stones will be of high attenuation on CT, even stones that are lucent on IVP and plain films (see below), whereas a TCC will show as a low-density mass. A suspected TCC can also be further investigated by retrograde or antegrade pyelogram. Once a filling defect suspicious of a TCC has been diagnosed on IVP, imaging by US and CT can be performed to further delineate tumour extent, assess complications like hydronephrosis, and assess local invasion, lymphadenopathy and other metastases.

A renal mass found on IVP will be investigated as

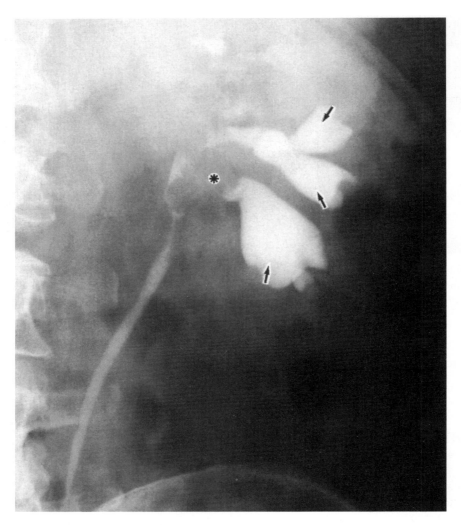

Figure 11.5 *Transitional cell carcinoma (TCC) of the renal pelvis – IVP. Irregular filling defect in renal pelvis (*). Dilated and blunted calyces (arrows) due to obstruction.*

above in the previous section, i.e. US followed by further imaging as indicated.

If IVP and/or cystoscopy show a bladder tumour, CT is used for staging, i.e. to assess perivesical spread, lymphadenopathy and metastases to other sites.

US

For a renal mass to be visible on IVP it must distort the renal outline or deform/invade the collecting system. A small mass may therefore be missed on IVP. If IVP and cystoscopy are negative, US is warranted as it is more sensitive than IVP for showing small renal masses lying outside the collecting system.

CT urography

'CT urography' is a term that is appearing more frequently in the imaging literature. It describes a contrast-enhanced CT examination of the kidneys, followed by one or more abdominal radiographs. The abdominal radiographs are performed immediately after the CT so that the collecting systems and ureters are outlined by the contrast material. As stated above, imaging assessment of both renal parenchyma and urothelium is required in the patient with haematuria. CT urography fulfils these requirements and at the time of writing, is replacing IVP in the investigation of painless haematuria.

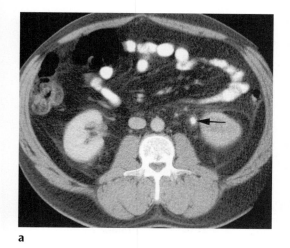
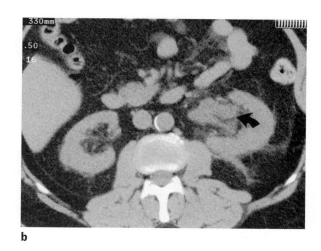

a   b

Figure 11.6 *Acute flank pain – CT.*
(a) Ureteric calculus. A calculus of the upper left ureter is seen as a high-attenuation focus on CT (arrow). (b) Urinary tract obstruction. The left renal collecting system is dilated (curved arrow). Note also soft tissue strands extending from the surface of the left kidney into the perinephritic fat. This is due to dilated lymphatics.

Renal biopsy

If all imaging is negative then medical causes of haematuria such as glomerulonephritis should be considered. After exclusion of coagulopathy a renal biopsy may be performed, most safely under US control.

Renal colic and acute flank pain

Acute flank pain describes pain of the posterolateral abdomen from the lower thorax to the pelvis. The most common cause of acute flank pain is ureteral obstruction caused by an impacted renal calculus. For this reason, the terms acute flank pain and renal colic are often used interchangeably. I prefer the term 'acute flank pain' as I believe that it more accurately reflects the fact that non-renal causes may produce similar symptoms to genuine renal colic.

Common renal causes of acute flank pain include:

- Ureteric calculus.

- Renal calculus.

- Pelvi-ureteric junction obstruction.

- Acute pyelonephritis.

- Ureteric stricture.

- TCC of the ureter causing obstruction.

- Clot colic, i.e. colic due to a blood clot complicating haematuria.

Non-renal causes of acute flank pain include:

- Appendicitis.

- Torsion or haemorrhage of ovarian cyst.

- Choledocholithiasis.

- Diverticulitis.

- Inflammatory bowel disease.

- Pancreatitis.

In the patient with acute flank pain, initial assessment is directed towards confirming or excluding urinary tract obstruction secondary to a ureteric calculus. Until recently, plain films and IVP have been the imaging tests of choice. Helical CT without contrast enhancement is now the imaging test of choice for acute flank pain.

Unenhanced helical CT

A helical CT is performed from the tops of the kidneys to the bladder base. The helical acquisition means that the whole length of the urinary tract can be scanned without the possibility of missing small ureteric stones. Contrast material injection causes opacification of the renal collecting systems and ureters. This would obscure most renal or ureteric stones. For this reason, scans are done without contrast material, i.e. unenhanced.

Unenhanced helical CT has a number of advantages over IVP in the assessment of acute flank pain:

- Speed:
  (i)   CT usually takes about 5 min.
  (ii) IVP may take several hours where there is delayed renal function.

- Contrast material is not required.

- Virtually all stones are identified:
  (i)   The only exceptions are stones due to precipitation of Indinavir crystals in HIV patients taking this medication.
  (ii) Cystine, urate, xanthine and matrix stones are all well seen as high-attenuation foci.

- Stone position and size are accurately assessed.

- Non-renal causes of acute flank pain may be identified.

CT signs of urinary tract obstruction are as follows:

- Direct visualization of the ureteric calculus.

- Dilatation of the ureter above the level of obstruction.

- Dilatation of renal pelvis and collecting system.

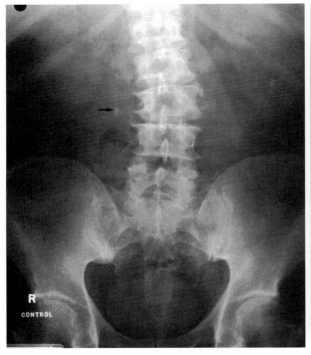

a

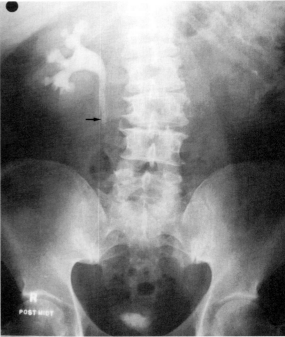

b

Figure 11.7 *Renal calculus.*
(a) Plain film. Note:
- *stones in both kidneys*
- *calculus seen projected over the tip of the right transverse process of L3 (arrow).*
(b) IVP. Note:
- *dilatation of the right collecting system with 'hold-up' of contrast; compare with the normal left side.*
- *right ureter dilated down to the level of the calculus at L3 (arrow).*

- Soft tissue stranding in the perinephritic fat due to distended lymphatic channels (*Fig. 11.6*).

Plain films

Despite the growing use of CT as above, plain films and IVP are still widely used. This is particularly true where there is limited availability of helical CT services.

Ninety per cent of renal calculi contain sufficient calcium to be radio-opaque, i.e. visible on plain films (*Fig. 11.7*). Cystine stones (3%) are faintly opaque. Urate stones (5%) are lucent, and not able to be seen. Xanthine and matrix stones are rare and lucent. Note that opacities seen on plain films thought to be renal or ureteric calculi need to be differentiated from other causes of calcification, such as arterial calcification, calcified lymph nodes and pelvic phleboliths.

IVP

Following plain films, IVP is performed for the following reasons:

- To prove that an opacity seen on plain films lies within the urinary tract.
- To diagnose lucent calculi not seen on plain films.
- To identify other causes of renal colic, as above, and guide further actions.

An obstructing ureteric calculus shows all or some of the following signs on IVP (*Fig. 11.7*):

- Delayed uptake of contrast by the involved kidney.
- Persistent contrast outlining the renal cortex, i.e. delayed nephrogram.
- Delayed appearance of contrast in the collecting system.
- Dilated collecting system above the calculus.
- Leakage of contrast with severe obstruction.
- Increased pain following injection of contrast.

Dilatation of the entire length of the ureter with no apparent obstructing opacity is most commonly due to oedema of the vesico-ureteric junction secondary to recent passage of a calculus.

Acute pyelonephritis may show no changes on IVP or a focal deformity in the event of inflammatory mass or abscess formation.

Pelvi-ureteric junction obstruction shows dilatation of the collecting system with marked dilatation of the renal pelvis and failure to opacify the ureter. Percutaneous nephrostomy may be required to salvage renal function prior to surgery.

Renal calculi may be amenable to extracorporeal shock wave lithotripsy (ESWL) which uses highly focused, high-intensity US to shatter calculi into small fragments able to be passed or removed percutaneously.

Adrenal imaging

CT is the investigation of choice for imaging of the adrenal glands. This includes fine sections pre- and postcontrast injection. Whilst adrenal masses may be seen on US, CT is more accurate for diagnosis and characterization. Scintigraphy may occasionally be useful. More specialized techniques, such as adrenal vein sampling and percutaneous biopsy, may rarely be required.

Indications

- Endocrine syndromes:
  (i)   Cushing syndrome.
  (ii) Conn syndrome.
  (iii) Phaeochromocytoma.
  (iv) Primary adrenal insufficiency.
- Neoplasms with a high incidence of metastatic spread to the adrenals, especially lung and breast.
- Miscellaneous indications:
  (i)   Investigation of calcification seen on abdominal X-ray (AXR).
  (ii) Neonatal haemorrhage.
  (iii) Palpable mass.

CT of adrenal masses

In the above situations, and in incidental adrenal masses seen on CT, it is important to differentiate

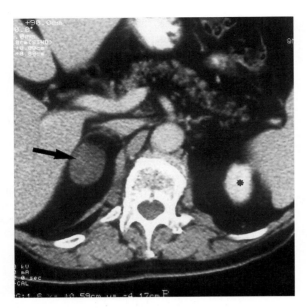

Figure 11.8 *Adrenal adenoma – CT.*
There is an adenoma of the right adrenal gland (arrow).
The upper pole of the left kidney is also seen on this
section (*). Note the CT features of adrenal adenoma:
* *small size*
* *smooth contour*
* *low attenuation.*

benign from malignant, specifically adrenal adenoma from adrenal metastasis or carcinoma. It should be noted that about 50% of adrenal masses seen in patients with primary carcinoma elsewhere are in fact benign adenomas, not metastases.

CT features of benign non-hyperfunctioning adrenal adenomas

* Size <3 cm.

* Well-defined, smooth contour.

* Low density on unenhanced scans (*Fig. 11.8*).

CT features of adrenal carcinoma

* Size >5 cm.

* Higher density on unenhanced scans.

* Low density centrally due to necrosis.

* Direct evidence of malignancy: liver metastases, lymphadenopathy, venous invasion.

CT features of an adrenal metastasis

* Tend to be larger though size not a reliable indicator.

* Higher density on unenhanced scans.

* When an adrenal mass is the only evidence of metastasis in a patient with a lung, breast or other primary tumour, percutaneous biopsy under CT guidance is often required for definitive diagnosis.

Cushing syndrome

Bilateral adrenal hyperplasia (70%)

* Normal appearance or diffuse thickening of limbs of both adrenals.

Unilateral adrenocortical adenoma (20%)

* Small well-defined mass usually <5 cm.

Adrenal carcinoma (10%)

* Mass usually >5 cm.

* Central necrosis.

* Metastatic spread: liver metastases, lymphadenopathy.

Primary hyperaldosteronism (Conn syndrome)

* Solitary unilateral adenoma (70%): usually a small mass of 1–2 cm.

* Multiple adenomas (20%).

* Bilateral adrenal hyperplasia (10%).

* Adrenal carcinoma (rare).

When bilateral adrenal disease is seen on CT, or when CT is normal, bilateral selective adrenal vein sampling for aldosterone levels may be helpful to localize a small abnormality and therefore guide surgery.

Phaechromocytoma

Phaeochromocytoma presents in two situations:

- Symptomatology related to excess catecholamine production: paroxysmal or sustained hypertension, headaches, sweating, flushing, nausea and vomiting, abdominal pain.

- Part of a syndrome, e.g. multiple endocrine neoplasia, familial phaeochromocytomas, tuberous sclerosis, von Hippel–Lindau disease, neurofibromatosis.

The following features may be noted:

- 10% multiple.

- 10% malignant.

- 10% extra-adrenal.

- 90% occur in adrenal medulla.

- Usually large tumours up to 12 cm, average around 5 cm.

- When the adrenals are normal and phaeochromocytoma is suspected on clinical grounds, whole body scintigraphy with iodine-labelled metaiodobenzyl-guanidine (^{131}I-/^{123}I-MIBG) is useful.

Primary adrenal insufficiency (Addison disease)

Idiopathic adrenal atrophy most common cause (probably autoimmune)

- Adrenal glands reduced in size.

Bilateral adrenal haemorrhage

- Newborn: birth trauma, hypoxia, sepsis.

- Adults: anticoagulation therapy, sepsis, surgery, trauma.

- CT: high-attenuation mass in acute haemorrhage.

TB/sarcoid

- Soft tissue masses.

- Cysts.

- Calcification.

Myelolipoma

- Benign cortical neoplasm containing myeloid tissue and fat.

- Asymptomatic: usually incidental finding on US or CT.

US

- Well-defined hyperechoic mass.

CT

- Low-attenuation fat content well seen on CT.

Trauma to the urinary tract

Trauma to kidneys and ureters

Imaging is for two purposes:

- To delineate the nature of injuries.

- To detect pre-existing abnormalities, seen in up to 50% of traumatized kidneys.

CT with intravenous contrast material is the investigation of choice for imaging of renal trauma. It provides good definition of haematomas, lacerations, urine leaks and urinomas (*Fig. 11.9*), as well as functional information. A non-functioning kidney in a setting of acute trauma may be due to:

- Massive parenchymal damage.

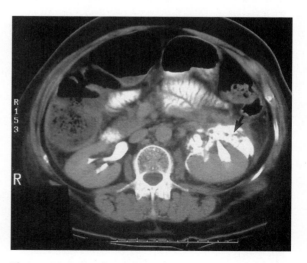

Figure 11.9 *Renal trauma – CT.*
There is leakage of contrast around the left kidney (arrow) indicating laceration of the collecting system.

- Vascular pedicle injury.

- Obstructed collecting system due to blood clot.

Plain-film findings suggestive of renal trauma include:

- Loss of fat planes around the kidney and psoas muscle.

- Fractures of the lower three ribs.

- Fractures of lumbar transverse processes.

- Overlying dilated loops of bowel.

- Pleural effusion.

Angiography may be used in selected cases, for example where marked haematuria is not explained by findings of other imaging modalities, or following percutaneous procedures (biopsy, nephrostomy, percutaneous stone removal). In these cases, angiography is used to define a bleeding point, arteriovenous fistula, or false aneurysm, which may then be embolized or undergo surgery.

Trauma to bladder and urethra

Plain films

Plain-film signs of bladder trauma:

- Fracture/dislocation of the pelvis (see Fig. 13.17).

- Soft tissue mass with obliteration of normal fat planes due to leakage of urine.

- Air may be seen in the bladder following penetrating injury.

Urethrogram (see above for technique)

Prior to performing a cystogram for suspected bladder damage, the urethra must be examined. Urethral catheterization should not be attempted prior to urethrogram in any patient with an anterior pelvic fracture/dislocation, or with blood at the urethral meatus following trauma. Urethrogram is a simple procedure that can be performed quickly in the emergency room (Fig. 11.10).

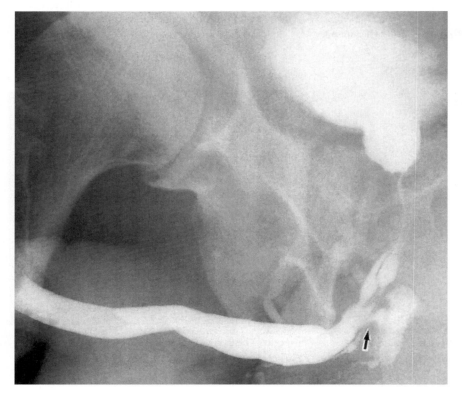

Figure 11.10 *Ruptured urethra – urethrogram. Leakage of contrast from the posterior urethra (arrow).*

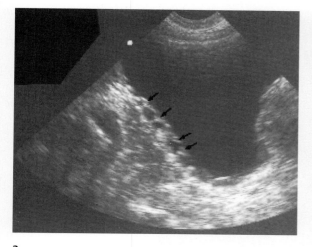
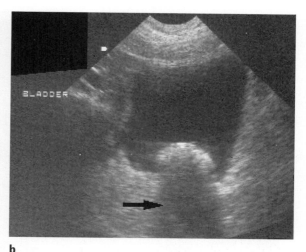

a

b

Figure 11.11 *Bladder changes in prostatism – US.*
(a) Bladder trabeculation. Note the hypertrophied muscle bands producing irregularity of the bladder wall (arrows).
(b) Bladder calculus. A bladder calculus is well seen as a large hyperechoic focus in the bladder lumen casting a prominent acoustic shadow (arrow).

Cystogram

If the urethra is normal on urethrogram, a catheter can be passed into the bladder and a cystogram performed. Bladder deformity may be seen. Leakage of contrast may be intraperitoneal, intrapelvic or extrapelvic.

Imaging in prostatism

The symptoms of prostatism include frequency, nocturia, poor stream, hesitancy, etc.

The primary imaging investigations in the assessment of prostatism are urinary tract US and plain AXR. IVP is no longer recommended for routine use in prostatism.

Urinary tract US

Bladder US

- Measure volume pre- and postmicturition.

- Calculate residual volume by the simple formula: volume = height × width × length × 0.50.
- Morphological changes indicating bladder obstruction include:
  (i)   Bladder wall thickening.
  (ii) Trabeculation and diverticula.
  (iii) Bladder calculi (*Fig. 11.11*)

Renal US

- Hydronephrosis.
- Asymptomatic congenital anomalies and tumours.
- Renal calculi (*Fig. 11.12*).

Prostate US

- Measure prostate volume = height × width × length × 0.50.

Plain AXR

For calculi in kidneys and ureters which may not be seen on US.

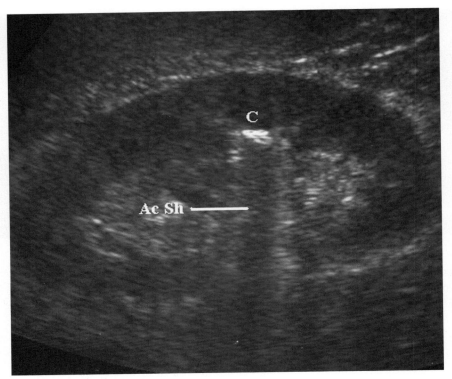

Figure 11.12 *Renal calculus – US.*
A calculus in the middle of the right kidney is well shown on US examination as a hyperechoic focus (C), which is casting an acoustic shadow (Ac Sh).

Adenocarcinoma of the prostate

Adenocarcinoma of the prostate is the second most common malignancy in males, its incidence increasing steadily with age. It may present clinically in several ways such as with signs of prostatism, haematuria or urinary tract infection. Bone metastases may be the initial finding due to a specific presentation like bone pain or spinal block. Multiple sclerotic metastases are occasionally picked up as an incidental finding on an X-ray performed for unrelated reasons, e.g. pre-anaesthetic chest X-ray. Autopsy studies have shown that a large percentage of prostate cancers remain asymptomatic.

The staging system for adenocarcinoma of the prostate is as follows:

- Stage A: non-palpable tumour, confined to the prostate.

- Stage B: palpable tumour, confined to the prostate.

- Stage C: invasion of the prostatic capsule, capsule penetration, seminal vesicle invasion.

- Stage D: distant metastases to lymph nodes and bone.

The finding of elevated serum levels of prostate specific antigen (PSA) in association with prostate cancer is currently the subject of debate. Some advocate the use of serum PSA levels as a screening test in elderly males. The premise is that stage A and B tumours, if detected, may be definitively treated with radical prostatectomy or radiotherapy. Others argue that the risks of surgery (incontinence and impotence) outweigh the benefits of treating small non-invasive cancers, at least some of which will remain asymptomatic. At the time of writing, these issues remain to be resolved.

Transectal ultrasound (TRUS) and biopsy

TRUS is particularly useful for Stage A and B tumours, which can not be seen on CT (*see Fig. 2.6*). Malignancies may appear as focal hypoechoic areas in the peripheral zone of the gland. However, a large percentage of Stage A and B malignancies are not seen, even with TRUS. For this reason, TRUS is usually accompanied by biopsy. TRUS-guided biopsy of hypoechoic lesions plus sextant biopsy are used for assessing extent and distribution of tumour within the prostate gland.

Where tumour is present, TRUS is highly sensitive for subtle signs of local invasion not detectable on CT, i.e. invasion of the gland capsule and early invasion of seminal vesicles.

CT

CT is unable to reliably visualize stage A and B carcinomas. CT signs of invasive prostate carcinoma include:

- Pelvic lymphadenopathy.

- Invasion of pelvic side wall.

- Invasion of seminal vesicles.

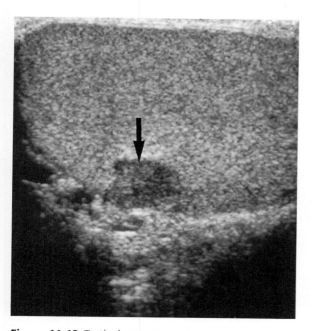

Figure 11.13 *Testicular tumour – US.*
A small seminoma is seen as a hypoechoic mass well outlined against normal surrounding hyperechoic testicular tissue (arrow).

MRI

MRI using an endorectal coil provides excellent visualization of the intraglandular architecture of the prostate gland and may be useful for Stage A and B tumours.

Further staging

Further imaging for staging of prostate carcinoma includes scintigraphy where bone metastases plus CT for liver metastases and lymphadenopathy. Bone metastases from prostate carcinoma are usually sclerotic. Common sites of spread include the pelvis and spine. Occasionally, a generalized increase in bone density may be seen with extensive skeletal spread (*see Figs 13.50 & 13.51*).

Investigation of a scrotal mass

US

US is the first investigation of choice for a scrotal mass. The primary role of US is to differentiate intra-testicular from extratesticular masses; in most cases this is sufficient to distinguish malignant and benign lesions. Most (over 90%) intratesticular masses are malignant. Exceptions include:

- Testicular abscess.

- TB.

- Testicular infarct.

- Benign tumour such as Sertoli–Leydig tumour.

- Sarcoidosis.

Most intratesticular tumours are hypoechoic compared with surrounding testicle, although some may be hyperechoic, particularly in the presence of haemorrhage or calcification. Seminomas are usually hypoechoic and may be seen as a localized hypoechoic mass well outlined by surrounding hyperechoic testicular tissue (*Fig. 11.13*). Occasionally with a large tumour the entire testicle is replaced by abnormal hypoechoic tissue. Other tumour types such as choriocarcinoma, embryonal cell carcinoma, teratoma and mixed tumours usually show a heterogeneous echotexture. Lymphoma of the testis is hypoechoic and homogeneous and may be focal or diffuse.

Further imaging for staging of testicular tumours consists of abdomen CT for retroperitoneal lymphadenopathy, and chest CT for mediastinal lymphadenopathy and pulmonary metastases.

Most (90%) extratesticular lesions are benign. The more common of these are outlined below.

Hydrocele

- Anechoic fluid surrounding the testicle.

- May be congenital, idiopathic, or secondary to inflammation, torsion, trauma or tumour.

Varicocele

- Dilated veins of the pampiniform plexus producing a tortuous nest of veins well seen on US.

- Vascular nature of the mass is confirmed with colour Doppler.

- Occur mostly on the left.

- Present with a clinically obvious mass or with infertility.

- Small varicoceles are often incidental findings on scrotal US.

- Caused by venous incompetence in most cases; rarely may be caused by obstruction of the left renal vein by tumour or thrombosis.

- May be amenable to therapeutic embolization (see below).

Spermatocele/epididymal cyst

- Well-defined anechoic simple cyst in the head of the epididymis, i.e. posterolaterally at the superior pole of the testis.

- Common incidental finding on scrotal US.

- May occasionally be large enough to present as a palpable mass.

Acute scrotum

The main differential diagnosis in this situation is torsion versus acute epididymo-orchitis. The need for early exploration in suspected torsion gives imaging a role only in doubtful cases and where it is quickly available. Acute epididymo-orchitis is usually caused by bacterial infection or mumps.

Scrotal haematoma, usually related to trauma, is the next most common cause of acute scrotum. Rarely, haemorrhage into a testicular tumour may present with acute pain.

US

Where imaging is required in the assessment of the patient with acute scrotum, US with colour Doppler is the investigation of choice. It is quick, non-invasive and highly accurate at differentiating torsion from inflammation.

Epididymo-orchitis

- Enlarged hypoechoic epididymis.

- Enlarged hypoechoic testis.

- Fluid around the testis.

- Increased blood flow in the testis/epididymis on colour Doppler.

- Abscess formation: intra- or extratesticular.

Torsion

- Testis may be normal in appearance or enlarged and hypoechoic.

- Epididymis usually enlarged and hypoechoic.

- Decreased spermatic cord Doppler signal.

- Lack of blood flow in the testis on colour Doppler.

Haematoma

- Hypoechoic collection with loculations and septations.

- Reduction in size over time.

- Chronic haematomas may calcify producing hyperechoic areas with shadowing.

Scintigraphy

- Very quick method (takes about 10 min).

- Inject ^{99m}Tc-pertechnetate, and take immediate images during perfusion plus serial static images for 10 min.

- Epididymo-orchitis shows increased uptake.

- Torsion shows a well-defined area of decreased uptake, sometimes with a surrounding 'halo' of increased uptake on the static images.

- Scintigraphy for the acute scrotum is now a rare examination given the high level of availability and accuracy of colour Doppler.

Once again, it should be emphasized that imaging should not hold up surgical exploration where torsion is suspected clinically.

Interventional radiology of the urinary tract

Percutaneous nephrostomy

Indications

- Relief of urinary tract obstruction, which may be caused by ureteric calculi, carcinoma of the bladder, ureteric TCC or carcinoma of the prostate.

- Pyonephrosis.

- Leakage of urine from upper urinary tract secondary to trauma or postsurgery.

Contraindications

- Bleeding diathesis.

Technique

- Local anaesthetic and sedation usually adequate; may require general anaesthetic in children or complicated cases.

- Antibiotic cover.

- Perform with US and fluoroscopic guidance, or under CT control.

- Puncture collecting system; pass wire; dilate tract; insert nephrostomy over wire.

Complications

- Haematuria: usually mild and transitory and occurs in most patients.

- Vascular trauma: very rare with imaging guidance.

Ureteric stents

Indications

- Malignant obstruction of urinary tract caused by carcinoma of the bladder, prostate or cervix.

- Pelviureteric junction obstruction.

- Other benign obstructions of the urinary tract, e.g. retroperitoneal fibrosis, radiotherapy.

- Postureteric surgery.

- Extracorporeal shock wave lithotripsy (ESWL) of large renal calculi, to promote passage of stone fragments and relieve ureteric obstruction by fragments.

Technique

- Either retrograde or antegrade insertion may be performed.

- Retrograde insertion via cystoscopy.

- Antegrade insertion: puncture kidney; guide wire passed down ureter into bladder; stent over guide wire pushed into position.

- The upper pigtail of the stent should lie in the renal pelvis or upper pole calyx.

- The lower pigtail should lie in the bladder.

Shock wave lithotripsy

Shock wave lithotripsy uses highly focused sound waves to fragment renal or ureteric stones. Where the shock waves are generated outside the body, the process is referred to as ESWL. Intracorporeal shock wave lithotripsy refers to shock waves generated inside the body through a ureteroscope. Shock wave lithotripsy is the technique of choice for most renal stones. Smaller stones <1 cm are usually easily fragmented with ESWL.

Percutaneous nephrolithotomy (PCNL)

Indications

- Failed ESWL.

- Staghorn calculus.

- Cysteine or matrix calculus.

Technique

- General anaesthetic.

- Insert retrograde catheter to opacify collecting system with contrast material and prevent calculus fragments passing down ureter.

- Puncture renal collecting system; pass guide wire; dilate tract; stone extracted by endoscopist.

Renal artery percutaneous transluminal angioplasty (PTA) and stent insertion (see Chapter 8)

Renal artery embolization

Indications

- Control of bleeding, which may occur postsurgery, postbiopsy or as a result of trauma.

- Treatment of arteriovenous malformation (AVM) and arteriovenous fistula, which are most commonly seen postbiopsy or as a complication of nephrostomy.

- Palliation/preoperative reduction of renal tumour.

Testicular vein embolization

Indications

- Varicocele associated with infertility.

- Large varicocele with normal fertility.

Technique

- Femoral vein puncture.

- Diagnostic venography of renal and testicular veins.

- Embolization of testicular vein and collateral channels, usually with steel coils.

12 Female reproductive system

First trimester ultrasound (US)

Biochemical screening, including serum human chorionic gonadotropin (hCG) levels, plus US form the basis of diagnosis in most first trimester patients with a variety of clinical presentations including vaginal bleeding, pain, uncertain dates, family history of multiple pregnancy, 'large for dates' etc. US in the first trimester is preferably performed with a transvaginal technique. The roles of US in the first trimester include:

- Detection of non-viable pregnancy.
- Diagnosis of ectopic pregnancy.
- Assess gestational age.
- Determine the number of embryos.
- Diagnosis of any obvious foetal anomalies.
- Diagnose relevant maternal abnormalities such as uterine fibromas or large ovarian cysts and masses.

Detection of non-viable pregnancy

US signs of a non-viable pregnancy include:

- Gestation measurements less than menstrual age.
- Lack of heartbeat in a defined foetus.
- Distorted gestational sac.
- Gestational sac occupies a low position in the uterus.
- Gestational sac of >25 mm diameter without an embryo.

First trimester bleeding with a viable foetus is termed a threatened miscarriage. US signs indicating a poor prognosis include:

- Reduced foetal activity.
- Subchorionic haematoma.
- Bradycardia, i.e. heart rate <85 beats/min at 5–8 weeks' gestation. (Normal foetal heart rate 100/min at 5–6 weeks, up to 140).

Diagnosis of ectopic pregnancy

Ectopic pregnancy rates are increasing. Factors associated with an increased risk of ectopic pregnancy include:

- Increasing maternal age and parity.
- Previous ectopic pregnancy.
- Previous fallopian tube surgery.
- Previous fallopian tube infection, i.e. salpingitis.

Clinical diagnosis of ectopic pregnancy is often difficult, with a history of a missed period present in only two-thirds of cases. Pain and vaginal bleeding with a palpable adnexal mass is the classic triad. Like most clinical classic triads, it occurs in a minority of cases. US findings correlated with serum hCG levels is often helpful in making or suggesting the diagnosis of ectopic pregnancy. US findings in ectopic pregnancy include:

- Complex mass in the adnexa with an empty uterus and a positive serum hCG.
- Foetal cardiac activity within an adnexal mass may be seen.

Note that the adnexal mass may be difficult to see. A normal pelvic US examination does not exclude ectopic pregnancy.

The visualization of an intrauterine pregnancy does not exclude ectopic pregnancy. The association of an ectopic pregnancy with an accompanying intrauterine gestation is estimated to occur in up to 1 in 4000 pregnancies, with a higher incidence in IVF patients.

Assess gestational age

A gestational sac can be visualized by transvaginal US at around 4 weeks. A foetus will be seen from around 6–7 weeks' gestation, with foetal heart activity also visible at this time.

Measurements used to estimate gestational age in the first trimester are gestational sac size and crown–rump length. As the gestational sac is often ovoid in shape an average sac diameter is used. Crown–rump length is the most accurate measurement.

Determine the number of embryos

It is important to recognize multiple pregnancies as early as possible as there are a number of associated risks, as well as the social implications (*Fig. 12.1*).

Risks to the foetuses include:

- Increased incidence of congenital anomalies.
- Intrauterine growth retardation and low birth weight.
- Premature labour.

There is also an increased risk of maternal complications including:

- Hyperemesis.
- Cholestasis.
- Antepartum haemorrhage.
- Polyhydramnios.
- Hypertension and pre-eclampsia.

When twin pregnancy is recognized on US examination, it is important to try to classify as follows:

Dichorionic diamniotic

- May be dizygotic or monozygotic.
- Dizygotic may be different sex; monozygotic are same sex.
- Separating membrane seen between the foetuses.
- Separate placentas may be identified.
- Mortality rate 9%.

Monochorionic diamniotic

- Monozygotic, therefore same sex.
- Separating membrane between the foetuses may be seen.
- Single placenta.
- Mortality rate 26%.

Monochorionic monoamniotic

- Monozygotic, therefore same sex.
- No separating membrane.
- Single placenta.
- Mortality rate 50%.

This classification is best performed in the first trimester as the separating membranes may be impossible to see in later pregnancy.

Diagnosis of any obvious foetal anomalies

Only some obvious anomalies may be seen in the first trimester. The most accurate US assessment of foetal morphology is obtained at around 18–19 weeks' gestation (see below).

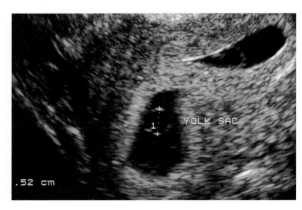

Figure 12.1 *Twin pregnancy: transvaginal US. A transvaginal US study was performed at about 6 weeks' gestation in a patient with a strong family history of twin pregnancies. US shows two separate gestational sacs in the uterus. Each gestational sac was seen to contain a yolk sac and an embryo.*

Recent interest has centred on the measurement of nuchal translucency thickness at 10–14 weeks' gestation as a screening test for chromosome disorders, in particular Down syndrome. The nuchal translucency is a hypoechoic layer between the soft tissue line over the posterior cervical spine and the overlying skin. Various reports have shown that thickening of this layer may be associated with chromosome disorders.

More traditional screening methods have relied on measurement of serum levels of biochemical markers correlated with maternal and gestational age. The most widely known is the triple test which measures serum levels of alpha feto-protein (AFP), hCG and unconjugated oestriol. At the time of writing, the role of nuchal thickness measurement is the subject of much debate and controversy, with its exact role yet to be defined.

Diagnose relevant maternal abnormalities such as uterine fibromas or large ovarian cysts and masses

The most commonly encountered maternal mass in early pregnancy is the corpus luteum cyst. Corpus luteum cysts may measure up to 10 cm in diameter, and may contain internal echoes due to haemorrhage. They usually regress by 18 weeks. Other ovarian cysts may present in early pregnancy due to torsion or haemorrhage or may be incidental findings on US examination performed for other reasons. Uterine fibromas may also be seen. Their size and position are important to assess as they may cause problems such as obstructed labour or foetal malposition. Some may enlarge in early pregnancy and be complicated by necrosis and haemorrhage causing pain.

The 'routine' obstetrical scan

The word 'routine' appears in inverted commas because there really is no such thing as a routine obstetrical scan. I say this despite the fact that in Western society the majority of pregnant women will have an ultrasound scan. The obstetrical scan should only be performed when the referring doctor and patient have a clear view of the benefits and limitations of the technique. The potential implications of an abnormal finding should be understood prior to the examination. Having said that, the best time for such a scan is at 18–20 weeks' gestation. This provides accurate dating, as well as a good assessment of foetal morphology.

The findings of obstetrical US scans are as follows.

Number of foetuses (see above)

Assessment of gestational age

- Measurements of biparietal diameter, head circumference, abdomen circumference and femur length.
- These measurements are accurate to +/- 1 week.

Position of the placenta

- Anterior or posterior.
- Relationship of lower placental edge to internal os, i.e. diagnosis of placenta praevia.
- If placenta praevia is diagnosed at 18 weeks, a follow-up scan is performed. Owing to increased growth of the lower uterine segment in later pregnancy, the majority of placenta praevia will resolve spontaneously.

Liquor volume

Common causes of oligohydramnios

- Intrauterine growth retardation, which may be due to a number of causes including placental insufficiency, chromosomal disorders, congenital infection and severe maternal systemic illness.
- Renal agenesis.
- Obstruction of the foetal urinary tract.

Common causes of polyhydramnios

- Idiopathic (most common cause).
- Maternal diabetes.
- Twin pregnancy.

- Neural tube defect.

- Foetal hydrops.

- Any disorder with impaired foetal swallowing, e.g. oesophageal atresia, duodenal atresia.

Foetal morphology as outlined below:

Head

- Outline of skull bones.

- Cerebral ventricles.

- Posterior fossa.

- Falx cerebri.

- Facial sections for cleft palate.

Spine

- Ossification centres.

- Overlying skin line.

- Nuchal fold thickness (may be increased in Down syndrome).

Thorax

- Cardiac activity.

- Four-chamber view of heart.

- Aortic arch.

- Diaphragm.

Abdomen

- Stomach (filled with fluid).

- Kidneys.

- Bladder.

- Umbilical cord insertion (exclude omphalocele).

- Ensure three vessels in cord, two arteries and one vein (two vessels associated with foetal anomalies).

Extremities

- Arms/legs.

- Hands/feet.

Detection of maternal pelvic masses or cysts

Scans may also be required later in pregnancy for a variety of reasons:

- Follow-up of placenta praevia.
  (i) Most cases of placenta praevia diagnosed on the 18–20 weeks' scan will resolve later in pregnancy with increased growth of the lower uterine segment producing apparent upward 'migration' of the placenta.

- Follow-up of foetal abnormality.

- Suspected growth retardation.

- Maternal problems such as diabetes.

- Guidance of amniocentesis or other interventions.

US in gynaecology

US is the primary imaging investigation of choice for assessment of gynaecological disorders. A variety of clinical presentations may occur including pelvic mass, postmenopausal bleeding and irregular or painful periods in premenopausal women.

Masses are characterized on US examination as cystic, solid or mixed. The organ of origin of a mass, i.e. uterus, ovary or other pelvic organ, may be ascertained.

Two types of US examination are performed:

Transabdominal

- Requires a full bladder to push small bowel loops out of the way and so provide an 'acoustic window' to the pelvic organs.

- Good for larger masses or cysts.

- May also assess complications of pelvic masses such as hydronephrosis, ascites and liver metastases.

Transvaginal

- Empty bladder required.

- Higher frequency probes are used giving better anatomical resolution of the uterus and ovaries.

- Major limitation is smaller field of view, so unable to fully assess large pelvic masses or kidneys for complications such as hydronephrosis.

- May be inappropriate for very young or elderly patients.

- Apart from these constraints, the transvaginal technique is more accurate than transabdominal scanning in early pregnancy (up to 12 weeks' gestation) and in most gynaecological conditions.

- Transvaginal US may be used to guide interventional procedures such as biopsy, cyst aspiration, abscess drainage and ovarian harvest, etc. in IVF programmes.

Classification of pelvic masses based on US appearances and organ of origin is as follows.

Simple ovarian cysts

Follicular cyst

- Unilocular simple cyst with anechoic contents and a thin well-defined wall.

- Usually 1–2 cm.

- Often multiple.

- Fine internal echoes may be seen with haemorrhage.

Polycystic ovarian disease

- Common cause of chronic anovulation and infertility.

- Refers to a spectrum of clinical disorders with the classic triad of oligomenorrhoea, obesity and hirsutism (Stein–Leventhal syndrome) being the best known.

- US findings include bilateral enlarged ovaries, each containing over five small simple cysts.

- A normal US does not exclude this condition.

Corpus luteum cyst (see above)

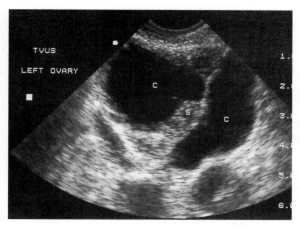

Figure 12.2 *Cystadenocarcinoma of the ovary – transvaginal US.*
Note cystic components (c), separated by a thick soft tissue septum (s).

Complex ovarian cysts, i.e. cysts with internal echoes or solid components such as soft tissue septae, wall thickening, or associated soft tissue mass

Ectopic pregnancy (see above)

Serous cystadenocarcinoma

- Commonest type of ovarian malignancy.

- Usually large, often >15 cm.

- Multiloculated cystic masses with thick, irregular septae and soft tissue masses (*Fig. 12.2*).

- May also see ascites, lymphadenopathy and liver metastases.

Other ovarian tumours

- Mucinous and serous cystadenoma, mucinous cystadenocarcinoma and endometroid carcinoma may all produce complex partly cystic ovarian masses.

Endometrioma

- Endometriosis is a common condition characterized by the presence of functioning endometrial tissue outside the uterus.

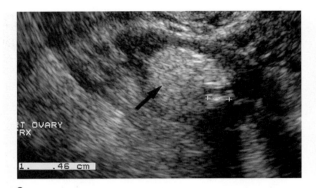

a

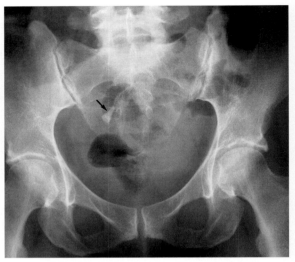

b

Figure 12.3 *Dermoid cyst.*
(a) Transvaginal US. US shows a hyperechoic mass (arrow). Note the more markedly hyperechoic focus with acoustic shadow indicating calcification. (b) Plain film. A plain film of the pelvis shows that the focus of calcification is in fact a well-formed tooth (arrow) within the dermoid cyst.

- Any part of the body may be affected with the most common sites being ovary, fallopian tube and broad ligament.

- Endometrioma refers to a focal lesion in the ovary.

- Cyst with a thick wall and variable internal echoes due to haemorrhage ('chocolate cyst').

Dermoid cyst

- Common tumours in young women.

- Bilateral in 10%.

- Contain fat, hair and sometimes teeth.

- Usually benign; malignant teratomas are rare.

- Complex cyst on US examination.

- Markedly hyperechoic areas due to fat content (*Fig. 12.3*).

Pelvic inflammatory disease

Solid ovarian masses

- Fibroma.

- Brenner tumour.

Uterine masses

- Fibroid.

- Uterine sarcoma/carcinoma.

Staging of gynaecological malignancies

Ovarian carcinoma

Ovarian carcinoma is the leading cause of death from gynaecological malignancy. This is due to the late stage at the usual time of diagnosis, with over 75% of patients having tumour spread beyond the ovaries.

The staging system used is as follows:

- Stage I: tumour confined to the ovary.

- Stage II: tumour involving one or both ovaries with pelvic extension.

- Stage III: intraperitoneal metastases and/or retroperitoneal or inguinal lymphadenopathy.

- Stage IV: distant metastases, e.g. liver metastases or malignant pleural effusion.

US

Most ovarian tumours are well seen with US. Pelvic US may be transabdominal or transvaginal; the two techniques are complementary (see above).

Malignant ovarian tumours are usually cystic with solid components such as septa, soft tissue masses or irregular wall thickening. Fluid contents may be clear (anechoic) or may have internal echoes due to mucin, haemorrhage or fat. Occasionally ovarian tumours are solid masses, e.g. fibroma and Brenner tumour.

Further staging

Further imaging for staging of ovarian malignancies consists of abdomen and pelvis CT to detect ascites, lymphadenopathy, and liver metastases, plus chest CT and chest X-ray (CXR) for pulmonary metastases and pleural effusion.

Carcinoma of the cervix

The majority of cervical carcinomas are squamous cell carcinoma. Peak age of incidence is 45–55 years. The mode of spread is by local invasion plus involvement of lymph nodes. The staging system is as follows:

- Stage 0: carcinoma *in situ*.
- Stage 1: confined to the cervix.
- Stage 2: local invasion beyond cervix, not involving the pelvic sidewall.
- Stage 3: more extensive invasion with involvement of pelvic sidewall or lower vagina.
- Stage 4: distant metastases, including pelvic and retroperitoneal lymph nodes.

Colposcopy is used for initial diagnosis and assessment. Further imaging is directed to assessing the extent of local invasion, as well as the presence of lymphadenopathy.

CT abdomen, pelvis and chest

- Invasion of surrounding structures and pelvic side wall.
- Pelvic lymphadenopathy.
- Retroperitoneal lymphadenopathy.

- Liver metastases.
- Pulmonary metastases.

MRI

Carcinoma of the cervix shows as a high signal mass on T2-weighted images. The multiplanar capabilities of MRI are particularly useful for staging of cervical carcinoma. Images obtained in the coronal and sagittal planes are particularly useful for assessing invasion of the pelvic sidewall and vaginal vault.

Endometrial carcinoma

Endometrial carcinoma is the most common gynaecological malignancy. Most tumours are adenocarcinomas, with a peak age of incidence of 55–65 years. The most common clinical presentation is postmenopausal bleeding. Fifteen per cent of women with postmenopausal bleeding will have endometrial carcinoma.

US

Transvaginal US is the imaging investigation of choice for the investigation of postmenopausal bleeding. The key finding is the thickness of the endometrium. An endometrial thickness of <6 mm would indicate endometrial atrophy, with no further assessment required. An endometrial thickness of >6 mm may indicate endometrial hyperplasia or carcinoma, and biopsy may be performed.

Sonohysterography

Saline infusion sonohysterography is a new technique which enhances the accuracy of US assessment of the endometrium. A small catheter is placed in the uterus. Under direct visualization with transvaginal US, a small volume of sterile saline is injected to give a degree of distension of the uterine cavity. This produces excellent delineation of the two layers of endometrium and allows differentiation of endometrial masses from generalized endometrial thickening.

Further staging

The staging system for endometrial carcinoma is as follows:

- Stage 0: carcinoma *in situ*.

- Stage I: tumour limited to the uterus.

- Stage IA: tumour limited to the endometrium.

- Stage IB: invasion of less than 50% of the myometrium.

- Stage IC: invasion of more than 50% of the myometrium.

- Stage II: invasion of the cervix with no extrauterine extension.

- Stage III: extension beyond the uterus.

- Stage IV: invasion of bladder or rectum, or distant metastases.

As can be seen from this staging system, the most important factor in early endometrial carcinoma is the degree of local invasion. This may be appreciated with transvaginal US. MRI may provide accurate staging, particularly in stage I tumours, with the degree of local invasion better shown than with US.

Investigation of a breast lump

Mammography

Mammography is the first investigation of choice for a breast lump in women over 30 years of age, though US is increasingly used in younger women. Diagnostic mammography may also be performed for other reasons such as nipple discharge, or to search for a primary breast tumour where metastases are found elsewhere. Screening mammography is performed to search for early cancers in asymptomatic women (see below).

The standard mammographic examination consists of two views: craniocaudad and lateral oblique. A range of further views may be used to delineate an abnormality seen on the two standard views. These include spot compression, magnification, and craniocaudad views angulated medially or laterally.

Mammographic features of a benign mass

The two most common benign masses seen on mammography are simple cyst and fibroadenoma.

They have the following features:

- Round or oval in shape.

- Well circumscribed.

- Homogeneous density.

- Usually low or medium density, i.e. normal structures can be seen through the mass.

- 'Halo': a lucent line around all or part of the boundary of a mass.

- Note that a halo may occasionally be seen with a malignant mass, so this sign must be interpreted with caution.

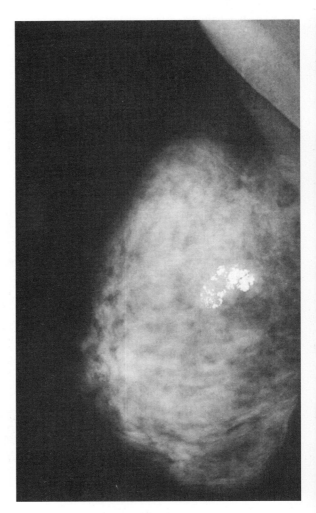

Figure 12.4 *Benign calcification. 'Pop corn' type calcification in a fibroadenoma.*

- Radiological size equal to, or greater than, clinical size.

- Benign calcification of which many patterns may be seen:
  (i) Large cyst: thin rim peripherally; fluid layer due to precipitated calcium in cyst fluid (milk of calcium).
  (ii) Fibroadenoma: calcification with involution after menopause; 'pop corn' calcification or well-defined peripheral calcification (*Fig. 12.4*).
  (iii) Arterial calcification.
  (iv) Duct ectasia (secretory disease): rod-like well-defined calcification in an obvious ductal orientation towards the nipple.
  (v) Small cysts, adenosis, hyperplasia: multiple, tiny, pinpoint calcifications; milk of calcium in tiny cysts with multiple small fluid levels on the oblique view ('tea cupping').

Mammographic features of a malignant mass

- Irregular outline with a spiculated (*Fig. 12.5*) or indistinct margin.

- Often high density, i.e. normal structures cannot be seen through the mass.

- Non-homogeneous.

- Disruption of surrounding architecture: architectural distortion.

- Radiological size less than clinical size.

- Secondary signs: increased vascularity, skin thickening, nipple retraction.

- Malignant microcalcification:
  (i) Irregular.
  (ii) Variable shape and size.
  (iii) Branching, ductal pattern, i.e. 'casting'.
  (iv) Grouped in clusters.
  (v) Variable density (*Fig. 12.6*).

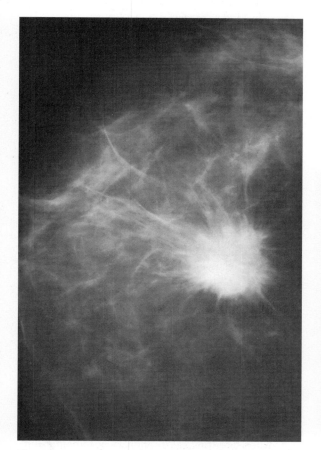

Figure 12.5 *Breast carcinoma – mammogram.*
Note the features of a malignant mass:
- *irregular margin*
- *high density.*

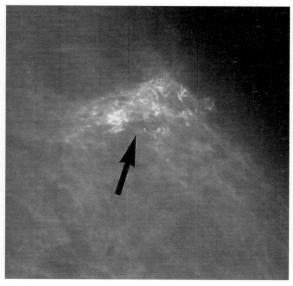

Figure 12.6 *Malignant microcalcification – mammogram.*
Dense cluster of irregular, branching-type calcification (arrow).

US

High-resolution US now has multiple roles in breast imaging. It is the first investigation of choice for a palpable breast lump in a woman under 30 years of age. The traditional role for US has been differentiating cystic from solid lesions seen on mammography or found on palpation. As well as diagnosing cysts, breast US is useful for providing further definition of solid masses. US is also useful for assessment of mammographically dense breasts where small masses or cysts may be obscured by overlying breast tissue.

Cyst aspiration, needle biopsy and drainage placement are all easily and safely performed under US guidance.

US features of a simple cyst

- Anechoic contents.

- Low-level internal echoes may be seen due to infection, haemorrhage, or cellular and proteinaceous debris.

- Smooth walls.

- Sharp anterior and posterior borders.

- Posterior acoustic enhancement; this sign may be absent with deep cysts near the chest wall (*see Fig. 2.2*)

US features of an intracystic tumour (benign or malignant)

- Soft tissue mass.

- Cyst wall thickening and irregularity.

- Soft tissue septum.

US features of a carcinoma

- Irregular infiltrative margin.

- Central hypoechoic or heterogeneous nidus.

- Surrounding hyperechoic halo.

- Acoustic shadow (*Fig. 12.7*).

US features of a fibroadenoma

- Well-defined, oval, lobulated mass.

- Mostly hypoechoic.

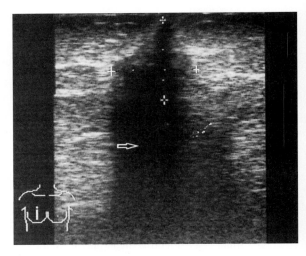

Figure 12.7 *Carcinoma – US. Hypoechoic lesion with an irregular margin. Note acoustic shadow (arrow).*

- Variable acoustic enhancement.

Breast biopsy

Fine-needle aspiration (FNA)

- Minimally invasive.

- 20–25 gauge needle.

- Quick, relatively inexpensive.

- Requires experienced cytopathologist.

- Often non-specific report such as 'no malignant cells seen'.

Core biopsy

- Best results obtained with 14-gauge core biopsy needle used with automated core biopsy 'gun'.

- When biopsying calcification, may combine with specimen radiography to confirm calcifications within the specimen.

- Definitive histological diagnosis usually obtained.

Mammotome

A mammotome consists of a probe that is positioned under mammographic control in or near a breast mass or area of calcification. A vacuum pulls a small sample of breast tissue into the probe. This is cut off and transported back through the probe into a specimen chamber. This technique is particularly useful for microcalcification.

Open surgical biopsy

Non-palpable masses may be localized under US or mammographic control prior to surgery. Suspicious microcalcifications may be localized under mammographic control.

A needle containing a hook-shaped wire is positioned in or near the breast lesion. Once correct positioning is attained, the needle is withdrawn leaving the wire in place. US or mammography of the excised specimen is performed to ensure that the mass or calcifications have been removed.

Imaging guidance

The mammotome is positioned using stereotactic mammography. FNA or core needles may be positioned using mammography or US. For most masses, US is the quickest and most accurate method. With the 'freehand' technique, the US probe is held in one hand and the needle in the other. The needle is guided into the mass under direct US visualization (*Fig. 12.8*). Cysts may be aspirated under US control; FNA of any soft tissue component may be performed at the same time. US is unable to visualize microcalcification. Therefore, for biopsy of microcalcification, mammographic guidance is used.

Investigation of nipple discharge

Radiological investigation is particularly useful if the discharge is either unilateral, from a single duct, or bloodstained. First, mammography and US should be

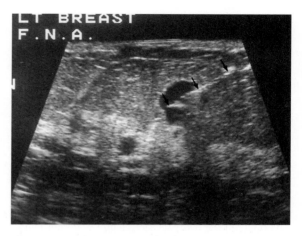

Figure 12.8 *Fine-needle aspiration (FNA).*
FNA of a breast cyst. The needle is well seen with its tip positioned in the cyst (arrows).

performed to exclude any obvious mass or suspicious microcalcification. If these are negative, galactography may be required.

Galactography is a procedure whereby the mammary duct orifice is gently cannulated and a small amount of contrast injected. A small amount of fluid can usually be 'milked' as a guide to which duct to inject.

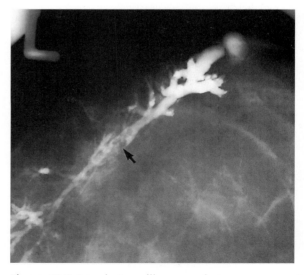

Figure 12.9 *Intraduct papilloma – galactogram.*
Note:
- *contrast-filled duct system*
- *papilloma shows as an irregular filling defect (arrow).*

Also, the discharging duct is usually slightly dilated. Intraduct papilloma shows as a smooth or irregular filling defect (*Fig. 12.9*); these may be multiple. Invasive carcinoma shows as an irregular duct narrowing with distal dilatation.

Brief notes on breast screening

Mammographic screening is of benefit in reducing mortality in the over-50-year age group. Recent literature would suggest a benefit also for the 40–49-year age group. The aim of a screening programme is to reduce mortality in the 55–69-year age group. A dedicated team is essential comprising radiographer, radiologist, surgeon, pathologist and counselling nurse. X-ray mammography is the initial screening test of choice and strict quality control over equipment, film processing and training of personnel is essential to provide optimum images and maximize diagnostic efficiency.

An abnormality on initial screening leads to recall of the patient and a second stage of investigation comprising:

- US.
- Further mammographic views including magnification.
- Clinical assessment.
- FNA or core biopsy.
- Radiological localization and surgical biopsy where percutaneous techniques are unhelpful, especially areas of suspicious microcalcification.

If, after this second stage, a lesion is found to be malignant, the patient is referred for surgery. If benign, she is brought back for routine screening. Indeterminate lesions would usually undergo open biopsy, or be reassessed after 1 year.

13 Musculoskeletal system

Fractures and dislocations: general principles

Anatomy of a growing bone (Fig. 13.1)

Before exploring the general principles of bony trauma, it is important to understand some of the anatomical terms used in the skeletal system. This is particularly true when describing fractures occurring in the growing bones of children.

Bones develop and grow through primary and secondary ossification centres. Virtually all primary centres are present at birth. The part of bone ossified from the primary centre is termed the *diaphysis*. In long bones the diaphysis forms most of the shaft. Secondary ossification centres occur later in growing bones, most appearing after birth. The secondary centre at the end of a growing long bone is termed the *epiphysis*. The epiphysis is separated from the shaft of the bone by the epiphyseal growth cartilage or physis. An *apophysis* is another type of secondary ossification centre that forms a protrusion from the growing bone. Examples of apophyses include the greater trochanter of the femur and the tibial tuberosity. The *metaphysis* is that part of the bone between the diaphysis and the physis. The diaphysis and metaphysis are covered by periosteum, and the articular surface of the epiphysis is covered by articular cartilage.

Classification of fractures

Fractures may be classified in a number of ways and are usually described by using a combination of the following terminology.

Complete or incomplete

- Complete fractures are described as transverse, oblique or spiral.

- Incomplete fractures occur in children and are classified as buckle or torus, greenstick, and plastic or bowing (see below).

Bone involved and position

Comminution

- A comminuted fracture is a fracture associated with more than two fragments.

Closed or open (compound)

Degree of deformity

- Angulation.

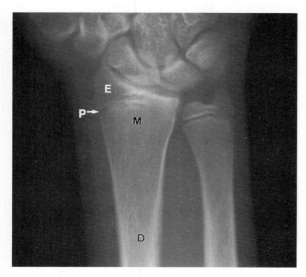

Figure 13.1 *Anatomy of a growing bone.*
Note:
- *epiphysis (E)*
- *epiphyseal cartilage or growth plate (P)*
- *metaphysis (M)*
- *diaphysis (D).*

- Displacement of fracture fragments.
- Rotation.
- Associated joint subluxation or dislocation.

Complications of fractures

Delayed union

Occurs due to incomplete immobilization, infection at the fracture site, pathological fractures, i.e. fractures through an underlying bone lesion, vitamin C deficiency, or in elderly patients.

Malunion

Union has occurred, though in a poor position leading to bone or joint deformity, and often to early osteoarthritis (*Fig. 13.2*).

Non-union

This term implies that the bone will never unite without some form of intervention.

Two appearances may be seen:

- Sclerosis (increased density) of the bone ends with a lucent margin between them.

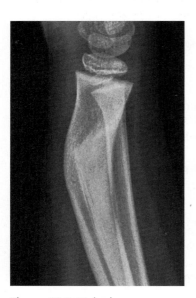

Figure 13.2 *Malunion.*
A fracture of the radius has united with considerable residual angulation and deformity.

- Fracture line able to be seen through surrounding callus.

Avascular necrosis

- Occurs most commonly in three sites: proximal pole of scaphoid (*Fig. 13.3*), femoral head, and body of talus.
- Due to interruption of blood supply as may occur in fractures of the waist of the scaphoid, femoral neck, and neck of talus.
- The non-vascularized portion of bone becomes sclerotic over 2–3 months; this is due to new bone being laid down on necrosed bone trabeculae.
- Due to weight bearing, the femoral head and talus may show deformity and irregularity as well as sclerosis.

Reflex sympathetic dystrophy (Sudeck's atrophy)

- Reflex sympathetic dystrophy may be considered as

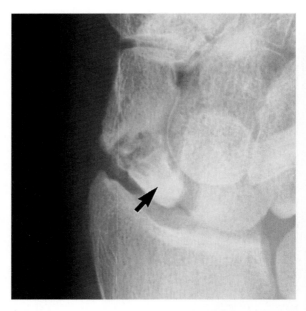

Figure 13.3 *Avascular necrosis complicating scaphoid fracture.*
Note:
- *non-union of a fracture through the waist of the scaphoid*
- *increased density of the proximal pole of the scaphoid indicating avascular necrosis (arrow).*

a severe form of disuse osteoporosis, which may follow trivial bone injury.

- Occurs in bones distal to the site of injury.

- Associated with severe pain and swelling.

- X-ray changes include a marked decrease in bone density distal to the fracture site with thinning of the bone cortex.

- Scintigraphy shows increased tracer uptake in the limb distal to the trauma site.

Myositis ossificans

- Refers to post-traumatic non-neoplastic formation of bone within skeletal muscle.

- Usually forms within 5–6 weeks of trauma.

- May occur at any site though the muscles of the anterior thigh are most commonly affected.

- Seen on X-ray as bone formation in the soft tissues; this bone has a striated appearance conforming to the structure of the underlying muscle.

Subtle fractures

Obvious fractures are just that – obvious – and can often be diagnosed by the patient holding their X-ray up to the ceiling light! The diagnosis of fractures that display subtle X-ray changes is important and often difficult. There is no substitute for careful history and examination followed by close perusal of the tender region on X-ray. Fractures may be difficult to see for a number of reasons as below.

Minimal displacement

These are often referred to as 'hairline' fractures. Oblique fractures of the long bones can be especially difficult, particularly in paediatric patients. A classic example of this is the undisplaced spiral fracture of the tibia in the 1–3-year age group, the so-called 'toddler's fracture'.

Fractures through the waist of the scaphoid can also be difficult in the acute phase. Owing to the risk of avascular necrosis of the proximal pole of the scaphoid it is recommended that regardless of the initial X-ray result, all patients with clinically suspected scaphoid fracture be treated and have a repeat X-ray

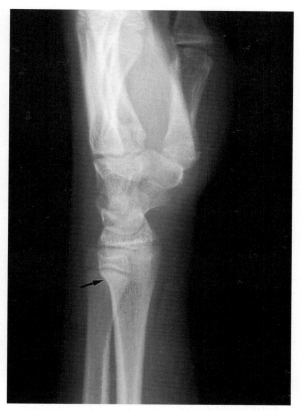

Figure 13.4 *Buckle (torus) fracture.*
There is a buckle in the posterior cortex of the distal radius without a definite cortical break (arrow).

in 7–10 cases. Bone scintigraphy is useful in doubtful cases.

Paediatric fractures

- Children tend to have softer, more malleable bones, which may not completely fracture.

- Buckle (torus) fracture: bend in the cortex without actual cortical break; common in the distal radius (*Fig. 13.4*).

- Greenstick fracture: only one cortex is broken with bending of the other cortex (*Fig. 13.5*).

- Plastic or bowing fracture: bending of a long bone without angular deformity (*Fig. 13.6*).

Growth plate fractures

Fractures in and around the epiphysis may be difficult

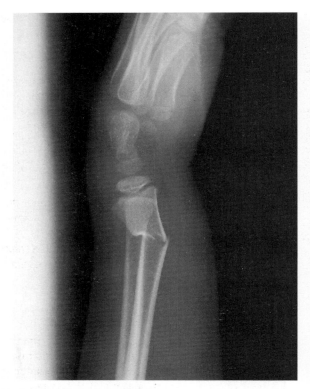

Figure 13.5 *Greenstick fracture.*
Note:
- *buckling of posterior cortex*
- *break in anterior cortex.*

to see and are classified by the Salter–Harris system, as follows:

- Salter–Harris 1: epiphyseal plate (cartilage) fracture (*Fig. 13.7*).

- Salter–Harris 2: fracture of metaphysis with or without displacement of the epiphysis (*Fig. 13.8*).

- Salter–Harris 3: fracture of epiphysis only.

- Salter–Harris 4: fracture of metaphysis and epiphysis.

- Salter–Harris 5: impaction and compression of the epiphyseal plate.

Type 2 is the most common form. Types 1 and 5 are the most difficult to appreciate as the bones themselves are intact. They are important to diagnose, however, as untreated disruption of the epiphyseal plate may lead to problems with growth of the bone.

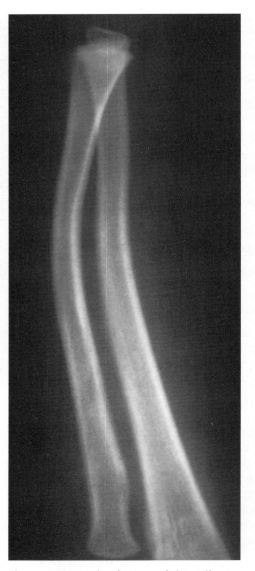

Figure 13.6 *Bowing fracture of the radius.*
Note that the radius is bowed without a visible lucent fracture line. This type of fracture occurs in children, as the bones are more malleable.

Fractures in complex areas

These fractures are difficult to diagnose radiographically due to overlapping structures. Examples include the pelvis, especially the acetabulum; the feet, particularly the tarsal bones; and the wrist, particularly less common fractures such as fracture of the hook of the hamate.

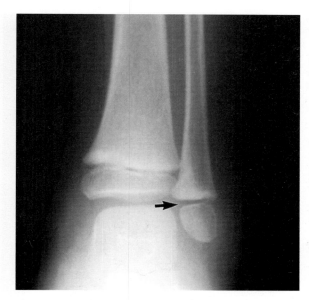

Figure 13.7 *Salter–Harris Type 1 fracture.*
There is angulation of the distal epiphysis of the fibula
with widening of the epiphyseal plate medially (arrow).

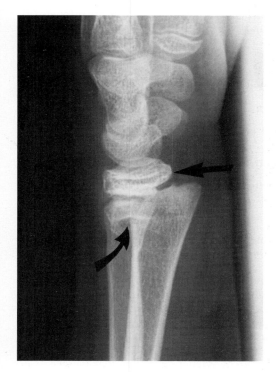

Figure 13.8 *Salter–Harris Type 2 fracture.*
There is a fracture of the posterior surface of the
metaphysis of the distal radius (curved arrow), with
posterior displacement of the epiphysis (straight arrow).

Strategies for diagnosis of suspected fractures in these regions include:

- Further radiographic views: obliques, stress views.

- Recognition of joint effusions. Effusions are easily recognized in the elbow, knee and ankle joints. Elbow effusion and lipohaemarthrosis of the knee joint have a very high incidence of associated fractures.

- Scintigraphy, i.e. bone scan with ^{99m}Tc-MDP. Will be positive within 24 h of a fracture.

- CT with fine sections through the area of interest. CT is particularly useful for giving further anatomical detail prior to surgery. This function is especially applicable to the calcaneus and acetabulum where 3D reconstruction may also be useful.

Stress fractures

A stress fracture is a fracture occurring in a normal bone due to prolonged, repetitive muscle action on that bone. Stress fractures are particularly common in people engaged in sports, ballet and gymnastics and a wide range of stress fractures has been described occurring in particular activities.

- X-rays are often normal at the time of initial presentation. After 7–10 days, periosteal thickening is usually visible, as well as a faint fracture line.

- Scintigraphy with ^{99m}Tc- MDP is usually positive at the time of initial presentation.

- CT is useful for stress fractures in complex areas difficult to see with conventional X-rays, e.g. navicular.

Fractures and dislocations: specific areas

In the following section X-ray signs of the more common fracture/dislocations are discussed. Those lesions that may cause problems with diagnosis are emphasized. Most fracture/dislocations are diagnosed with conventional X-rays. Other imaging modalities are described where applicable.

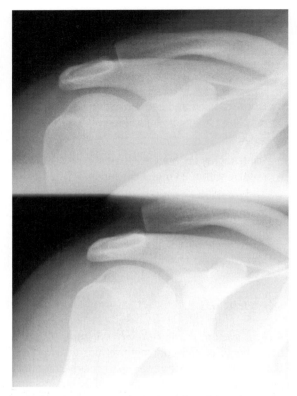

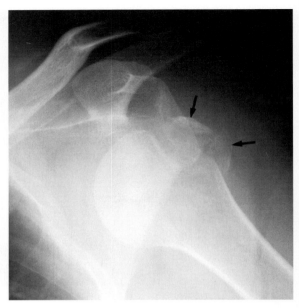

Figure 13.10 *Anterior dislocation of the shoulder joint. With anterior shoulder joint dislocation, the humoral head moves downwards and medially to lie in front of the sternum. Note in this case there are associated fractures of the greater tuberosity (arrows).*

Figure 13.9 *Acromio-clavicular joint dislocation: weight-bearing view.*
The upper view shows the acromio-clavicular joint in normal position. The lower view is taken with the patient holding a weight. This shows the dislocation.

Shoulder

Fractured clavicle

- Usually involves the middle third.

- The outer fragment usually lies at a lower level than the inner fragment with the acromio-clavicular joint intact.

Acromio-clavicular joint dislocation

- Widening of the joint space.

- Elevation of the outer end of the clavicle.

- Increased distance between the undersurface of the clavicle and the coracoid process.

- X-ray signs may be subtle; weight-bearing views may be useful in doubtful cases (*Fig. 13.9*).

Sterno-clavicular joint dislocation

- Very difficult to see on conventional X-rays.

- CT is the modality of choice.

Anterior dislocation of the shoulder

- Antero-posterior film: head of humerus overlaps the lower glenoid and the lateral border of the scapula (*Fig. 13.10*).

- Lateral film: head of humerus lies anterior to the glenoid fossa.

- Associated fractures: wedge-shaped defect in the posterolateral humeral head (Hill–Sachs deformity), fracture of the inferior rim of the glenoid (Bankart lesion), fracture of the greater tuberosity, fracture of the surgical neck of the humerus.

- Recurrent anterior dislocation may be seen associated with fracture of the glenoid, fracture of the anterior cartilage labrum, and laxity of the joint capsule and glenohumeral ligaments: investigate with CT-arthrogram or MRI.

Posterior dislocation of the shoulder

Posterior shoulder dislocation is a rare injury, representing only 2% of shoulder dislocations. It is easily missed on X-ray examination.

Signs on the AP film are often subtle and include:

- Loss of parallelism of articular surface of humeral head and glenoid fossa.

- Medial rotation of the humerus so that the humeral head looks symmetrically rounded like an ice cream cone or an electric light bulb (*Fig. 13.11*).

On the lateral film the humeral head is seen posterior to the glenoid fossa.

Humerus

Proximal fractures

- Surgical neck; displaced or impacted.
- Greater tuberosity.

- Lesser tuberosity.
- Combination of above.

Humeral shaft fracture

- Transverse; oblique; simple; comminuted.

Elbow

Elbow joint effusion

Fat pads lie on the anterior and posterior surfaces of the distal humerus at the attachments of the synovium of the elbow joint. On a lateral view of the elbow these fat pads are usually not visualized, though occasionally the anterior fat pad may be seen applied to the anterior surface of the humerus. With an elbow joint effusion the fat pads are lifted off the humeral surfaces and are seen on lateral X-rays of the elbow as dark grey triangular structures. There is a high rate of association of elbow joint effusion with fracture. Recognition of such effusions is therefore very

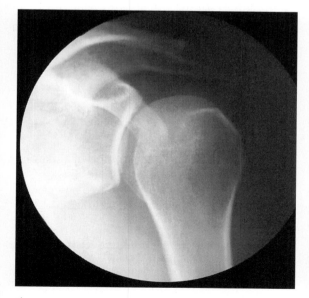

Figure 13.11 *Posterior dislocation of the shoulder. The signs of posterior shoulder dislocation on the frontal X-ray may be remarkably subtle. Note that the humeral head has a rounded symmetrical configuration and that there is loss of visualization of the normal joint space. This is because the humeral head is rotated with the articular surface facing posteriorly.*

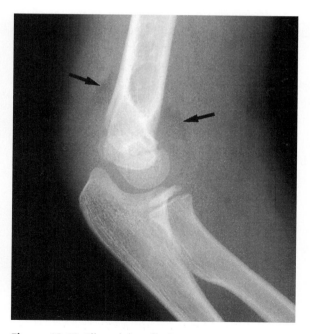

Figure 13.12 *Elbow joint effusion. The anterior and posterior fat pads are elevated from the lower shaft of the humerus (arrows) indicating the presence of a joint effusion. This was associated in this case with an undisplaced supracondylar fracture.*

important (*Fig. 13.12*) in the diagnosis of subtle elbow fractures. Where an elbow joint effusion is present in a setting of trauma and no fracture can be seen on standard elbow films, consider an undisplaced fracture of the radial head or a supracondylar fracture of the distal humerus. In this situation, either perform further oblique views, or treat and repeat X-rays in 7–10 days.

Supracondylar fracture (*Fig. 13.12*)

- May be undisplaced, or displaced anteriorly or posteriorly.
- Posterior displacement is the most common.
- May be associated with injury to brachial artery and median nerve.
- Anterior displacement is very rare.

Fracture and separation of the lateral condylar epiphysis

This fracture is a problem for two reasons:

- The fracture may be missed on X-ray or may look deceptively small as, depending on the age of the child, the growth centre may be predominantly cartilage.
- Adequate treatment is vital as this fracture may damage the growth plate and the articular surface leading to deformity.

Fracture of the head of the radius

Three patterns of radial head fracture are commonly seen:

- Vertical split.
- Small lateral fragment.
- Multiple fragments.

These may be difficult to see; joint effusion may be the only X-ray sign initially.

Fracture of the olecranon

Two patterns of olecranon fracture are commonly seen:

- Single transverse fracture line with separation of fragments due to unopposed action of the triceps muscle.

- Comminuted fracture.

Other elbow fractures

- 'T'- or 'Y'-shaped fracture of the distal humerus with separation of the condyles.
- Fracture and separation of the capitulum – the capitulum is sheared off vertically.
- Fracture and separation of the medial epicondylar epiphysis (*Fig. 13.13*).

Radius and ulna

Mid-shaft fractures

- Usually involve both radius and ulna.
- Transverse; oblique; angulated; displaced.
- Anteriorly angulated fracture of upper third of the shaft of the ulna is often associated with anterior dislocation of the radial head, i.e. Monteggia fracture (*Fig. 13.14*).
- Fracture of the lower third of the shaft of the radius may be associated with subluxation or dislocation of the distal radio-ulnar joint, i.e. Galeazzi fracture.

Fracture of the distal radius

- Most common site of radial injury.
- The classical Colle's fracture consists of a transverse fracture of the distal radius with the distal fragment angulated and/or displaced posteriorly, usually associated with avulsion of the tip of the ulnar styloid process.
- The less common Smith's fracture refers to anterior angulation of the distal radial fragment.

The distal radius is a common fracture site in children with the following patterns seen:

- Salter–Harris Type 2 fracture with posterior displacement and/or angulation of the distal fragment.
- Buckle fracture of the posterior cortex.
- Greenstick fracture.

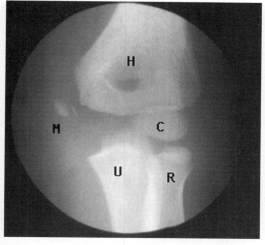

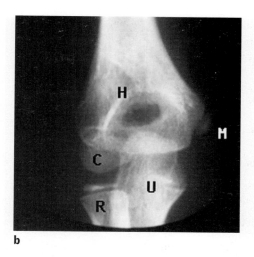

Figure 13.13 *Separation of the medial epicondyle.*
(a) There is a separation of the growth centre at the medial humeral epicondyle (M). Note the anatomy of the other bones of the elbow:

- *H, humerus*
- *C, capitellum*
- *U, ulna*
- *R, radius.*

(b) Normal elbow in a child the same age as (a). Note the normal position of the growth centre at the medial humeral epicondyle (M).

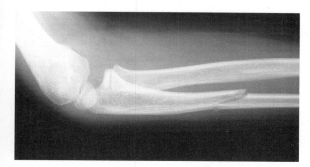

Figure 13.14 *Monteggia fracture.*
A fracture of the shaft of the ulna is associated with dislocation of the radial head. The dislocation is best seen on the lateral view with the radial head lying above its normal articulation with the capitulum.

Wrist and hand

Scaphoid fracture

Two common patterns of scaphoid fracture are seen:

- Transverse fracture of the waist of the scaphoid.

- Fracture and separation of the scaphoid tubercle.

Fracture of the waist of the scaphoid is a problem for the following reasons:

- May be difficult to see on X-ray at initial presentation, even on dedicated oblique views.

- High incidence of avascular necrosis of the proximal pole due to interruption of its blood supply (*see Fig. 13.3*).

Further investigations may be required to confirm the diagnosis:

- Repeat X-ray after 10 days to 3 weeks of treatment where scaphoid fracture is suspected clinically though not seen on initial X-rays.

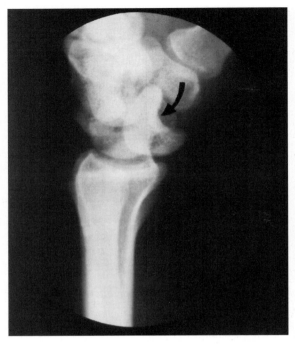

Figure 13.15 *Lunate dislocation.*
Note that the lunate is rotated anteriorly (arrow) while the remainder of the carpal bones align normally with the radius.

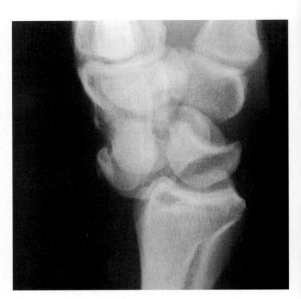

Figure 13.16 *Perilunate dislocation.*
The lunate is seen in normal alignment with the radius, while the other carpal bones are dislocated posteriorly. Compare this appearance with Fig. 13.15.

- Scintigraphic bone scan: positive 24 h following fracture.

Lunate dislocation

- Anterior dislocation of the lunate.
- May be difficult to appreciate on the frontal film.
- Easily seen on a lateral film with the lunate rotated and displaced anteriorly (*Fig. 13.15*).

Perilunate dislocation

In perilunate dislocation, the lunate remains attached to radius with the remainder of the carpal bones displaced posteriorly.

Frontal film

- Abnormal overlap of bone shadows.
- Dissociation of articular surfaces of the lunate and capitate.

Lateral film

- Minimal, if any, rotation of the lunate.
- Posterior displacement of the remainder of the carpal bones (*Fig. 13.16*).

Perilunate dislocation may be associated with scaphoid fracture (trans-scaphoid perilunate dislocation), or fracture of the radial styloid.

Other carpal fractures

- Avulsion fracture of the posterior surface of the triquetral; this is seen only on the lateral view as a small fragment of bone adjacent to the posterior surface of the triquetral.
- Fracture of the hook of hamate:
  (i) Common injury in golfers and tennis players.
  (ii) May see on a carpal tunnel view.

Ligament and cartilage injuries

The wrist is an anatomically complex area with several

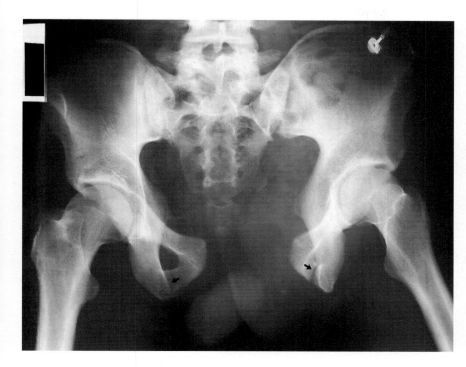

Figure 13.17 *Pelvic trauma.*
Note:
- *separation of the pubic symphysis*
- *widening of the left sacro-iliac joint*
- *fractures of the inferior ischiopubic rami (arrows)*
- *soft tissue mass on the left due to haematoma.*
Injuries such as this have a high incidence of associated urinary tract damage.

important ligaments and cartilages supporting the carpal bones. The most commonly injured structures are:

- Scapholunate ligament.
- Triquetrolunate ligament.
- Triangular fibrocartilage complex.

Ligament and cartilage injuries may be investigated with:

- Stress X-rays to demonstrate carpal instability.
- MRI.

Fractures of the base of the first metacarpal

Fractures of the base of the first metacarpal are usually unstable. Two patterns of fracture are seen:

- Transverse fracture of the proximal shaft with lateral bowing.
- Oblique fracture extending to the articular surface at the base of the first metacarpal.

Pelvis

Pelvic ring fracture

In general, fractures of the pelvic ring occur in two separate places though there are exceptions. Three common patterns of injury are seen:

- Separation of the pubic symphysis with widening of a sacro-iliac joint, or fracture of the posteromedial aspect of the iliac bone (*Fig. 13.17*).
- Fractures of the superior and inferior pubic rami, which may be uni- or bilateral.
- Unilateral fracture of the pubic rami anteriorly, and the iliac bone posteriorly.

Pelvic ring fractures have a high rate of association with urinary tract injury (see Chapter 11) and with arterial injury causing severe blood loss. Angiography and embolization may be required in such cases.

Hip dislocation

- Anterior dislocation is a rare injury easily recognized on X-ray and usually not associated with fracture.

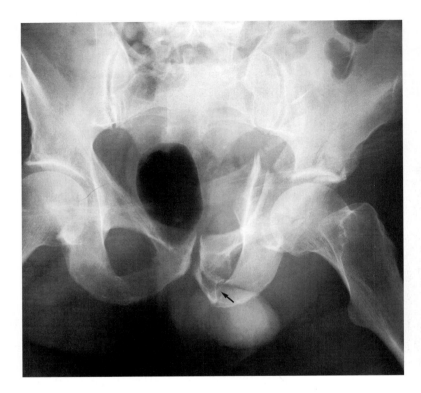

Figure 13.18 *Acetabular fracture. A comminuted fracture of the left acetabulum has resulted in central dislocation of the femoral head. There are associated fractures of the pubic bone and ischial tuberosity (arrow).*

- Posterior dislocation:
  (i)   Most common form of hip dislocation.
  (ii) Femoral head dislocates posteriorly and superiorly.
  (iii) Usually associated with small or large fractures of the posterior acetabulum, and occasionally fracture of the femoral head.

Fractures of the acetabulum

Three common fracture patterns are seen:

- Fracture through the anterior acetabulum associated with fracture of the inferior pubic ramus.

- Fracture through the posterior acetabulum extending into the sciatic notch associated with fracture of the inferior pubic ramus.

- Horizontal fracture through the acetabulum.

Acetabular fractures are difficult to define on X-rays owing to the complexity of the anatomy and overlapping bony structures (*Fig. 13.18*). CT with multiplanar and 3D reconstruction is useful for definition of fractures and for planning of operative reduction. Combinations of the above fracture patterns may be seen as well as extensive comminution, and central dislocation of the femoral head.

Femur

Upper femur

Fractures of the upper femur are particularly common in the elderly and have a strong association with osteoporosis.

- Femoral neck fracture:
  (i)   Usually consists of a fracture across the femoral neck with varying degrees of angulation and displacement.
  (ii) The occasional undisplaced or mildly impacted fracture may be difficult to recognize on X-ray; these fractures may be seen as a faint sclerotic band passing across the femoral neck.
  (iii) Complicated by avascular necrosis in 10% of cases with a higher rate for severely displaced fractures.

- Intertrochanteric fracture: varies in appearance from an undisplaced oblique fracture to commin-

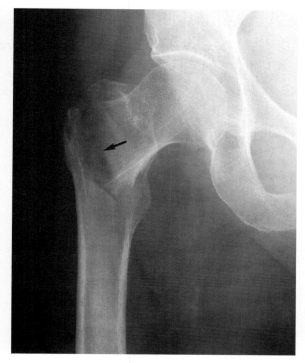

Figure 13.19 *Intertrochanteric fracture.*
A fracture line is seen extending from the greater trochanter downward to the base of the lesser trochanter (arrow).

uted fractures with marked displacement of the lesser and greater trochanters (*Fig. 13.19*).

- Subtrochanteric fracture: refers to fracture below the lesser trochanter.

Femoral shaft

These fractures are easily recognized on X-ray. Common patterns include transverse, oblique, spiral and comminuted fractures with varying degrees of displacement and angulation. Femoral shaft fractures are often associated with severe blood loss, and occasionally with fat embolism.

Knee

Lower femur

Supracondylar fracture

- Usually consists of a transverse fracture above the femoral condyles with posterior angulation of the

distal fragment best appreciated on the lateral X-ray.

Fractures of the femoral condyles

- Fracture and separation of a femoral condyle with varying degrees of vertical displacement.
- 'T'- or 'Y'-shaped fracture with a vertical fracture line extending upwards from the articular surface causing separation of the femoral condyles.

Patella

Three common patterns of patellar fractures are seen:

- Undisplaced fracture.
- Displaced transverse fracture.
- Complex comminuted fracture.

All patterns may be associated with haemarthrosis.

Fracture of the patella should not be confused with bipartite patella. This is a common anatomical variant with a fragment of bone separated from the superolateral aspect of the patella. Unlike an acute fracture, the bone fragments in bipartite patella are corticated; i.e. they have a well-defined white margin.

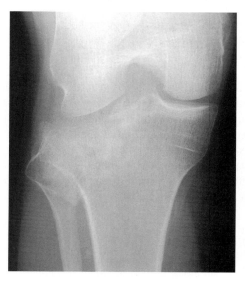

Figure 13.20 *Lateral tibial plateau fracture.*
An AP view shows a comminuted fracture of the lateral tibial plateau. This is associated with considerable collapse, plus deformity of the articular surface.

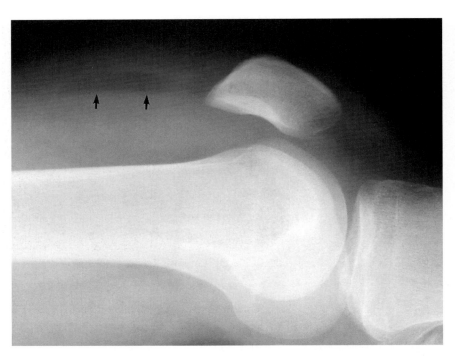

Figure 13.21 *Knee joint lipohaemarthrosis. Note low-density fat floating on higher-density blood in the suprapatellar pouch of the knee joint. This produces a fluid level (arrows) and indicates release of fat into the knee joint from a fracture. In this case, there was a fracture of the upper tibia.*

Tibial plateau

Common patterns of upper tibial injury include:

- Crush fracture of the lateral tibial plateau (*Fig. 13.20*).

- Fracture and separation of one or both tibial condyles.

- Complex comminuted fracture of the upper tibia.

Minimally crushed or displaced fractures of the upper tibia may be difficult to recognize on X-ray. Often the only clue is the presence of a joint effusion or lipohaemarthrosis (*Fig. 13.21*). Oblique views may be required to diagnose subtle fractures, and CT with multiplanar reconstructions is often performed to define the injury and assist in the planning of surgical management.

Tibia and fibula

Fracture of the tibial shaft is usually associated with fracture of the fibula. Fractures may be transverse, oblique, spiral, and comminuted with varying degrees of displacement and angulation. Fractures of the tibia are often open (compound) with an increased incidence of osteomyelitis, compartment syndrome and vascular injury. In particular, injury to the popliteal artery and its major branches requires emergency angiography and treatment.

Isolated fracture of the tibia is a relatively common injury in children aged 1–3 years (Toddler's fracture). These fractures are often undisplaced and therefore very difficult to see. They are usually best seen as a thin oblique lucent line on the lateral X-ray. Scintigraphic bone scan may be useful in difficult cases.

Tibial stress fracture is a common injury in athletes.

Ankle and foot

Common ankle fractures

Injuries may include fractures of the distal fibula (lateral malleolus), fractures of distal tibia medially (medial malleolus) and posteriorly, talar shift and displacement, fracture of the talus, separation of the distal tibio-fibular joint, and ligament rupture with joint instability. Salter–Harris fractures of the distal tibia and fibula are common in children. The pattern of fracture seen on X-ray depends on mechanism of injury.

Adduction

- Vertical fracture of the medial malleolus, avulsion of the tip of the lateral malleolus, medial tilt of the talus.

Abduction

- Fracture of the lateral malleolus, avulsion of the tip of the medial malleolus, separation of the distal tibio-fibular joint.

External rotation

- Spiral or oblique fracture of the lateral malleolus, lateral shift of the talus.

Vertical compression

- Fracture of the distal tibia posteriorly or anteriorly, separation of the distal tibio-fibular joint.

Fractures of the talus

Small avulsion fractures of the talus are commonly seen in association with ankle fractures and ligament damage.

Osteochondral fractures of the upper articular surface of the talus are common sports-related injuries. These fractures may be difficult to see on X-ray and often require assessment with scintigraphy and CT (*Fig. 13.22*).

Fracture of the neck of the talus:

- May be widely displaced and associated with disruption of the subtalar joint.

- Complicated by avascular necrosis of the body of the talus, particularly when the fracture is displaced.

Fractures of the calcaneus

Fractures of the calcaneus may show considerable displacement and comminution, and may involve the subtalar joint.

Boehler's angle is the angle formed by a line tangential to the superior extra-articular portion of the calcaneus and a line tangential to the superior intra-articular portion.

- Boehler's angle normally measures 25–40°.

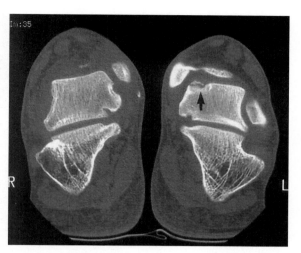

Figure 13.22 *Talar dome fracture – CT.*
An osteochondral fracture of the articular surface of the talus is well shown on this CT in the coronal plane. Note the defect in the articular surface with a small irregular bone fragment (arrow).

- Reduction of this angle is a useful sign of a displaced intra-articular fracture of the calcaneus as these fractures may be difficult to see on X-ray (*Fig. 13.23*).

- CT is useful to define fractures and to assist in planning of surgical reduction.

- Calcaneal fractures, particularly when bilateral, have a high association with spine and pelvis fractures.

Other fractures of the foot

Fractures of the other tarsal bones are less common than fractures of the talus and calcaneus. Tarsal fractures are often quite complex and associated with ligament disruption and dislocations.

Metatarsal fractures are usually transverse (*Fig. 13.24*). The growth centre at the base of the fifth metatarsal lies parallel to the shaft and should not be mistaken for a fracture; fractures in this region usually lie in the transverse plane.

Stress fractures of the foot are common particularly involving the metatarsal shafts, and less commonly the navicular and talus.

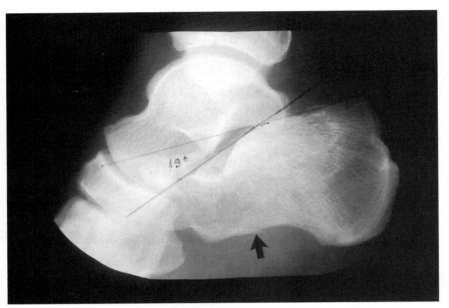

Figure 13.23 *Fracture of the calcaneus. Lines drawn as shown form Boehler's angle. It should measure 25–40°. In this case it is abnormal at 19°. This indicates a fracture of the intra-articular portion of the calcaneus. A fracture line can be seen inferiorly (arrow).*

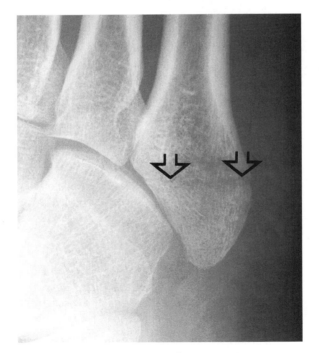

Figure 13.24 *Fracture of the 5ᵗʰ metatarsal. There is an undisplaced fracture of the base of the 5ᵗʰ metatarsal. As is usually the case in this location, the fracture line lies in the transverse plane.*

Facial trauma

For notes on head trauma and skull fractures, see Chapter 14.

Inadequate facial detail is seen on normal skull X-rays and separate facial views must be requested if facial fractures are suspected.

Maxillary fractures

The Le Fort classification provides a useful descriptive guide only; different degrees of fracture may exist on either side of the face (*Fig. 13.25*).

- Le Fort I: fracture line through the lower maxillary sinuses and nasal septum with separation of the lower maxilla.

- Le Fort II: fracture lines extend from the nasal bones in the midline through the medial and inferior walls of the orbits and the lateral walls of the maxillary sinuses, giving a large triangular separate fragment.

- Le Fort III: fracture lines run horizontally through the orbits and the zygomatic arches, causing complete separation of the facial bones from the cranium.

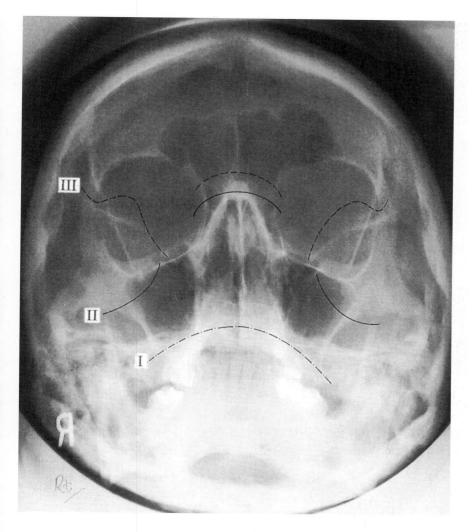

Figure 13.25 *Le Fort fracture.*
A diagrammatic representation of the Le Fort classification of facial features.
Le Fort I – · — · — · –
Le Fort II ————————
Le Fort III – – – – – –

CT may provide better anatomical definition prior to surgery (*Fig. 13.26*).

Zygomatic fractures

Zygomatic fractures occur classically in four places:

- The inferior orbital margin.
- The lateral wall of the maxillary sinus.
- The anterior end of the zygomatic arch.
- The lateral wall of orbit (usually diastasis of the zygomatico-frontal suture) (*Fig. 13.27*).

Other X-ray signs associated with facial fractures:

- Soft tissue swelling.
- Opacification or fluid level of the maxillary or other sinuses.
- Air in the orbit or other soft tissues.

Orbital trauma

The commonest type of orbital fracture seen is a blow-out type fracture. This is usually the result of a direct blow with sudden increase of intraorbital pressure producing a fracture of the orbital floor. Plain films may show a soft tissue mass in the shape of a 'teardrop' in the roof of the maxillary sinus (*Fig. 13.28*). This is due to downward herniation of orbital fat

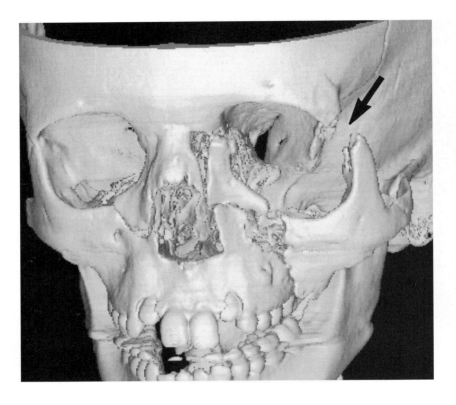

Figure 13.26 *Complex facial fracture: CT.*
CT with 3D reconstructions allows accurate delineation of complex facial fractures. Note the bilateral orbital floor fractures, fractures of the left maxilla, and wide separation of the articulation between the left frontal bone and zygoma (arrow).

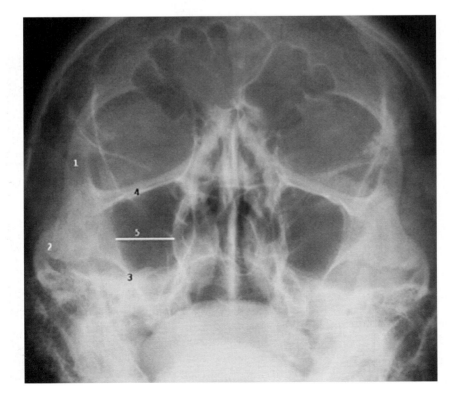

Figure 13.27 *Zygomatic fractures.*
Diagrammatic representation of points to look for in suspected zygomatic fractures:
1. Diastasis of the zygomatico-frontal articulation in the lateral orbital wall.
2. Fracture of the anterior zygomatic arch.
3. Fracture of the lateral wall of the maxillary sinus.
4. Fracture of the orbital floor.
5. Fluid level in the maxillary sinus.

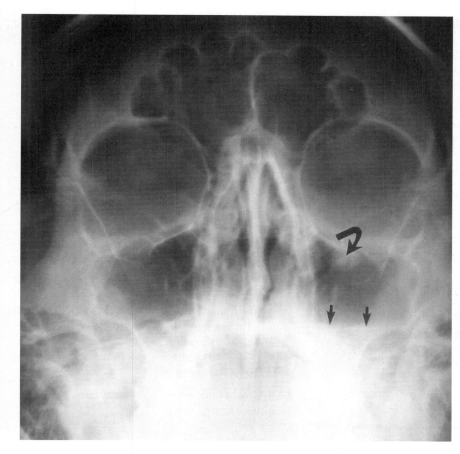

Figure 13.28 *'Blow-out' orbital fracture.*
Note:
- *teardrop-shaped mass in the roof of the maxillary sinus (curved arrow)*
- *fluid level in the sinus due to haemorrhage (straight arrows).*

Figure 13.29 *'Blow-out' orbital fracture – CT.*
Note:
- *fracture of the orbital floor (arrow) with downward herniation of orbital fat producing the teardrop-shaped mass in the roof of the maxillary sinus*
- *blood in the sinus.*

through the orbital floor fracture. The actual fracture is usually quite difficult to see unless displaced.

CT performed in the coronal plane shows the fractures as well as herniation of orbital structures into the maxillary sinus (*Fig. 13.29*). Usually only orbital fat is involved however other structures such as the inferior rectus and inferior oblique muscles may herniate with resultant diplopia.

CT signs of direct ocular trauma include:

- Deformity of the eyeball.

- Intraocular haemorrhage seen as an irregular area of raised attenuation in the vitreous.

CT signs of extraocular trauma include:

- Optic nerve separation from the globe.

- Optic nerve transection.

- Retrobulbar haematoma.

- Extraocular muscle damage.

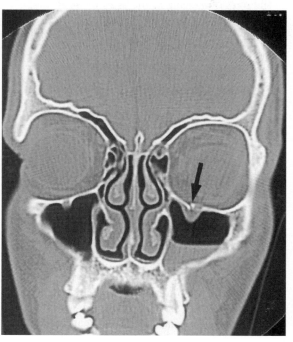

Orbital foreign bodies

Plain films may be used to diagnose radio-opaque foreign bodies and to localize these with respect to the bony margins of the orbit. Eye movement films give an idea of the position of a foreign body.

US may also be used for foreign bodies. It provides accurate localization except for very small bodies lying posteriorly in the orbit. A foreign body shows as a dense localized echo, usually with shadowing.

CT provides accurate localization of orbital foreign bodies.

Mandibular fractures

Numerous views may be needed, including OPG (orthopantomogram) which gives a panoramic view of the tooth-bearing part of the mandible. Being U-shaped the mandible often fractures in two places. The following areas must be fully imaged in suspected mandibular trauma: midline, body, angle, ramus, condyle, and coronoid process.

Spine trauma

The roles of imaging in the assessment of spinal trauma are:

- Diagnosis of fractures/dislocation.

- Assessment of stability/instability.

- Diagnosis of damage to, or impingement on, neurological structures.

- Follow-up:
  (i)   Assessment of treatment.
  (ii) Diagnosis of long-term complications, e.g. post-traumatic syrinx or cyst formation.

Cervical spine

Plain films

Plain-film assessment of the cervical spine should be performed in all trauma patients with neck pain or tenderness, other signs of direct neck injury, or abnormal findings on neurological examination. Cervical spine films should also be performed in all patients with severe head or facial injury or following high velocity blunt trauma or near-drowning.

The following films should be performed:

- Lateral view with patient supine showing all seven cervical vertebrae:
  (i)   Traction on the shoulders may be used.
  (ii) Traction on the head must never be used.

- AP.

- AP open mouth view to show the odontoid peg.

- Oblique views to show the facet joints and intervertebral foramina.

- Functional views, i.e. lateral views in flexion and extension with the patient erect:
  (i)   Performed where no fractures are seen on the neutral views to diagnose posterior or anterior ligament damage.
  (ii) Patient must be conscious and co-operative and must themselves perform flexion and extension, i.e. the head must not be moved passively by doctor or radiographer.

Films should be checked in a logical fashion for the following factors:

Vertebral alignment

- Disruption of anterior and posterior vertebral body lines, i.e. lines joining the anterior and posterior margins of the vertebral bodies on the lateral view.

- Disruption of the posterior cervical line, i.e. a line joining the anterior aspect of the spinous processes of C1, C2 and C3; disruption of this line may indicate upper cervical spine fractures, especially of C2 (*Fig. 13.30*).

- Facet joint alignment at all levels; abrupt disruption at one level may indicate locked facets.

- Widening of the space between spinous processes on the lateral film.

- Rotation of spinous processes on the AP film.

- Widening of the predental space, i.e. >5 mm in children; >3 mm in adults.

Bone integrity

- Vertebral body fractures.

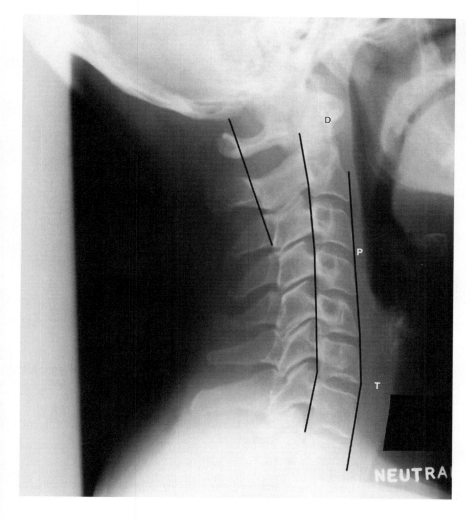

Figure 13.30 *Normal cervical spine.*
Note:

- *anterior vertebral body line*
- *posterior vertebral body line*
- *posterior cervical line*
- *alignment of the facet joints*
- *equal spaces between spinous processes*
- *normal predental space (D)*
- *normal retropharyngeal space (P)*
- *normal retrotracheal space (T).*

- Fractures of posterior elements, i.e. pedicles, laminae, spinous processes.

- Integrity of odontoid peg: anterior/posterior/lateral displacement.

Disc spaces: narrowing or widening

Soft tissue changes

- Prevertebral swelling: widening of the retrotracheal space, i.e. posterior aspect of trachea to C6: >14 mm in children; >22 mm in adults.

- Widening of the retropharyngeal space, i.e. posterior aspect of pharynx to C2: >7 mm in adults and children.

Common patterns of cervical spine injury are as follows:

Flexion, i.e. anterior compression with posterior distraction (*Fig. 13.31*)

- Vertebral body compression fracture.

- 'Teardrop' fracture, i.e. small triangular fragment at lower anterior margin of vertebral body.

- Disruption of posterior vertebral line.

- Disc space narrowing.

- Widening of facet joints.

- Widening of space between spinous processes.

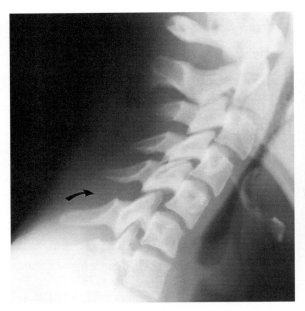

Figure 13.31 *Soft tissue flexion injury at C5/C6.*
Note:
- *disruption of the posterior vertebral body line*
- *slightly narrowed C5/C6 disc space*
- *increased space between spinous processes of C5 and C6 indicates interspinous ligament damage (arrow).*

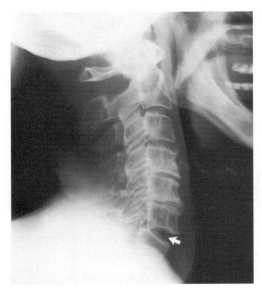

Figure 13.32 *Extension injury at C6/C7.*
Note:
- *disruption of posterior and anterior vertebral body lines*
- *widening of C6/C7 disc space (arrow).*

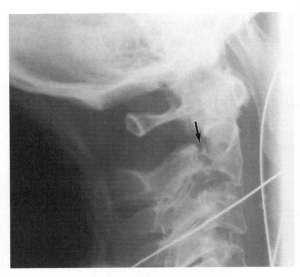

Figure 13.33 *Hangman's fracture.*
Note:
- *disruption of posterior cervical line*
- *fractures of the pedicles of C2 (arrow).*

Extension, i.e. posterior compression with anterior distraction (*Fig. 13.32*)

- 'Teardrop' fracture of upper anterior margin of vertebral body: indicates severe anterior ligament damage.

- Disc space widening.

- Retrolisthesis with disruption of anterior and posterior vertebral lines.

- Fractures of posterior elements, i.e. pedicles, spinous processes, facets.

- 'Hangman's' fracture: bilateral C2 pedicle fracture (*Fig. 13.33*).

Rotation (*Fig. 13.34*)

- Anterolisthesis with disruption of posterior vertebral line.

- Lateral displacement of upper vertebral body on AP view.

- Abrupt disruption of alignment of facet joints: locked facets.

Instability implies the possibility of increased spinal deformity or neurological damage occurring with continued stress.

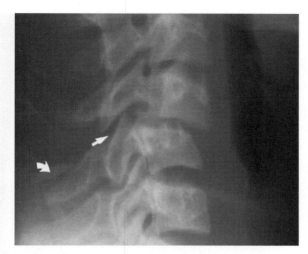

Figure 13.34 *Flexion – rotation injury at C4/C5.*
Note:
* *disruption of posterior and anterior cervical lines*
* *narrowed C4/C5 disc space*
* *disruption of facet joint alignment (straight arrow)*
* *increased space between spinous processes of C4 and C5*
* *avulsion fracture of upper surface of C5 spinous process (curved arrow).*

Signs of instability are:

* Displacement of vertebral body.

* 'Teardrop' fractures of vertebral body.

* Odontoid peg fracture.

* Widening or disruption of alignment of facet joints including locked facets.

* Widening of space between spinous processes.

* Fractures at multiple levels.

CT

CT is used for further delineation of fractures and associated deformity. It provides more accurate assessment of bony injuries, especially those of the neural arches and facet joints, as well as an accurate estimation of the dimensions of the spinal canal.

MRI

MRI has replaced myelography for the following:

Assessment of spinal cord damage (*Fig. 13.35*)

* Transection.

* Swelling/oedema/haemorrhage.

* Cyst and syrinx formation.

Soft tissue changes

* Disc lesions.

* Spinal canal haematoma.

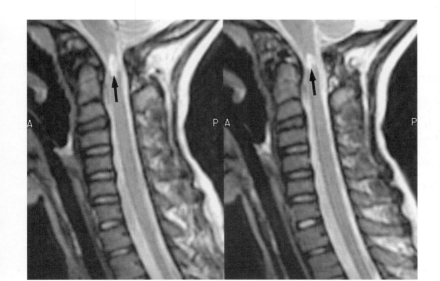

Figure 13.35 *Cervical cord injury: MRI.*
This child presented with ongoing neurological problems several months after a neck injury. A T2-weighted MRI image shows cyst formation in the upper cervical cord (arrows).

Thoracic and lumbar spine

Plain films

Assessment of plain films of the thoracic and lumbar spine following trauma is similar to that outlined for the cervical spine with particular attention to the following factors:

- Vertebral alignment.

- Vertebral body height.

- Disc space height.

- Facet joint alignment.

- Space between pedicles on AP film: widening at one level may indicate a burst fracture of the vertebral body.

Common patterns of injury are:

Burst fracture

- Fractures of the vertebral body with a fragment pushed posteriorly into the spinal canal.

Compression fracture

- Loss of height of vertebral body.

Fracture/dislocation

- Vertebral body displacement.

- Disc space narrowing or widening.

- Fractures of neural arches, including facet joints.

- Widening of facet joints or space between spinous processes.

Chance fracture (seatbelt fracture)

- Fracture of posterior vertebral body.

- Horizontal fracture line through spinous process, laminae, pedicles and transverse processes.

- Most occur at thoracolumbar junction.

- High association with abdominal injury, i.e. solid organ damage, intestinal perforation, duodenal haematoma.

CT

CT is more accurate for delineation of fractures and

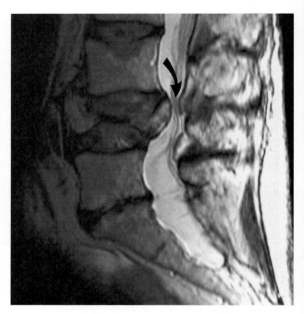

Figure 13.36 *Crush fracture lumbar spine: MRI. Sagittal T2-weighted MRI. This image shows a burst fracture of L4. It is particularly useful for showing the degree of encroachment on the spinal canal with compression of the thecal sac (arrow). Note that there is also a small crush fracture of the upper vertebral end plate of L3.*

deformity. The spinal canal is well visualized in cross-section. Posterior vertebral fragments impinging on spinal canal are well seen.

MRI

As in the cervical spine, MRI is useful in the assessment of the spinal cord and soft tissues, and for the diagnosis of long-term complications (*Fig. 13.36*).

Joint disease: methods of investigation

Wrist

Imaging methods for the wrist include:

- Plain films, including stress views.

- Scintigraphy.

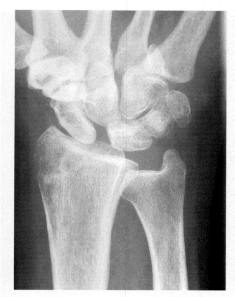

Figure 13.37 *Scapho-lunate ligament tear.*
Note the increased space between the radius and ulna in a patient with wrist pain persisting several months after an injury. This indicates a tear of the scapho-lunate ligament, which may be confirmed with MRI or wrist arthrography.

- CT.
- Arthrography.
- MRI.

Suspected fracture

- Plain films.

Scaphoid fracture

- Plain films – oblique views; films at 7–10 days.
- Scintigraphy in doubtful cases.

Carpal instability (e.g. post-trauma)

- Plain films with stress views (*Fig. 13.37*).
- MRI.
- Arthrography.

Triangular fibrocartilage complex injury

- MRI.
- Arthrography.

Shoulder

Imaging methods available for assessment of the shoulder are as follows:

- Plain films.
- US.
- Arthrography.
- Arthrography with CT.
- MRI.

Rotator cuff disease

Plain films

- Diagnose calcific tendonitis (*Fig. 13.38*).
- Exclude underlying bony pathology as a cause of shoulder pain.
- Assess acromio-clavicular joint and acromion: downward-projecting osteophytes may cause impingement on the rotator cuff.

US

- Very useful as an accurate, non-invasive screening test for rotator cuff tear.
- US of the rotator cuff is highly accurate when performed by radiologists experienced in the technique and using appropriate equipment.

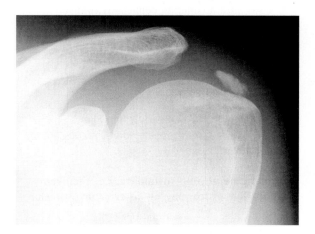

Figure 13.38 *Rotator cuff calcification.*
Calcification above the greater tuberosity indicates calcific tendonitis of the supraspinatus tendon. This is the most common site for calcific tendonitis.

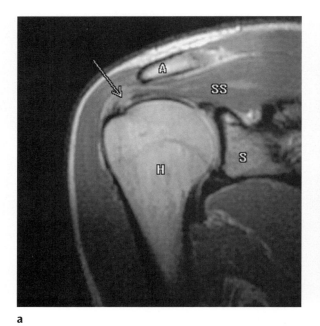
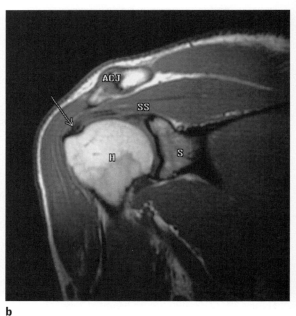

a   b

Figure 13.39 *Supraspinatus tendon tear: MRI.*
(a) A tear of the supraspinatus tendon (arrow) is well shown on a coronal MRI scan. Compare this appearance with the normal supraspinatus tendon in (b). Note the adjacent anatomy:

- *A, acromion*
- *SS, supraspinatus muscle*
- *H, humerus*
- *S, scapula.*

(b) Intact supraspinatus tendon.

- US is most accurate in delineating complete thickness tears; it is less accurate for partial thickness tears.

MRI

- MRI provides excellent views of the muscles and tendons of the rotator cuff.

- Its ability to image in any plane allows oblique coronal views to show the supraspinatus tendon and muscle (*Fig. 13.39*).

Gleno-humeral joint instability, i.e. recurrent dislocation which may be anterior or posterior

Plain films

- Used to diagnose the initial dislocation injury and to confirm joint position postreduction.

- Exclude fractures associated with dislocation:

greater tuberosity of humerus; surgical neck of humerus; inferior rim of glenoid.

- Exclude bony damage in recurrent dislocation: defect in postero-superior aspect of humeral head (Hill–Sachs deformity); fracture of glenoid rim (Bankart lesion).

Arthrography with CT

- CT performed immediately following double-contrast arthrography provides excellent views of the anterior and posterior cartilaginous labrum.

- Labral tears not visible on plain films may be diagnosed.

MRI

- MRI for shoulder instability is best combined with an intra-articular injection of dilute gadolinium.

Hip

Imaging methods available for assessment of the hip are as follows:

- Plain films.

- CT.

- Scintigraphy.

- MRI.

- US.

Fractured neck of femur

- Plain films.

- Tomography may be helpful for undisplaced or slightly impacted femoral neck fractures.

Acetabular fractures

- Plain films including oblique views.

- CT with 3D reconstruction may assist in planning surgery.

Avascular necrosis

- Plain films.

- Scintigraphy.

- MRI.

Hip problems in children: see Chapter 16.

Knee

Imaging methods available for assessment of the knee are as follows:

- Plain films.

- Depending on local availability and practice, arthroscopy or MRI, or a combination of the two, are used in the assessment of most knee conditions including meniscus injury, cruciate ligament tear, collateral ligament tear, osteochondritis dissecans, etc.

- Knee arthrography, once a common procedure, is now rarely performed where the above modalities are available.

- US is useful in the assessment of popliteal cysts, and patellar tendonopathy.

Approaches to arthropathies

Many classifications of joint diseases are available based on differing criteria (e.g. X-ray appearances, aetiology, etc.). I find it most useful to decide first whether there is involvement of a single joint, i.e. monoarthropathy, or multiple joints, i.e. polyarthropathy. This is fine as long as one remembers that a polyarthropathy may present early with a single painful joint.

Monoarthropathy

Trauma

- Usually an obvious history.

- Associated fracture and joint effusion.

Septic arthritis

- Joint may be radiographically normal at time of initial presentation.

- Later a joint effusion and swelling of surrounding soft tissues may occur, followed by bone erosions and destruction.

- Scintigraphy (^{99m}Tc-MDP): usually positive at time of presentation.

Gout

- See below.

Osteoarthritis

- See below.

Early presentation of rheumatoid arthritis

- See below.

Polyarthropathy

Polyarthropathies may be divided into three large categories:

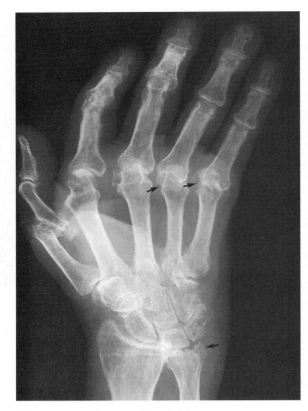

Figure 13.40 *Rheumatoid arthritis.*
Note:
* *decreased bone density*
* *erosion of the metacarpophalangeal and proximal interphalangeal joints, and of the ulnar styloid (arrows)*
* *subluxation of the metacarpophalangeal joints.*

* Inflammatory.
* Degenerative.
* Metabolic.

Inflammatory

Inflammatory arthropathies present with painful joints with associated soft tissue swelling.

Rheumatoid arthritis (RA) (*Fig. 13.40*)

* Symmetrical distribution.
* Affects predominantly the small joints, especially metacarpophalangeal (MCP), metatarsophalangeal (MTP), carpal, proximal interphalangeal.

* Soft tissue swelling overlying joints is an early sign.
* Bone erosions:
  (i) Occur earlier in the feet than the hands.
  (ii) Affect metatarsal and metacarpal heads, articular surfaces of phalanges, and carpal bones.
* Periarticular osteoporosis.
* Abnormalities of joint alignment:
  (i) Subluxation of MCP joints: ulnar deviation.
  (ii) Subluxation of MTP joints: lateral deviation of toes.
* Axial involvement is rare apart from the cervical spine where erosion of the odontoid peg is the most significant feature.

Other connective tissue (seropositive) arthropathies

* Systemic lupus erythrematosis (SLE).
* Systemic sclerosis.
* CREST.
* Mixed connective tissue disease.
* Polymyositis.
* Dermatomyositis.

These arthropathies tend to present with symmetrical arthropathy involving the peripheral small joints, especially the MCP and proximal interphalangeal joints. X-ray signs may be subtle and include soft tissue swelling and periarticular osteoporosis. Erosions are less common than with RA. Soft tissue calcification is common, especially around joints. Generalized osteoporosis and avascular necrosis of the hip may complicate steroid therapy.

Resorption of distal phalanges and joint contractures are prominent features of systemic sclerosis.

Seronegative inflammatory arthropathies

The seronegative arthropathies are asymmetrical polyarthropathies usually involving few joints. They have a predilection for the spine and sacro-iliac joints, especially ankylosing spondylitis. They most commonly occur in HLA-B27-positive patients.

Ankylosing spondylitis (Fig. 13.41)

Ankylosing spondylitis most commonly occurs in HLA-B27-positive male patients. It may also be associated

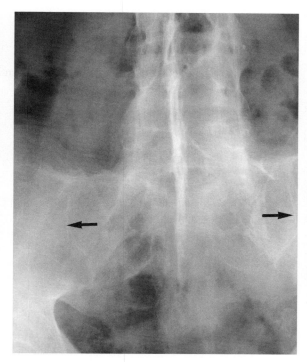

Figure 13.41 *Ankylosing spondylitis.*
There is ankylosis of the lumbar spine ('bamboo spine'),
including fusion of the spinous processes. Note also
fusion of the sacro-iliac joints (arrows).

with ulcero-inflammatory bowel diseases, i.e. Crohn's
disease or ulcerative colitis.

Spine changes include:

- Syndesmophytes: vertically orientated bony spurs
  arising from the vertebral bodies.

- Ankylosis giving 'bamboo spine'.

Sacro-iliac joint changes include:

- Early erosions producing an irregular joint margin.

- Later sclerosis and joint fusion.

Reiter syndrome

Reiter syndrome most commonly affects HLA-B27-
positive males and consists of arthritis, uveitis and
urethritis. It affects the joints of the lower limb with
an asymmetrical arthropathy. Achilles tendonopathy
and plantar fasciitis are common features.

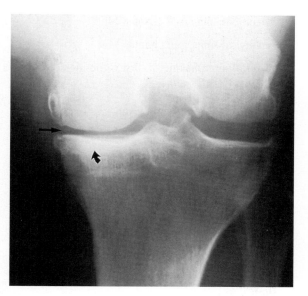

Figure 13.42 *Osteoarthritis of the knee.*
Note:
- *joint space narrowing most severe medially (straight*
  arrow)
- *osteophyte formation*
- *peri-articular sclerosis (curved arrow).*

Psoriatic arthropathy

Psoriatic arthropathy is an asymmetrical arthropathy,
predominantly affecting the small joints of the hands
and feet. X-ray changes seen in the peripheral joints
include:

- Asymmetrical distribution.

- Periarticular erosions.

- Periosteal new bone formation.

- Osteoporosis is less prominent than with RA.

Degenerative: osteoarthritis (OA) (*Fig. 13.42*)

Primary OA refers to degenerative arthropathy with no
apparent underlying or predisposing cause. Secondary
OA refers to degenerative change complicating underlying arthropathy such as RA, trauma or Paget's
disease.

Distribution of primary OA:

- Asymmetric.

- Large weight-bearing joints: hips, knees.

- Lumbar spine (see Chapter 14).
- Cervical spine (see Chapter 14).
- Distal interphalangeal, first carpo-metacarpal, and lateral carpal joints.

X-ray signs of OA include:

- Joint space narrowing.
- Osteophyte formation.
- Periarticular sclerosis.
- Periarticular erosion and cyst formation.
- Loose bodies due to detached osteophytes and ossified cartilage debris.

Metabolic

Gout

Distribution of gouty arthropathy:

- First MTP joint in 70%.
- Other joints of lower limbs: ankles, knees, inter-tarsal joints.
- Asymmetric, often monoarticular.

Acute gout refers to soft tissue swelling, with no visible bony changes.

Chronic gouty arthritis occurs with recurrent acute gout. X-ray features include:

- Bone erosions: para-articular erosions medially and dorsally around the first MTP joint.
- Calcification of articular cartilages, especially the menisci of the knee.
- Tophi: soft tissue masses in the synovium of joints, the subcutaneous tissues of the lower leg, Achilles' tendon, olecranon bursa, helix of the car; calcification is an uncommon feature.

Other crystal deposition disorders

Calcium pyrophosphate deposition disease

- May occur in young adults as an autosomal dominant condition, or sporadically in older patients.
- Presents with intermittent acute joint pain and swelling.

- May affect any joint, most commonly knee, hip, shoulder, elbow, wrist and ankle.
- X-ray: calcification of intra-articular cartilages, especially the menisci of the knee and the triangular fibrocartilage complex of the wrist.
- Secondary degenerative change with subchondral cysts and joint space narrowing is common.

Calcium hydroxyapatite crystal deposition disease

- Peak age 40–70 years.
- Presents with monoarticular or polyarticular joint pain, with reduced joint motion.
- Most common site is the shoulder ie. calcific tendonitis of the supraspinatus tendon (*see Fig. 13.38*).
- Virtually any other tendon in the body may be affected, though much less commonly than supraspinatus.
- X-ray: calcification in the supraspinatus tendon.
- In acute cases, the calcification may be semi-liquid and difficult to see on X-ray.

Other less common metabolic arthropathies include

- Amyloidosis.
- Multicentric reticulohistiocytosis.
- Hyperlipidaemia.

Some common bone conditions

Radiological features of some of the more common general bone conditions are outlined below.

Paget disease

Paget disease is an extremely common bone disorder, occurring in elderly patients, characterized by increased bone resorption followed by new bone formation. The new bone thus formed has thick trabeculae, and is softer and more vascular than

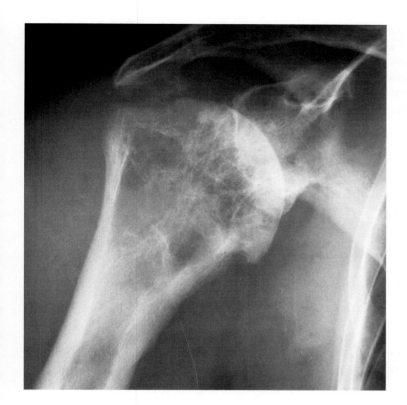

Figure 13.43 *Paget disease of the humerus.*
Note general enlargement of the upper humerus with thickening of the cortex and a coarse trabecular pattern.

normal bone. Common sites include the pelvis and upper femur, spine, skull, upper tibia and proximal humerus. Paget disease is often asymptomatic and seen as an incidental finding on X-rays performed for other reasons. The clinical presentation may otherwise be quite variable and falls into three broad categories:

General symptoms

- Pain.

- Fatigue.

Symptoms related to specific sites

- Cranial nerve pressure; blindness, deafness.

- Increased hat size.

- Local hyperthermia of overlying skin.

Complications

- Pathological fracture.

- Secondary osteoarthritis.

- Sarcoma formation (rare).

X-ray changes of Paget disease reflect an early active phase of bone resorption, an inactive phase of sclerosis and cortical thickening, and most commonly, a mixed lytic and sclerotic phase.

X-ray features include:

- Well-defined reduction in density of the anterior skull: osteoporosis circumscripta.

- V-shaped lytic defect in long bones extending into the shaft of the bone from the subarticular region.

- Thick cortex and coarse trabeculae with enlarged bone. (*Fig. 13.43*).

- Bowing of long bones.

Osteoporosis

Osteoporosis may be defined as a condition in which the quantity of bone per unit volume, i.e. bone mineral density (BMD) is decreased in amount. Osteo-porosis may be generalized or localized, primary or secondary such as in RA. BMD is the most important determinant of bone fragility. Accurate measurement of BMD is therefore important in the early diagnosis of osteoporosis and in follow-up of therapy.

Dual X-ray absorptiometry (DEXA)

DEXA is widely accepted as a highly accurate, low radiation dose technique for measuring BMD. It uses an X-ray source, which produces X-rays of two differ-ent energies. The lower of these energies is absorbed almost exclusively by soft tissue. The higher energy is absorbed by bone and soft tissue. Calculation of the two absorption patterns gives an attenuation profile of the bone component from which BMD may be estimated. Measurements are usually taken from the lumbar spine (L2–L4) and the femoral neck.

Dual photon absorptiometry

This technique uses a radionuclide source with two different energies (^{153}Gd). The same principles apply as for DEXA.

Its disadvantages are that it is more expensive than DEXA, plus it presents greater logistical difficulties with handling of the radionuclide.

Quantitative CT

Quantitative CT is a much more complex technique than DEXA. It is more expensive with a higher radia-tion dose, and is no longer commonly used.

Osteomyelitis

Osteomyelitis may be due to various causes. It is mainly caused by haematogenous spread in infants and children with multisite involvement common. The most common organism is *Staphylococcus aureus*, with group B *Streptococcus* common in neonates. The vascular anatomy is crucial to the distribution of bone infection in children. In infants metaphyseal infection with epiphyseal extension occurs. In children older than 18 months metaphyseal infection predominates.

In adults, osteomyelitis may occur from a number of causes including:

- Trauma, especially compound fractures.

- Adjacent infection, e.g. skin, paranasal sinuses.

- Postoperative.

- Diabetes.

- Intravenous drug use.

Imaging

X-ray

- Usually normal for up to 7–14 days following infec-tion.

- Metaphyseal destruction and periosteal reaction.

- Soft tissue swelling, loss of fat planes.

- Epiphyseal lucency in infants.

Bone scintigraphy

- Positive within 24–72 h of infection.

Gallium scintigraphy

- May help to confirm bone infection.

- Particularly useful in chronic osteomyelitis.

Brodie abscess

- Chronic circumscribed osteomyelitis.

- Focal lucency with marginal sclerosis.

- Most common in the lower extremity.

Histiocytosis X

Histiocytosis X describes a spectrum of disorders, the common feature being histiocytic infiltration of tissues and aggressive bone lesions. The three forms are described below.

Eosinophilic granuloma (*Fig. 13.44*)

- 75% of cases.

- Focal skeletal lesions.

- Peak age of incidence 5–10 years, though may be seen in older patients.

- Common sites: skull, spine and femur.

- Usually seen as a lytic lesion with periosteal reaction.

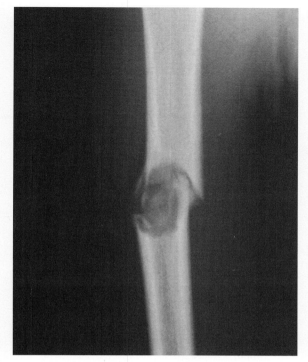

Figure 13.44 *Eosinophilic granuloma.*
An eosinophilic granuloma in an 8-year-old girl
presented with a pathological fracture. Note the
following features of the eosinophilic granuloma:

- *lytic*
- *mildly expansile*
- *well-defined, though non-sclerotic margin*
- *narrow zone of transition to normal bone.*

Hand–Christian–Schuller disease

- 15% of cases.
- Chronic disseminated form of histiocytosis.
- Usually manifest by the age of 5 years.
- High mortality and morbidity.
- Multiple skeletal lesions, which have similar appearances to eosinophilic granuloma.

Letterer–Siwe disease

- 10% of cases.
- Acute fulminant form of histiocytosis.
- Most cases manifest before the age of 2 years and are fatal.

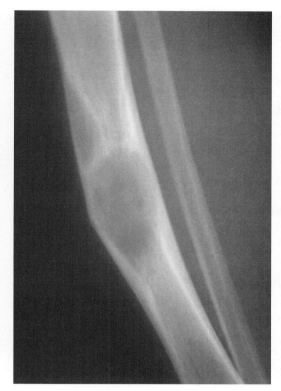

Figure 13.45 *Fibrous dysplasia.*
A 2-year-old boy presents with minor deformity of the
right leg. X-ray shows a homogeneous lytic lesion in the
tibia with expansion and cortical thinning. This is a
common appearance for fibrous dysplasia. Occasionally,
these lesions may present with a pathological fracture
following minor trauma.

- Poorly defined, diffuse skeletal involvement.
- Also involves skin, liver, spleen and lymph nodes.

Fibrous dysplasia

Fibrous dysplasia refers to a common condition characterized by single or multiple benign bone lesions composed of a fibrous stroma with islands of osteoid and woven bone. It may occur up to the age of 70 years, though is usually recognized from 10 to 30 years. Bone lesions are solitary in 75% of cases. Fibrous dysplasia most commonly involves the lower extremity or skull. It usually presents with local swelling, pain or pathological fracture.

X-ray signs include:

- Expansile lytic lesion with cortical thinning (*Fig. 13.45*).

- A homogeneously dense 'ground glass' matrix may also be seen.

Associated syndromes may also occur:

McCune–Albright syndrome

- Polyostotic fibrous dysplasia.

- Patchy cutaneous pigmentation.

- Sexual precocity.

Leontiasis ossea ('lion's face')

- Asymmetric sclerosis and thickening of skull and facial bones.

Cherubism

- Expansile lesions of the jaws in children under 4 years old.

Osteochondritis dissecans

Osteochondritis dissecans affects males more than females, most commonly in the 10–20 year age group. The knee is most commonly affected with other sites including the dome of the talus and the capitellum. In the knee the lateral aspect of the medial femoral condyle is involved in 75–80% of cases, with the lateral femoral condyle in 15–20% and the patella in 5%. Trauma is thought to be the underlying cause in most cases. Subchondral bone is first affected, then overlying articular cartilage. Subsequent revascularization and healing occur, though a necrotic bone fragment may persist. This may become separated and displaced as a loose body in the joint.

Imaging

Plain film

- Lucent defect and separate bone fragment.

- Differentiate from normal irregularities in children.

MRI

- Define bone and cartilage abnormality.

- Establish prognosis: fluid around bone fragment makes separation and loose body formation likely.

- Confirm healing.

An approach to bone tumours

General principles

Bone tumours are relatively rare, representing less than 1% of all malignancies. Imaging, particularly plain X-ray assessment, is vital to the diagnosis and delineation of bone tumours and a basic approach is outlined here, along with a summary of the roles of the various modalities.

In the analysis of a solitary bone lesion, a couple of things need to be borne in mind:

- In adult patients, a solitary bone lesion is more likely to be a metastasis than a primary bone tumour.

- A number of conditions may mimic bone tumour in children and adults including:
  (i)   Osteomyelitis.
  (ii) Fibrous dysplasia.
  (iii) Bone cyst.
  (iv) Histiocytosis.
  (v)   Intraosseous ganglion.
  (vi) Stress fracture.

Before examining the X-ray it is vital to know the age of the patient. Osteogenic sarcoma and Ewing sarcoma occur in the 2nd–3rd decades while chondrosarcoma and multiple myeloma occur in older patients.

Next, it is important to know which bone is involved. Chondrosarcoma and Ewing sarcoma tend to involve flat bones such as the pelvis, while osteogenic sarcoma most commonly involves the metaphysis of long bones. Chondroblastoma and giant cell tumour arise in the epiphyses of long bones.

Finally, the X-ray is examined and a number of parameters assessed:

Type of bone lesion

- Lytic, i.e. lucent.

- Sclerotic, i.e. dense.

Zone of transition

- The part of bone between the lesion itself and normal bone.

- May be wide and irregular, or narrow.

Effect on surrounding bone

- Penetration of cortex.

- Periosteal reaction and new bone formation.

Associated features

- Soft tissue mass.

- Pathological fracture.

Imaging assessment of a bone tumour

X-ray (*Figs 13.46 & 13.47*)

- Multiple projections may be required.

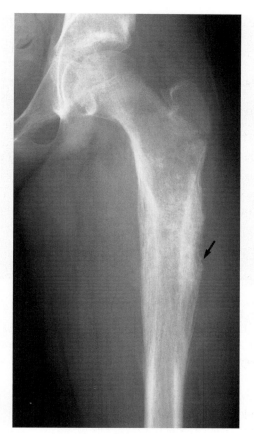

Figure 13.47 *Osteogenic sarcoma upper femur. Note the following features:*
- *extensive features with ill-defined margins*
- *marked subperiosteal new bone formation*
- *elevation of the periosteum at the margins of the lesion forming a triangle of new bone, i.e. 'Codman's triangle' (arrow)*

- Assessment of parameters as above.

- Most diagnostic information as to tumour type comes from clinical assessment plus the plain film.

- The other imaging modalities add further information on staging and complications.

CT

- Accurate localization.

- Sensitive for cortical destruction and soft tissue mass.

- Biopsy guidance.

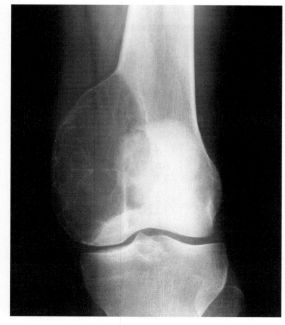

Figure 13.46 *Giant cell tumour. Note the following features:*
- *lytic lesion with marked expansion*
- *involvement of the end of the bone with extension to the articular surface.*

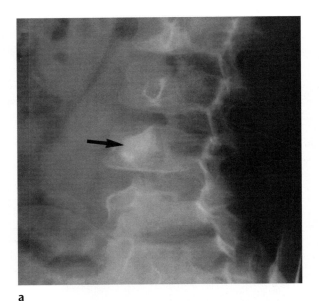

a

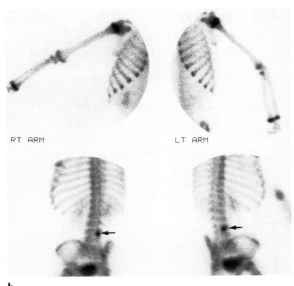

b

Figure 13.48 *Osteoid osteoma.*
(a) An 8-year-old boy presented with a history indicative of osteoid osteoma: back pain, worse at night, relieved by aspirin. An oblique view of the lumbar spine shows focal sclerosis of the right pedicle of L4 (arrow). (b) Bone scan shows a focus of intensely increased activity, typical of osteoid osteoma (arrows).

• Detection of distant metastases, e.g. lung.

Scintigraphy (*Fig. 13.48*)

• Assess activity of bone lesion.

• Detect multiple lesions.

MRI (*Fig. 13.49*)

• Accurate definition of tumour extent within marrow cavity of bone, and beyond into soft tissues.

Skeletal metastases

Almost any primary tumour may metastasize to bone. The most common primary sites are:

• Breast.

• Prostate.

• Kidney.

• Lung.

• Gastrointestinal tract.

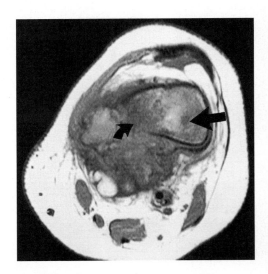

Figure 13.49 *Osteogenic sarcoma: MRI.*
This T1-weighted MRI provides information useful for staging and treatment planning. Note the following features:
• *replacement of normal bone marrow by low signal tumour (straight arrow)*
• *cortical destruction (curved arrow)*
• *tumour invading the soft tissues outside the bone.*

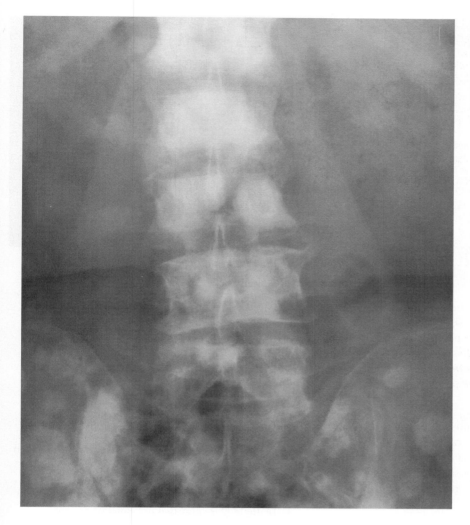

Figure 13.50 *Bone metastases – plain film. There are multiple dense sclerotic lesions throughout the pelvis and spine, in this case due to metastases from a prostate primary.*

- Thyroid.

- Melanoma.

Bone metastases are often clinically occult, or they may present with bone pain, pathological fracture or hypercalcaemia. They usually have the following X-ray features:

- Most commonly lytic.

- Sclerotic metastases occur with prostate (*Fig. 13.50*), stomach and carcinoid tumour.

- Usually arise in the medulla.

- Cortical destruction, without periosteal reaction.

- Most common sites are spine, pelvis, ribs, proximal femur and proximal humerus.

- Uncommon distal to knee and elbow.

Scintigraphy with ^{99m}Tc-MDP usually shows multiple areas of increased uptake (*Fig. 13.51*). Given that a large percentage of skeletal metastases are clinically occult at the time of diagnosis of the primary tumour, scintigraphy is often used for staging. This is especially true for tumours that have a high incidence of metastasizing to bone, such as prostate, breast and lung.

Multiple myeloma

Multiple myeloma is a common malignancy of plasma cells characterized by diffuse infiltration or multiple nodules in bone. It occurs in elderly patients, being rare below the age of 40 years. Multiple myeloma may

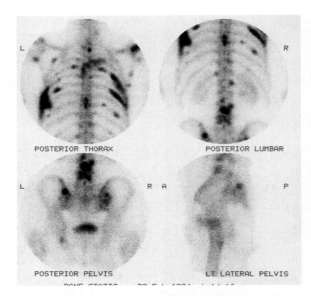

Figure 13.51 *Bone metastases – scintigraphy.*
Note multiple areas of increased uptake of radiopharmaceutical in the pelvis, spine and ribs. This indicates multiple sites of increased osteoblastic activity in a pattern typical of disseminated skeletal metastases, in this case from a prostate primary.

present in a number of non-specific ways including bone pain, anaemia, hypercalcaemia or renal failure. Unlike most other bone malignancies, bone scintigraphy is relatively insensitive so that it is particularly important to recognize the plain-film findings.

Common sites of involvement include:

• Spine.

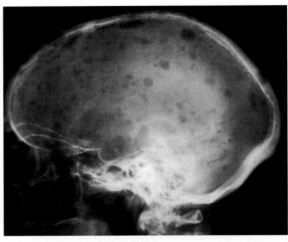

Figure 13.52 *Multiple myeloma.*
Multiple well-defined, 'punched out' lytic lesions. Metastatic carcinoma can also produce this appearance.

• Ribs.

• Skull (*Fig. 13.52*).

• Pelvis.

• Long bones.

Several different patterns of involvement may be seen on X-rays including:

• Generalized severe osteoporosis.

• Multiple lytic, punched-out defect.

• Multiple destructive and expansile lesions.

14 Central nervous system

Head trauma

CT

CT is the investigation of choice for the patient with head trauma. CT has replaced skull X-ray in the initial imaging assessment of all significant head trauma.

Indications

- Fractured skull.

- Confusion/impaired consciousness.

- Focal neurological signs or fits.

- Coma, with or without fracture.

- Deterioration in level of consciousness or development of further neurological signs.

- Confusion or other neurological disturbance for more than 6–8 h.

- Compound/depressed vault fracture.

- Signs of fractured base of skull, i.e. discharge of blood/cerebrospinal fluid (CSF) from nose/ear.

Common CT findings of head trauma

Acute intracranial haematoma

- Acute intracranial haematoma is of high attenuation (white).

- Over 7–10 days the attenuation gradually decreases to approximately that of adjacent brain tissue; a subdural haematoma of this age may therefore be difficult to see.

- Over the ensuing couple of weeks the attenuation decreases further to approximately that of CSF (black).

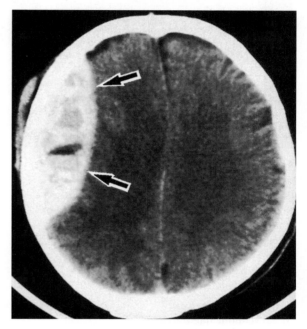

Figure 14.1 *Acute extradural haematoma. Peripheral collection of high attenuation. Convex inner margin (arrows) implies that the collection is extradural.*

Extradural haematoma

- High-attenuation peripheral lesion.

- Convex inner margin (*Fig. 14.1*).

Subdural haematoma

- High-attenuation peripheral lesion often spreading over much of the cerebral hemisphere.

- Concave inner margin (*Fig. 14.2*).

- Usually has severe associated mass effect due to swelling of the underlying damaged brain.

- Decreases in density with time, so that after 2–3 weeks is of lower attenuation than underlying brain.

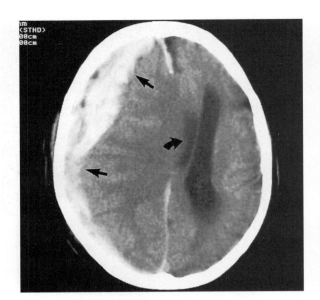

Figure 14.2 *Acute subdural haematoma – CT.*
Note:
- *high attenuation indicates acute haemorrhage*
- *concave inner margin follows the surface of the brain (straight arrows)*
- *marked mass effect with shift of the lateral ventricles to the left (curved arrow).*

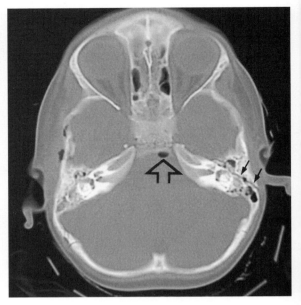

Figure 14.3 *Fractured base of skull – CT.*
There is a fracture of the left petrous temporal bone involving the middle ear (small arrows). Note a small amount of air in the posterior fossa of the skull (open arrow).

Subarachnoid haemorrhage

- High-attenuation material in the basal cisterns, Sylvian fissures, cerebral sulci, and ventricles.

Intracerebral haematoma

- High-attenuation area in the brain tissue, usually with a low-attenuation surrounding rim of oedema.

- Decreases in density with resolution to be of lower attenuation than surrounding brain after about 4 weeks.

Other CT signs of brain damage

- Cerebral oedema: low-attenuation areas which may be focal, multifocal or diffuse; associated mass effect with compression and distortion of ventricles and basal cisterns.

- Cerebral contusion: areas of mixed high and low attenuation which may be focal or multifocal; with time the haemorrhagic component resolves leaving irregular areas of low attenuation; variable associated oedema and mass effect.

- Diffuse axonal (shearing) injuries: small haemorrhagic areas at grey–white matter junction, brainstem and corpus callosum.

Other CT signs of head trauma

- Fractures: CT is especially useful for defining base of skull fractures and all traumatic scans must be perused on bone windows (*Fig. 14.3*).

- Scalp swelling.

- Pneumocephalus: subdural, subarachnoid, intraventricular.

- Opacification and/or fluid levels in sinuses.

- Foreign bodies.

Skull X-ray (SXR)

In view of the wide availability of CT, the indications for SXR in a setting of trauma are limited to the following:

- Penetrating injuries.

- Foreign bodies.

- Clinical suspicion of a depressed fracture.

- CT not readily available.

The appearance of skull fractures on SXR

Fractures need to be differentiated from normal lucent linear markings in the skull, i.e. sutures and vascular markings.

Sutures

Position is more reliable than appearance.

Sutures tend to be constant in position so this is the more important parameter. They may appear as straight or zigzag lucent lines. The following sutures are seen on a lateral SXR:

- Coronal suture between frontal and parietal bones.

- Lambdoid suture between parietal and occipital bones.

- May also see temporo-parietal and temporo-occipital sutures.

The following sutures are seen on an antero-posterior (AP) SXR:

- Sagittal suture between parietal bones.

- Lambdoid suture.

The lambdoid suture is also well seen on a Towne's view, i.e. an AP view angled to show the occipital bones.

Vascular markings

Appearance is more reliable than position.

Vascular markings are quite variable in position and as such their appearance is the most important parameter. Vascular markings have the following features:

- Tortuous and branching.

- Well-defined corticated (white) margins.

- Become smaller as they pass upwards.

- May cross sutures (*Fig. 14.4*).

Fractures have the following features:

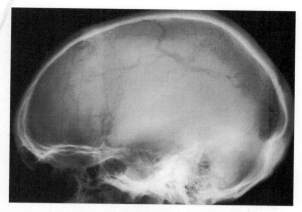

Figure 14.4 *Vascular markings – skull X-ray. Prominent vascular markings demonstrate the following features:*
- *tortuous*
- *branching*
- *cross sutures.*
Compare these features with the fractures shown in Fig. 14.6.

- Usually linear and well defined (*Fig. 14.5*).

- Non-corticated margins.

- Rarely branch.

- Usually do not cross sutures; a linear fracture extending to a suture is more often associated with separation of the suture.

- In children isolated separation of a suture may occur without an associated fracture; this most commonly involves the lambdoid and coronal sutures.

- Depressed fracture may show as a sharply defined area of high density due to overlapping of bone fragments.

- Depressed fragment best seen on tangential views (*Fig. 14.6*).

Other signs of trauma on SXR:

- Air in the cranial vault indicating penetration or base of skull/sinus fracture (*Fig. 14.7*).

- Air in the ventricles and subarachnoid spaces.

- Air collection (aerocele) anterior to the frontal lobes.

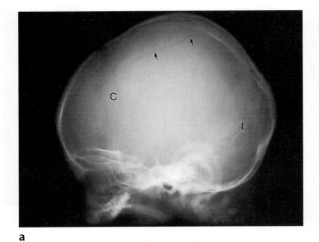

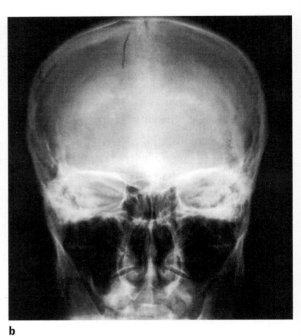

a

Figure 14.5 *(a) Linear skull fracture.*
Note the typical features of a skull fracture (arrows):
- *linear, non-branching*
- *able to be differentiated from the coronal (C) and lambdoid (L) sutures.*

(b) Skull fracture.
Linear fracture of the left frontal bone.

b

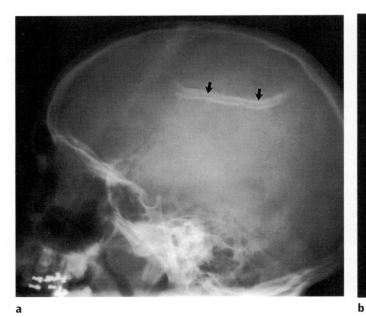

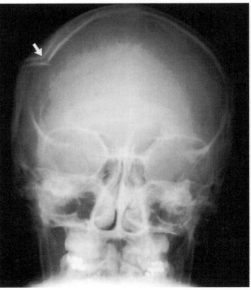

a   b

Figure 14.6 *Depressed skull fracture.*
(a) Lateral view. The fracture is seen as a white band (arrows) due to overlapping bone fragments. (b) AP view. The configuration of the depressed fracture fragments (arrow) is well shown in this projection.

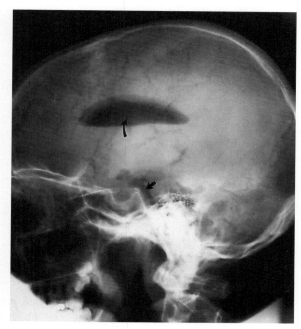

Figure 14.7 *Traumatic pneumocephalus.*
Air is seen in the basal cisterns (straight arrow) and
lateral ventricles (curved arrow) following a base of skull
fracture involving the sinuses.

- Opaque sinus or fluid levels in sinuses.

- Opaque middle ear cavities.

- Shift of pineal calcification (an extremely unreliable sign).

MRI

Owing to relatively poor visualization of acute haemorrhage, time of examination, and logistical problems with monitoring equipment, MRI has not been recommended for initial screening of acute head trauma. MRI is most useful in the non-acute situation of an otherwise stable patient with an ongoing neurological deficit. In particular, MRI is highly sensitive for the detection of diffuse axonal injury and 'old' blood products.

Cervical spine: see Chapter 13

In all major trauma and head injury cases, the importance of obtaining at least a lateral cervical spine X-ray showing all seven cervical vertebrae cannot be overstated.

Facial trauma: see Chapter 13

Subarachnoid haemorrhage

Subarachnoid haemorrhage may be seen in association with trauma (see above).

The most common causes of non-traumatic subarachnoid haemorrhage include:

- Ruptured aneurysm: 80–90%.

- Cranial arteriovenous malformation (AVM): 5%.

Less common causes include:

- Spinal AVM.

- Coagulopathy.

- Tumour.

- Venous/capillary bleeding.

The vast majority of cerebral aneurysms are congenital 'berry' aneurysms. They occur in 2% of the population and are multiple in 10% of cases. There is an increased incidence of berry aneurysms in association with coarctation of the aorta and autosomal dominant polycystic kidney disease. The majority of berry aneurysms occur around the circle of Willis, the most common sites being:

- Anterior communicating artery.

- Posterior communicating artery.

- Middle cerebral artery.

- Bifurcation of internal carotid artery.

- Tip of basilar artery.

The imaging investigation of suspected subarachnoid haemorrhage consists of CT to confirm the diagnosis, followed by angiography to define the cause and direct subsequent management.

CT

CT is the primary imaging investigation of choice in suspected subarachnoid haemorrhage.

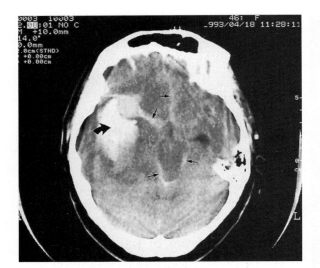

Figure 14.8 *Subarachnoid haemorrhage – CT. Subarachnoid blood is seen as high-attenuation material in the interhemispheric fissure, Sylvian fissures, and in the basal cisterns around the brain stem (straight arrows). Note also the large intracerebral haematoma in the right temporal lobe (curved arrow). Haemorrhage, in this case, was caused by rupture of an aneurysm of the right middle cerebral artery.*

The roles of CT are as follows:

- To confirm diagnosis:
  (i)   Acute subarachnoid haemorrhage shows as high-attenuation material (fresh blood) in the basal cisterns, Sylvian fissures, ventricles, and cerebral sulci (*Fig. 14.8*).

- To suggest possible site of bleeding and/or cause:
  (i)   By localizing the greatest concentration of blood a possible site of haemorrhage can be suggested, e.g. blood mainly in the Sylvian fissure: middle cerebral artery.
  (ii) Occasionally the cause may be seen, e.g. large aneurysm, AVM, tumour.

- To diagnose complications:
  (i)   Hydrocephalus is commonly seen, often within hours of the haemorrhage.
  (ii) Areas of low attenuation due to ischaemia and infarction secondary to vasospasm may also be present.
  (iii) Large aneurysms show as well-defined areas of high attenuation with dense contrast enhancement.

A normal CT does not exclude a small subarachnoid bleed; 5% of patients with a proven subarachnoid haemorrhage have a normal CT. In such cases diagnostic lumbar puncture *must* be performed.

AVM accounts for 5% of subarachnoid bleeds. CT signs of AVM:

- Poorly defined, irregular areas of mixed attenuation, often with calcification.

- Enhancement with contrast.

- Large feeding arteries.

- Large tortuous draining veins.

Angiography

Angiography with selective catheterization of the carotid and vertebral arteries is required to assess the patient with subarachnoid haemorrhage. The timing of angiography varies from centre to centre. The aims of angiography are:

- Show the aneurysm (*Fig. 14.9*).

- Demonstrate the relationship of its neck to the vessel of origin.

- Diagnose multiple aneurysms if present (10% of cases).

In the case of multiple aneurysms, the one responsible for the bleed may be predicted by the CT as above,

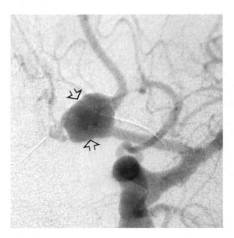

Figure 14.9 *Berry aneurysm – angiogram. A large aneurysm is seen arising from the right middle cerebral artery (arrows).*

may be associated with local vasospasm, and is usually the largest. Bleeding seen at angiogram by actively leaking contrast is very rare, bears a poor prognosis, and necessitates immediate cessation of the procedure.

Other intracranial vascular lesions, most commonly AVMs, will also be shown by angiography and may be amenable to embolization. Large aneurysms unsuitable for surgery may also be amenable to embolization techniques. Negative angiograms occur in up to 15% and may be due to clotting of the aneurysm or non-filling due to severe local vasospasm; in these cases a repeat angiogram may be worthwhile. If the repeat angiogram is negative, a spinal site of bleeding should be considered and MRI of the spine performed. MRI will usually show any spinal AVMs and act as a guide for spinal angiography, and possible embolization. MRI will also occasionally turn up an unexpected finding such as a spinal tumour, which may rarely present with a subarachnoid haemorrhage.

Helical CT angiography (CTA) and magnetic resonance angiography (MRA)

CTA and MRA may be used to image the cerebral vessels. Both techniques are of comparable sensitivity to conventional angiography for displaying aneurysms of 3 mm or greater; below this size CTA and MRA are significantly less sensitive than angiography. Conventional angiography therefore remains the technique of choice for proven subarachnoid haemorrhage though this may change in the future.

CTA and MRA may be used for screening purposes or for specific clinical problems. Indications include:

- Screening in 'at risk' patients.

- Family history of aneurysm and/or subarachnoid haemorrhage.

- Coarctation of the aorta.

- Autosomal dominant polycystic kidney disease.

- Isolated third cranial nerve palsy to exclude aneurysm of the posterior communicating artery.

- Assess possible aneurysm seen on conventional CT or MRI.

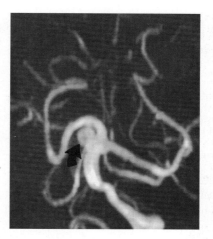

Figure 14.10 *Berry aneurysm – MRA.*
An MRA study of the vertebral and basilar circulation shows the arteries as bright structures on a dark background. There is an aneurysm arising from the tip of the basilar artery (arrow).

CTA and MRA each have relative advantages and disadvantages that influence selection of technique in individual patients.

MRA (*Fig. 14.10*):

- Non-invasive.

- Contrast material not required.

- Relatively long scan times: problem in restless or claustrophobic patients.

- Contraindicated by pacemakers, ferromagnetic clips and implants, ocular metal foreign bodies.

CTA:

- Short scan times (30–40 s), therefore better tolerated in restless patients.

- Claustrophobia is less of a problem.

- Requires use of iodinated contrast material.

Stroke/transient ischaemic attack (TIA)

The term 'stroke' refers to an acute neurological event. Broadly speaking, strokes are caused by either decreased blood flow to the brain (ischaemia and infarction) or by intracerebral haemorrhage. The common aetiologies are as follows:

- Cerebral ischaemia and infarction: 80%.

- Primary intracranial haemorrhage: 15%.

- Non-traumatic subarachnoid haemorrhage: 5% (see above).

- Venous occlusion: <1%.

A TIA is an acute neurological deficit that resolves completely within 24 h. TIAs are caused by transient reduction of blood flow to the brain or eye caused by emboli, or underlying stenosis of the carotid or cerebral arteries.

Primary intracerebral haemorrhage is most commonly due to hypertension. Rupture of a berry aneurysm or arteriovenous malformation may also cause intracerebral haemorrhage. The most common sites for primary intracerebral haemorrhage are the basal ganglia, brainstem, cerebellum, and deep white matter of the cerebral hemispheres.

Haemorrhagic infarction usually occurs secondary to embolic brain infarction. It is due to revascularization of damaged brain secondary to lysis of the occluding embolus.

The principal roles of imaging in the investigation of stroke/TIA are:

- To exclude haemorrhage in the acute situation:
  (i)   CT.

- Identify source of emboli, or nature of vascular occlusion:
  (i)   Doppler ultrasound (US) of carotid arteries.
  (ii) MR angiography of carotid and cerebral arteries.
  (iii) Carotid and cerebral angiography.
  (iv) Echocardiography.

- Identification of hyperacute ischaemia and early intervention:
  (i)   MRI: diffusion-weighted imaging and perfusion-weighted imaging.

CT

CT is used in the assessment of acute stroke mainly to exclude haemorrhage in patients being considered for

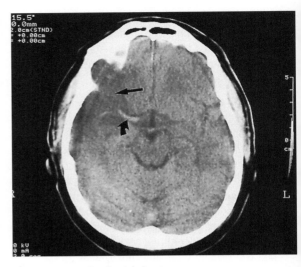

Figure 14.11 *Cerebral infarct.*
Note:
- *Cerebral infarct seen as a low-attenuation area in the right temporal lobe in the distribution of the right middle cerebral artery (straight arrow)*
- *High attenuation in the right middle cerebral artery due to thrombosis (curved arrow).*

anticoagulant therapy. It will also exclude other causes of stroke such as primary intracranial haemorrhage, subarachnoid haemorrhage, or haemorrhage into a tumour.

Whilst CT is highly sensitive for acute haemorrhage, it is relatively insensitive in the diagnosis of early infarction and ischaemia. Changes on CT depend on the size of the stroke, and the degree of associated oedema (*Fig. 14.11*). Up to 12 h following stroke onset, CT scans are often normal. Even where the CT is abnormal, the signs are often extremely subtle and difficult to detect and include:

- Early cerebral swelling with mild mass effect.

- Mild loss of grey–white matter differentiation.

- Decreased attenuation of affected brain tissue.

- Increased density of middle cerebral artery.

From 12–24 h and over the next 3 days there is increased oedema with more obvious flattening of cerebral gyri and mass effect.

As stated in the section on trauma, acute primary intracerebral haemorrhage shows as an area of

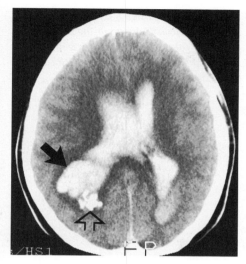

Figure 14.12 *Cerebral haemorrhage – CT.*
This patient suffered sudden loss of consciousness. There is a primary cerebral haemorrhage in the white matter of the right posterior parietal lobe (arrow). This has ruptured into the cerebral ventricles. Note also a densely calcified focus at the posterior margin of the haemorrhage (open arrow).This is a densely calcified AVM, which is the cause of the haemorrhage.

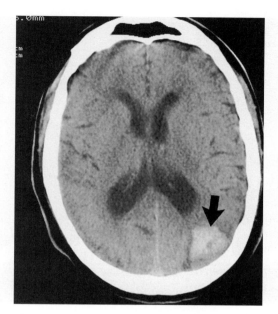

Figure 14.13 *Haemorrhagic infarct – CT.*
There is a small haemorrhagic infarct in the distribution of a posterior branch of the middle cerebral artery. Note the following features:
- *high attenuation indicates acute haemorrhage*
- *wedge-shaped*
- *involves the peripheral cortex.*

increased attenuation. Intracerebral haemorrhage may rupture into the cerebral ventricles, producing secondary subarachnoid haemorrhage (*Fig. 14.12*). Haemorrhagic infarct can usually be distinguished from primary intracerebral haemorrhage in that it is normally wedge-shaped, conforms to a vascular territory and involves the cerebral cortex (*Fig. 14.13*).

In a patient with stroke or TIA, the CT may show other signs of ischaemia as follows:

- Generalized low attenuation in the periventricular tissues.
- Old infarcts: well-defined peripheral areas of low attenuation associated with shrinkage.
- Lacunar infarcts: small well-defined low-attenuation lesions in the basal ganglia and deep white matter.

Doppler US (carotid duplex sonography)

Indications for imaging of the carotid arteries include:

- Cerebral infarction: Most cerebral infarcts are due to large vessel disease including occlusion, stenosis, and ulcerated plaques in the internal carotid arteries, and occlusion of the middle cerebral arteries.
- TIA: 30% of patients with TIA will eventually have an infarct.
- Miscellaneous indications including coronary artery disease, severe peripheral artery disease, bruit in the neck.

Doppler US examination of the carotid arteries is a useful screening test able to visualize most atheromatous lesions at the carotid bifurcation. Blood flow velocity is measured in the common carotid artery and internal carotid artery. A stenosis will be indicated by:

- Increased flow rate.
- Turbulent flow giving an abnormal Doppler wave pattern (spectral broadening).

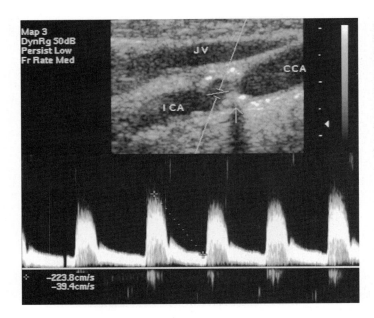

Figure 14.14 *Carotid stenosis – duplex US. There is calcified plaque in the origin of the internal carotid artery (arrow). Doppler US shows an increased blood flow velocity indicating stenosis of 50–69%.*

Based on the US appearance of the carotid arteries, plus the blood flow velocities measured, the degree of stenosis may be classified as follows:

- 0–15%
- 16–49%
- 50–69%
- 70–79%
- 80–99%
- Complete occlusion.

This classification is clinically relevant as carotid endarterectomy is beneficial in stenosis of 70–99%, with no definite benefit shown for stenoses of <70%, and complete occlusion considered to be inoperable (*Fig. 14.14*).

Increased experience with the use of US in vascular disease, plus improvements in equipment, have led to greater accuracy with respect to classification of atheromatous plaques. This includes the presence of calcification and ulceration.

Magnetic resonance angiography (MRA)

MRI is highly sensitive for detection of changes in acute cerebral ischaemia (see below).

MRA is able to provide accurate images of the carotid arteries, and of the circle of Willis and cerebral circulation. With increased availability, MRI of the head with MRA of the carotid arteries may largely replace other imaging tests in the assessment of the stroke patient.

Angiography

Study of the aortic arch is followed by selective catheterization of the common carotid arteries. Angiography is usually performed to assess stenoses of greater than 50% diameter reduction as assessed by US. Angiography may also be used to confirm complete occlusion of the internal carotid artery as shown with Doppler US as this diagnosis has profound implications for patient management.

Other imaging

In a stroke/TIA patient with normal carotid arteries a search for another site of embolus may be undertaken, typically a chest X-ray and an echocardiogram.

Recent advances in management and imaging of stroke

There have been a number of recent advances in the

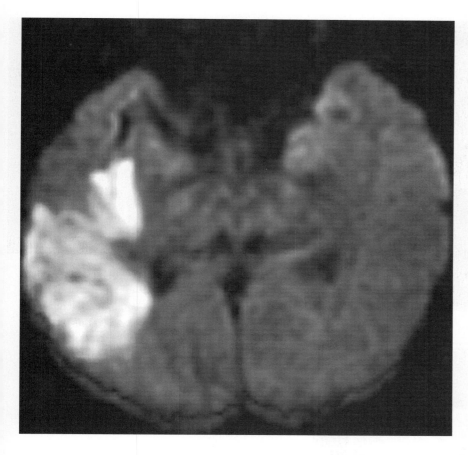

Figure 14.15 *Cerebral infarct – diffusion-weighted MRI.*
A diffusion-weighted scan was performed 6 h after the sudden onset of left-sided weakness. There is an area of relatively high signal in the right cerebral hemisphere. This involves grey and white matter and extends to the surface of the brain. This appearance indicates an area of cytotoxic oedema in a right middle cerebral artery infarct.

potential treatment of acute ischaemic stroke. These have involved the intravenous and intra-arterial infusion of thrombolytic agents including strepto-kinase, urokinase, and most promisingly, tissue plasminogen activator (tPA). In particular, early studies have suggested that the use of tPA within the first few hours following stroke onset may reverse ischaemia and salvage brain tissue. The role of imaging in acute ischaemia is therefore increasing with much research currently directed at the following:

- Early recognition of acute ischaemia.

- Identification of salvageable brain tissue.

- Exclusion of contraindications to thrombolytic therapy including haemorrhage or underlying tumour.

- Intervention: carotid and cerebral arteriography followed by intra-arterial infusion of tPA, carotid stent and angioplasty.

As noted above, CT is not sensitive for the diagnosis of acute infarction. MRI, especially diffusion-weighted imaging (DWI), now has an important role in the identification of hyperacute infarction and ischaemia. DWI is sensitive to diffusion of water molecules within tissue. The greater the amount of diffusion, the greater the signal loss on DWI. Areas of acute ischaemia show reduced diffusion of water molecules. This is thought to be due to an increase in the amount of intracellular water, referred to as cytotoxic oedema, seen in association with ischaemia. An acute infarct therefore has less loss of signal on DWI and shows as an area of relatively high signal (*Fig. 14.15*).

Perfusion-weighted imaging (PWI) can also be used to calculate the relative blood supply to a particular volume of brain. The brain is rapidly scanned following injection of a bolus of Gadolinium. The data obtained may be represented in a number of ways including maps of regional cerebral blood volume and mean transit time.

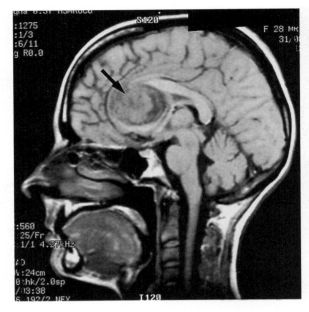

a

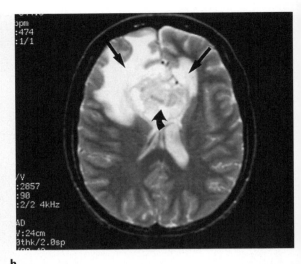

b

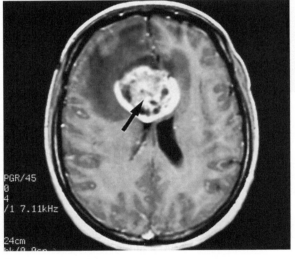

c

Figure 14.16 *Glioma MRI.*
(a) Sagittal T1-weighted scan. Note the large mass (arrow) arising from the anterior portion of the corpus callosum. (b) Axial T2-weighted scan. Note:
- *high-signal tumour mass (curved arrow)*
- *high-signal oedema adjacent to the tumour in the frontal lobes (straight arrows).*
(c) Axial T1-weighted contrast scan. Enhancing tumour (arrow) can be differentiated from low-signal oedema in the frontal lobes.

Studies have shown that, in general, the perfusion defects identified with PWI are larger than the diffusion abnormalities shown on DWI. The difference between these scans is referred to as the ischaemic penumbra. This term describes an area of non-infarcted brain that has reduced perfusion and is therefore at risk. The ischaemic penumbra is the centre of much current research as it is felt that early intervention such as intra-arterial injection of tPA may reduce the amount of brain tissue that eventually becomes infarcted.

Interventional radiology may also have an increasing role in the management of stroke patients including:

- Intra-arterial injection of tPA.
- Carotid angioplasty.
- Carotid stent deployment.
- Cerebral artery angioplasty.

Space-occupying lesions

Intracranial space-occupying lesions may present clinically with:

- General effects:
  (i)   Raised intracranial pressure with headaches, confusion and papilloedema.

- Local effects:
  (i)   Hemiparesis.
  (ii) Focal seizures.
  (iii) Visual field defects.
  (iv) Hormonal effects in the case of functioning pituitary tumours.

The aims of imaging in suspected intracranial space-occupying lesions are as follows:

- Detection of a mass and differentiation from other abnormalities such as hydrocephalus.

- Delineation of the nature of a mass:
  (i)   Site.
  (ii) Density: demonstration of specific contents such as calcification or fat may aid in differential diagnosis.
  (iii) Enhancement pattern.
  (iv) Compression or displacement of adjacent structures.

- Indicate and plan appropriate therapy such as surgery or radiotherapy:
  (i)   Includes biopsy and surgical guidance with stereotaxis.

- Follow-up:
  (i)   Assess efficacy of treatment.
  (ii) Diagnose postoperative complications such as haemorrhage or infarction.

MRI (*Fig. 14.16*)

If available, MRI would be considered the imaging investigation of choice for suspected intracranial space-occupying lesions.

Advantages of MRI over CT include:

- Better soft tissue contrast.

- Multiplanar imaging.

- No image degradation due to artefact in the pituitary and posterior fossae.

- No radiation.

CT

Despite some limitations related to artefact in the posterior and pituitary fossae, CT remains a superb modality for assessment of suspected intracranial masses.

Angiography

Since the advent of CT and MRI, angiography is now only occasionally used for the following:

- Further characterization of a mass, such as haemangioblastoma.

- To outline the vascular anatomy and provide a surgical 'roadmap'.

- As a precursor to embolization or other interventional procedures.

US

Though not useful in primary diagnosis, US has a minor role in localizing small cerebral lesions during craniotomy when the probe can be placed directly on the brain surface.

Other imaging for specific situations

- Drop metastases, i.e. metastases via CSF to the spine seen most commonly with medulloblastoma and ependymoma:
  (i)   MRI of the spine.

- Syndromes:
  (i)   The most common example would be von Hippel–Lindau syndrome where the diagnosis of intracranial haemangioblastoma in combination with retinal angioma should lead to abdominal imaging (CT or US) to exclude an associated renal cell carcinoma.

Neck pain

Seventy per cent of episodes of acute neck pain resolve within 1 month. Most of the remaining 30% resolve over the longer term. Only a minority go on to have chronic neck problems. There are three major sources of diagnostic difficulty. First, multiple structures in the neck are capable of producing pain. These include:

- Vertebral bodies.
- Ligaments.
- Muscles.
- Intervertebral discs.
- Vascular structures.
- Neural structures.

Second, pain may be referred to the neck from other areas:

- Shoulder.
- Heart.
- Diaphragm.
- Mandible.
- Temporomandibular joints.

Third, pain from the neck may be referred to other areas based on dermatomal, myotomal, or sclerotomal distributions.

Osteoarthritis of the cervical spine

Osteoarthritis is a major cause of neck pain. Disc degeneration is most common at C5/6 and C6/7 and is increased in incidence in old age. Degenerate discs have an increased incidence of herniation into the spinal canal or intervertebral foramina. More commonly, disc degeneration leads to abnormal stresses on the vertebral bodies, and on the intervertebral joints, i.e. the facet and uncovertebral joints. These abnormal stresses lead to osteophyte formation. These osteophytes may project into the spinal canal causing compression of the cervical cord, or into the intervertebral foramina causing nerve root compression.

Osteoarthritis uncomplicated by compression of neural structures may cause episodic neck pain. This pain tends to be increased by activity, may be associated with shoulder pain or headache, and usually resolves over 7–10 days.

Cervical cord compression presents clinically with neck pain associated with a stiff gait and brisk lower limb reflexes. Nerve root compression produces local neck pain plus pain in the distribution of the compressed nerve.

Other causes of cervical spine cord compression

As stated above, osteoarthritis is the most common cause of cervical spinal cord compression. Other less common causes may occur as follows:

- Syrinx.
- Spinal cord tumours, e.g. ependymoma, glioma, neurofibroma, meningioma.
- Vertebral body tumours, e.g. metastases, giant cell tumour, chordoma.

Imaging of the patient with neck pain

The goals of imaging should be as follows:

- Exclude conditions requiring urgent attention.
- Diagnose a treatable condition.
- Direct management.

With these goals in mind and given the fact that most neck pain resolves spontaneously, it follows that the majority of patients do not require imaging. Imaging should be reserved for those cases where symptoms are severe and persistent, or where there are other relevant factors on history or examination such as trauma or a known primary tumour.

Initial imaging in the majority of cases will be a plain film examination of the cervical spine. This should include oblique views to assess the intervertebral foramina. Plain-film signs of osteoarthritis include:

- Disc space narrowing, most common at C5/6 and C6/7 (*Fig. 14.17*).
- Osteophyte formation on the vertebral bodies and facet joints.

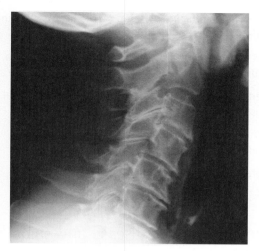

Figure 14.17 *Osteoarthritis – cervical spine.*
Note disc space narrowing and osteophyte formation at multiple levels in the cervical spine.

- Osteophytes projecting into the intervertebral foramina (*Fig. 14.18*).

MRI is the investigation of choice where further imaging is required for persistent nerve root pain, or for assessment of a possible spinal cord abnormality.

CT is used where fine bone detail is required such as in the assessment of vertebral body tumour. CT also has a major role in trauma (see Chapter 13).

Low back pain

Causes of low back pain

Many of the comments on neck pain may also be applied to the lower back. There are many structures that may cause back pain including:

- Vertebral bodies.

- Ligaments.

- Muscles.

- Intervertebral discs.

- Neural structures.

The first step in the assessment of low back pain is to try to classify it as mechanical or non-mechanical.

Mechanical back pain refers to pain that is aggravated by activity such as bending or lifting, and relieved by rest.

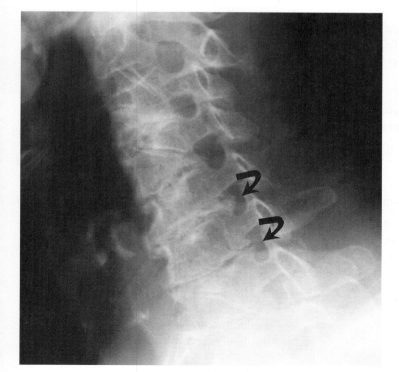

Figure 14.18 *Osteoarthritis – cervical spine.*
An oblique view of the cervical spine shows osteophytes projecting into the C5/6 and C6/7 intervertebral foramina (arrows). Compare these with normal foramina at C3/4 and C4/5.

Mechanical back pain syndromes may be further classified as follows:

Mechanical low back pain (i.e. back pain which does not extend below the iliac crests)

Common causes of mechanical back pain include:

- Soft tissue injuries such as ligament and muscle strains and tears.
- Osteoarthritis.
- Intervertebral disc herniation.
- Spondylolisthesis.

Unilateral acute nerve root compression (i.e. sciatica)

This refers to pain confined to a nerve root distribution with the leg pain being more severe than back pain. It is accompanied by other neurological symptoms such as paraesthesia, and by signs of nerve root irritation such as positive straight leg raise test. Sciatica is usually caused by a focal disc protrusion or spondylolisthesis.

Bilateral acute nerve root compression (i.e. cauda equina syndrome)

This refers to the sudden onset of bilateral leg pain accompanied by bladder and/or bowel dysfunction and is usually caused by a massive disc protrusion or sequestration.

Unilateral chronic nerve root compression (i.e. typical nerve root pain lasting for months)

This is usually caused by disc protrusion or spinal stenosis.

Bilateral chronic nerve root compression

This refers to vague bilateral pain aggravated by walking and slowly relieved by rest. The usual cause is spinal canal stenosis. A common difficulty is differentiating neural compression from vascular claudication. Helpful clinical pointers to a vascular cause include:

- Absent peripheral pulses.
- Pain is in the exercised muscles.
- Pain relief with rest is usually rapid.

The differential diagnosis of non-mechanical back pain includes:

- Vertebral tumour, e.g. metastases, osteoid osteoma, multiple myeloma.
- Vertebral infection, which includes discitis, epidural abscess and vertebral osteomyelitis.
- Other vertebral conditions such as Paget's disease and ankylosing spondylitis.
- Referred pain, e.g. pyelonephritis, aortic aneurysm, inflammatory bowel disease.

Degenerative disc disease and spinal canal stenosis

The two major risk factors for degenerative disc disease of the lumbar spine are age and trauma. Each intervertebral disc is composed of a tough outer layer, the annulus fibrosis, and a softer semi-fluid centre, the nucleus pulposus. With degeneration of the disc, small microtears appear in the annulus fibrosis allowing generalized bulging of the nucleus pulposus. This causes the disc to bulge beyond the margins of the vertebral bodies with narrowing of the spinal canal.

Secondary effects of degenerative disc disease include abnormal stresses on the vertebral bodies leading to osteophyte formation, as well as facet joint sclerosis and hypertrophy. These changes may lead to further narrowing of the spinal canal producing spinal canal stenosis.

The next step in disc degeneration is a localized tear in the annulus fibrosis through which the nucleus pulposus may herniate. This produces a focal protrusion of disc material that may project centrally into the spinal canal or posterolaterally into the intervertebral foramen.

A disc herniation that penetrates the posterior longitudinal ligament is referred to as an extruded disc. Usually, these extruded discs will separate from the parent disc and migrate superiorly or inferiorly in the spinal canal. This is referred to as a free fragment or sequestration. The use of the terms *annular bulge, protrusion, extrusion* and *sequestration* to describe the various stages and types of intervertebral disc pathology is to be encouraged as the development of a standard terminology will assist in the understanding and management of degenerative disc disease.

Imaging of low back pain

The need for imaging in the management of low back pain and sciatica remains controversial. Plain-film examination of the lumbar spine is one of the most frequently requested radiological examinations, despite its consistently demonstrated low impact on clinical management. The majority of patients with low back pain require no imaging at all, as most will respond to conservative management within 6 weeks. Imaging is recommended for the minority of patients in whom symptoms persist or in whom there is diagnostic uncertainty. An initial plain-film examination of the lumbar spine is reasonable in these patients (*Fig. 14.19*). This will help exclude obvious bony causes of pain as well as delineate any other relevant factors such as scoliosis.

The major limitations of plain films of the lumbar spine are:

- Soft tissue structures such as ligaments, muscles, nerve roots and intervertebral discs are not imaged.

- Relative insensitivity for bone conditions such as infection.

- The cross-sectional dimensions of the spinal canal are not assessed.

Cross-sectional imaging techniques, MRI and CT, are recommended for the following:

- True radicular symptoms are present, with leg pain being more severe than back pain.

- Evidence of nerve root irritation, e.g. positive straight leg raise test.

- Failure of conservative management.

- Persistent non-mechanical back pain.

- Other historical factors such as evidence of infection, or known primary malignancy, or severe osteoporosis.

MRI (*Fig. 14.20*)

MRI is the investigation of choice for most applications for the following reasons:

- Superior soft tissue contrast resolution. Nerve roots and the distal spinal cord and conus can be imaged without the use of contrast material.

- Multiplanar capabilities. The sagittal and occasionally the coronal planes are used as well as the transverse plane.

- Highly sensitive to tissue water content. Disc dehydration is an early sign of degenerative disease and is seen as reduced disc signal on T2-weighted images.

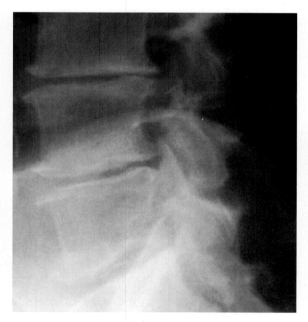

Figure 14.19 *Osteoarthritis of the lumbar spine.*
Note:
- *narrowing of the lower three disc spaces*
- *osteophyte formation at the corners of the vertebral bodies.*

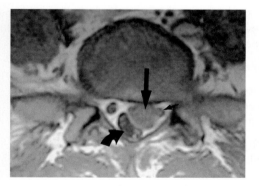

Figure 14.20 *Lumbar disc sequestration – MRI. T1-weighted axial image. There is a large disc fragment in the left side of the spinal canal (arrow). This is compressing the left S1 nerve root (small arrow), and the thecal sac (curved arrow). The disc fragment has migrated inferiorly from the L5–S1 disc.*

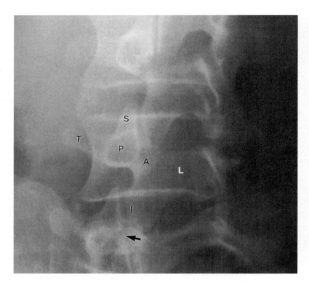

Figure 14.21 *Pars interarticularis defect at L5. Identify the following structures which form the outline of a Scottish terrier dog at L2, L3 and L4:*
- *transverse process (T)*
- *superior articular process (S)*
- *pedicle (P)*
- *pars interarticularis (A), i.e. the bar of bone seen medial to the pedicle*
- *inferior articular process (I)*
- *lamina (L).*

CT

CT is a reasonable alternative for investigation of back pain and sciatica where MRI is not available. Scintigraphy is used in those patients in whom a bony cause of pain is to be excluded. It is particularly useful for the following:

- Infection.

- Suspected neoplasm, especially to exclude spinal metastases where there is a known primary tumour.

- Pars interarticularis fractures. These may be difficult to see on plain films, particularly in young patients with subtle stress fractures.

Pars interarticularis defects and spondylolisthesis

Pars interarticularis defects are most common at L5.

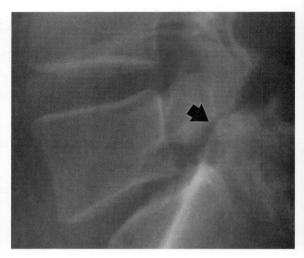

Figure 14.22 *Spondylolisthesis.*
Note:
- *bilateral pars interarticularis defects (arrow)*
- *forward shift of L5 on SI.*

Common aetiologies include:

- Congenital, associated with other developmental anomalies of the lumbar spine, especially spina bifida occulta.

- Post-traumatic, i.e. fractures.

- Stress fractures associated with sports such as gymnastics and fast bowling (cricket).

Bilateral pars defects may be associated with spondylolisthesis, i.e. anterior shift of L5 on S1.

Plain films

Pars interarticularis defects are best seen on oblique views of the lower lumbar spine. The complex of overlapping shadows from the superior and inferior articular processes, the pars interarticularis, and the transverse process forms an outline resembling that of a Scottish terrier dog (*Fig. 14.21*). A pars defect is seen as a line across the neck of the 'dog' (*Fig. 14.22*).

CT

Pars interarticularis defects are well shown on CT. Scans using a specific angle to 'cut through' the length of the pars interarticularis are extremely sensitive and may also be used to assess healing following treatment.

15 Neck

Investigation of a neck mass

The roles of imaging in the investigation of neck masses are as follows:

Localization of the mass

- Arising from the thyroid.
- Arising from other organs such as the salivary glands.

Features of the mass

- Cystic or solid.
- Calcification.

Anatomical relations

- Position relative to the great vessels, thyroid gland, laryngeal cartilages.
- Retrosternal extension.

Evidence of malignancy

- Invasion of surrounding structures.
- Lymphadenopathy.

Ultrasound (US)

US is an accurate and non-invasive screening test for initial localization and characterization of a neck mass. It will usually differentiate cystic from solid lesions, although branchial and thyroglossal cysts may appear solid owing to infection and haemorrhage.

CT

CT is the investigation of choice for accurate assessment of neck masses. It provides good localization and definition of anatomical relations. Complications such as invasion or displacement of surrounding structures as well as lymphadenopathy are well seen.

MRI

MRI is an excellent technique for neck masses and in centres where it is freely available, it may replace CT.

The principal advantages of MRI in imaging masses of the neck are:

- No iodinated contrast is needed to delineate blood vessels.
- Multiplanar imaging allows easy assessment of anatomical relationships (e.g. retrosternal spread of a thyroid mass well seen in the sagittal plane).

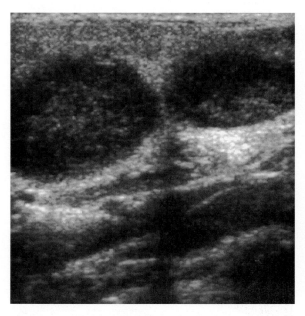

Figure 15.1 *Cervical lymphadenopathy – US. Enlarged cervical lymph nodes in a patient with lymphoma. The lymph nodes are seen as well-defined, round, hypoechoic masses.*

Table 15.1 *Imaging features of common neck masses arising outside the thyroid gland*

Mass	Clinical	CT	US
Abscess	Usually occur in close relation to the airway, i.e. parapharyngeal and retropharyngeal	Low-attenuation mass with thick enhancing wall. Swelling and obliteration of adjacent tissue planes	Irregular hypoechoic fluid collection
Malignant lymphadenopathy	Lymphoma Metastatic spread from head and neck tumours	Multiple round soft tissue masses	Multiple round hypoechoic masses (*Fig. 15.1*)
Second branchial cleft cyst	Usually presents in young adults with a mass of the upper neck, anterior to the sternomastoid muscle	Thin-walled low-attenuation cyst	Well-defined cyst
Thyroglossal duct cyst	Cyst of remnants of the thyroglossal duct. Usually located anteriorly in the midline	Well-defined low-attenuation cyst. Located in the midline, usually anterior to the hyoid bone (*Fig 15.2*)	Well-defined cyst. May have complex echogenic contents when complicated by infection
Cystic hygroma	Complex cyst of the lower neck, posterior to sternomastoid muscle. Associated with Turner's syndrome. Usually in young children under 2 years.	Low-attenuation mass, which may infiltrate soft tissue planes and extend into the superior mediastinum	Complex hypoechoic mass
Dermoid cyst	Midline cyst in the floor of the mouth	Well-defined mass. Low-attenuation fat content	Hyperechoic cystic mass
Carotid body tumour	Paraganglioma located in the carotid artery bifurcation	Well-defined mass between the internal and external carotid arteries. Dense enhancement with contrast material	Well-defined mass Highly vascular on colour Doppler examination

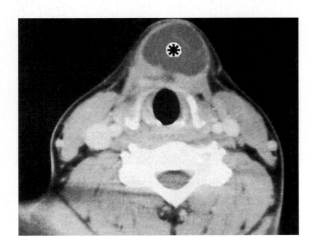

Figure 15.2 *Thyroglossal cyst – CT. Cystic lesion (*) anterior to the larynx.*

Investigation of a salivary gland mass

Common salivary gland tumours include:

Pleomorphic adenoma

• Benign.

- 70% of all parotid tumours.

Adenolymphoma (Warthin's tumour)

- Second most common benign parotid tumour.

- 10% bilateral.

Adenoid cystic carcinoma (cylindroma)

- Malignant.

- Usually arise in minor salivary glands.

Mucoepidermoid carcinoma

- Most common malignant tumour of the parotid gland.

Other soft tissue tumours may occur in the parotid gland:

- Lipoma, neuroma and melanoma.

Cross-sectional imaging with US and CT or MRI is usually sufficient prior to surgery.

Sialography and scintigraphy are used only in a few difficult or uncertain cases.

CT

CT is used to define the extent of tumour and, in the case of a parotid tumour, to establish its relationship to the facial nerve. Benign tumours tend to be well-defined. Malignant tumours often have irregular, ill-defined margins. Complicating factors such as lymphadenopathy and invasion of deep structures are well shown with CT.

MRI

MRI is useful for imaging tumours of the parotid gland because the facial nerve can be seen in the gland and hence a tumour's relationship to it can be demonstrated. Multiplanar imaging is also useful in this regard.

As with other modalities a specific histological diagnosis cannot be made, with the possible exception of adenolymphoma, which may appear as a multiloculated cystic mass.

US

US is of limited use, other than for defining if a lesion is cystic or solid.

Sialography

Masses show as filling defects in the gland surrounded by displaced ducts. Malignant masses may be more irregular with distortion of intraglandular ducts.

Scintigraphy

Most masses show as a photon deficient ('cold') filling defect, the exception being adenolymphoma, which may accumulate isotope.

Investigation of a salivary gland calculus

Plain films

Most salivary calculi are radio-opaque and therefore visible on plain films. Specific views are used for the gland of interest. These may include intra-oral films to show the submandibular ducts (*Fig. 15.3*).

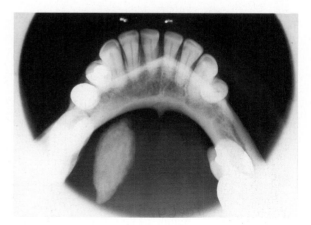

Figure 15.3 *Submandibular duct calculus.*
An intra-oral film of the floor of the mouth shows a large calculus in the anterior end of the right submandibular duct.

Sialography

Sialography is indicated for suspected salivary gland calculus in the parotid and submandibular ducts and glands. Plain films are first performed as above. The opening of the salivary duct is then cannulated with a fine catheter and oil-based or water-soluble contrast medium injected. A calculus appears as a filling defect within a localized expansion of the salivary duct, and the proximal duct may be dilated (*Fig 15.4*).

Other findings that may be seen on sialography include strictures and sialectasis, i.e. dilated ducts and cavities within the gland, some of which may contain calculi. Sialography is contraindicated in the presence of acute salivary gland infection.

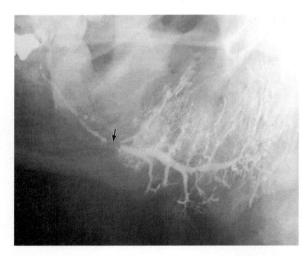

Figure 15.4 *Parotid sialogram – parotid duct calculus. Parotid duct calculus seen as a filling defect (arrow) in the contrast-filled parotid duct.*

US

When performed carefully by an experienced operator, US is a highly accurate technique for the non-invasive diagnosis of parotid calculi. A small US probe placed in the mouth may be used to diagnose calculi of the submandibular glands and ducts.

Staging of carcinoma of the larynx

Local growth

Laryngoscopy

Laryngoscopy is used for assessment of the mucosal surface. CT is required to assess submucosal and deeper tissues.

CT

CT is complementary to laryngoscopy for staging of laryngeal carcinoma. Carcinoma of the larynx appears as a high-attenuation mass causing asymmetry of the airway and anatomical distortion with obliteration of surrounding fat planes. Complicating factors that may be seen include:

- Invasion of surrounding fat planes.

- Invasion of surrounding structures such as laryngeal cartilages.

- Cervical lymphadenopathy.

Distant spread

Chest X-ray (CXR) and chest CT to demonstrate spread to the mediastinal lymph nodes or to the lungs.

Thyroid imaging

With the development of high-resolution US, fine-needle aspiration (FNA) techniques, and accurate laboratory tests including cytopathology, the diagnostic evaluation of thyroid disease has evolved over the past few years.

For diffuse thyroid diseases such as Grave's disease, Hashimoto's thyroiditis, subacute thyroiditis and multinodular goitre the diagnosis is often achieved by clinical history and examination, plus laboratory tests for thyroid function and antibodies. These may be complemented by thyroid scintigraphy and US including colour Doppler. CT may be required for intrathoracic goitre to show its location and extent, and to distinguish it from other causes of superior mediastinal mass.

Thyroid nodules and masses

FNA under direct palpation is often the first and only diagnostic procedure performed for a palpable thyroid nodule. US and scintigraphy may be used for further characterization of a thyroid nodule and US-guided FNA has several advantages over palpation-directed FNA. It is generally safer and more accurate. With the use of colour Doppler, the needle tip may be directed toward less vascular areas. This reduces the risk of haemorrhage following the procedure. It also provides a less bloodstained specimen, which increases the accuracy of cytology. CT is usually reserved for staging of thyroid carcinomas, and for assessment of large multinodular goitre.

The most common thyroid nodules are benign colloid nodules usually seen as partly cystic thyroid masses. Follicular adenoma is a true benign neoplasm of the thyroid gland. Thyroid carcinoma is usually of epithelial origin and is classified into papillary, follicular, medullary and anaplastic. Papillary carcinoma is the most common type (60%). Thyroid carcinoma has a high incidence of spread to regional cervical lymph nodes. Pulmonary and bone metastases are also common. For further notes on staging of thyroid carcinoma, see below.

US

The roles of US in assessment of thyroid nodules are:

*   Differentiate thyroid mass from non-thyroid mass or cyst (see above).

*   Characterize nodule.

*   Diagnose multiple nodules.

*   FNA guidance.

US is highly sensitive for nodules of 2 mm or greater.

US features of a benign thyroid nodule:

*   Hypoechoic with well-defined margins.

*   Cystic components:
    (i)   Malignant cysts are exceedingly rare.

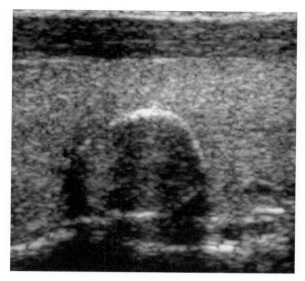

Figure 15.5 *Benign thyroid nodule – US. Well-defined hypoechoic nodule. Peripheral hyperechoic rim due to 'egg-shell' calcification. Note homogeneous hyperechoic texture of surrounding normal thyroid tissue.*

(ii)   Most thyroid cysts have some wall irregularity and contain echogenic debris.
(iii)   The majority of thyroid cysts are due to necrosis or haemorrhage complicating a colloid nodule.
(iv)   Simple epithelial cysts of the thyroid are rare.

*   Peripheral 'egg shell' calcification (*Fig. 15.5*).

*   Hyperechoic nodules, though rare, are usually benign.

US features of a malignant mass:

*   Hypoechoic.

*   Ill-defined margins.

*   Fine internal calcifications.

*   Heterogeneity due to haemorrhage and necrosis.

There is considerable overlap in the US appearances of benign and malignant nodules so FNA is often required for diagnosis.

US-guided FNA

US-guided FNA has several advantages over palpation-directed FNA:

- With high-resolution US the needle can be selectively directed into cystic and solid components.

- With colour Doppler the needle is directed away from blood vessels; a highly bloodstained specimen is a common cause of non-diagnostic FNA.

- Small, non-palpable nodules may also be aspirated.

A 22–25 gauge needle is generally used. The 'free hand' method is quick, easy and safe. The US probe is held in one hand and the needle in the other. Under direct US visualization the needle tip is directed into the nodule. The needle is rapidly moved in and out through the area of interest.

FNA should be reported by the cytopathologist in one of four ways:

- Benign, i.e. no malignant cells seen.

- Malignant.

- Suspicious or equivocal.

- Non-diagnostic, usually due to a heavily blood-stained specimen.

Repeat FNA may be performed for cases reported as suspicious or non-diagnostic.

Scintigraphy

Thyroid scintigraphy uses ^{99m}Tc pertechnetate. It has a reduced role in the assessment of thyroid nodules with the increasingly widespread use of US and FNA. It is not sensitive for nodules of 5 mm or less. Nodules are described according to their level of uptake of isotope as 'hot', 'warm' or 'cold'. Only 1% of 'hot' nodules are malignant. 'Warm' nodules, i.e. those with a similar level of uptake to the surrounding thyroid gland, are usually benign, though up to 10% may be malignant. Approximately 20% of 'cold' nodules are malignant (Fig. 15.6).

Staging of thyroid carcinoma

Papillary carcinoma and medullary carcinomas have a high incidence of spread to local lymph nodes, with haematogenous metastases to lung and bone occurring less commonly. Follicular carcinoma tends to early haematogenous spread to lung and bone. Local invasion may be seen with all forms.

Local growth

CT

- Size of tumour.

- Invasion of surrounding structures: laryngeal cartilages, blood vessels and sternomastoid muscle.

- Compression/displacement of trachea/oesophagus.

- Cervical lymphadenopathy.

Distant spread

- Lung and mediastinum: chest CT and CXR.

- Bone: scintigraphy and plain films. Note that thyroid metastases to bone are usually lytic and often expansile.

Primary hyperparathyroidism

Primary hyperparathyroidism is the most common indication for imaging of the parathyroid glands. The causes of primary hyperparathyroidism are as follows:

- Solitary parathyroid adenoma: 80%.

- Multiple parathyroid adenoma: 7%.

- Parathyroid hyperplasia: 10%.

- Parathyroid carcinoma: 3%.

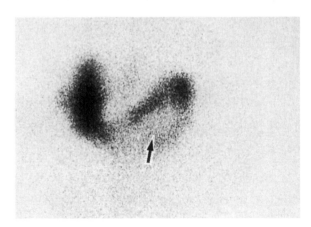

Figure 15.6 'Cold' thyroid nodule.
Area of decreased uptake in the left lobe of the thyroid, i.e. a 'cold' nodule (arrow), in this case due to a cyst. Other causes of this appearance include non-functioning thyroid adenoma and thyroid carcinoma.

Preoperative imaging for localization of parathyroid adenoma is not always performed, as in some centres it is felt unlikely to improve the rate of surgical success. However, where the surgeon requires preoperative localization, US is the investigation of first choice. US with high-resolution equipment has a high sensitivity (80–90%) for the detection of parathyroid adenoma.

The US appearance of parathyroid adenoma is a well-defined hypoechoic mass usually of around 1.0–1.5 cm in diameter (*Fig. 15.7*). The principal cause of a false-negative US is ectopic adenoma as may be present in up to 10% of cases. Where US is negative further imaging may be performed, i.e. scintigraphy, CT and MRI.

The imaging technique chosen will reflect local expertise and availability. CT and MRI are particularly useful for ectopic adenoma located in the mediastinum. Scintigraphy with ^{99m}Tc-sestamibi shows a high rate of uptake in parathyroid adenoma. It is especially useful for ectopic or multiple adenomas.

Postoperative imaging for recurrent or persistent hyperparathyroidism is best performed with US complemented by sestamibi scintigraphy.

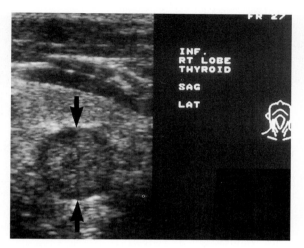

Figure 15.7 *Parathyroid adenoma – US. Adenoma of the right inferior parathyroid gland. Well-defined hypoechoic mass (arrows) deep to the inferior pole of the right lobe of the thyroid.*

16 Paediatrics

Neonatal respiratory distress: the neonatal chest

The normal neonatal chest X-ray (CXR) has the following features:

- Thymus may be prominent.

- Heart shadow is quite prominent and globular in outline; normal cardiothoracic ratio up to 65%.

- Air bronchograms may be seen in the medial third of the lung fields.

- Diaphragms normally lie at the level of the 6th rib anteriorly.

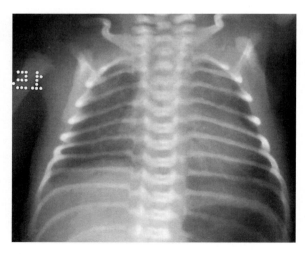

Figure 16.1 *Normal neonatal chest.*
Note:
- *prominent superior mediastinal shadow due to the thymus*
- *prominent cardiac shadow*
- *air bronchograms in the medial thirds of the lung fields.*

- Ossification of the proximal humeral epiphysis occurs at 36 weeks' gestation; visible ossification of this centre implies a term gestation (*Fig. 16.1*).

Most of us approach the CXR of a neonate with some trepidation. It should be borne in mind, however, that the differential diagnosis of neonatal respiratory distress involves only a few abnormalities, which tend to give quite typical radiographic patterns, as described below. Remember also that the clinical setting is important. For example, in the premature infant with respiratory distress, hyaline membrane disease will be the most likely diagnosis. In a distressed term infant following Caesarean delivery retained lung fluid will be most likely. For a term delivery with meconium-stained liquor, consider meconium aspiration syndrome.

Finally, the first step in assessing the CXR of a neonate is to check the position of the various tubes that may be present:

- Endotracheal tube: tip above carina.

- Umbilical artery catheter: tip in lower thoracic aorta away from renal artery origins.

- Umbilical vein catheter: tip in lower right atrium.

Hyaline membrane disease (HMD)

HMD is a generalized lung condition caused by insufficient surfactant production. It occurs most commonly in premature infants. The presentation is usually respiratory distress and cyanosis soon after birth. CXR changes of hyaline membrane disease include:

- Granular pattern throughout both lungs.

- Air bronchograms.

- Poor pulmonary expansion (*Fig. 16.2*).

Complications of HMD include:

- Pneumothorax (*Fig. 16.3*).

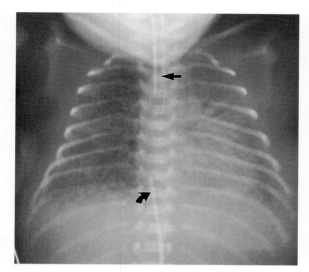

Figure 16.2 *Hyaline membrane disease.*
Note:
* *granular pattern through both lungs with air bronchograms*
* *endotracheal tube (straight arrow)*
* *umbilical artery catheter (curved arrow).*

* Pulmonary interstitial emphysema (PIE): air-filled bubbles throughout the lungs; high incidence of pneumothorax.

* Patent ductus arteriosus.

* Bronchopulmonary dysplasia (BPD).

BPD evolves over several days to months as a complication of HMD treated with positive pressure ventilation. A series of changes may be seen ranging from severe appearances of HMD to persistent poor pulmonary expansion and generalized opacity. These changes evolve over several weeks to a pattern of over-expansion with areas of collapse, fibrosis and bulla formation.

Retained foetal lung fluid

This condition is also known as transient tachypnoea of the newborn.

CXR signs include:

* Prominent interstitial pattern with thickening of lung fissures.

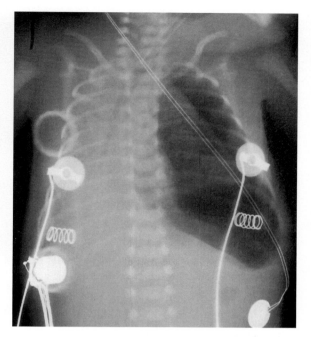

Figure 16.3 *Hyaline membrane disease and pneumothorax.*
Note:
* *left tension pneumothorax with enlarged left hemithorax and displacement of the heart to the right.*
* *complete opacification of the right lung with air bronchograms visible.*

* Small pleural effusions.

* Rapid resolution over 24 h.

Meconium aspiration syndrome

* Overexpanded lungs containing dense, patchy areas of linear atelectasis.

* May be complicated by pneumonia or pneumothorax.

Pulmonary oedema: cardiac failure

* Cardiomegaly (not a reliable sign in neonates).

* Combination of alveolar and interstitial opacification bilaterally.

Neonatal pneumonia

Range of appearances may be seen on CXR:

- Lobar consolidation.
- Patchy widespread consolidation.
- Dense, bilateral consolidation may mimic HMD.

Pulmonary dysmaturity (Wilson Mikity syndrome)

- Occurs in premature infants.
- Radiological changes and evolution similar to BPD, though with no history of ventilation.

Patterns of pulmonary infection in children

Most pulmonary infections in children are due to viruses such as respiratory syncitial virus (RSV), influenza, parainfluenza, and adenovirus, or *Mycoplasma* pneumonia. These infections tend to be seasonal and occur in epidemics.

Less commonly, bacterial infections may occur. These tend to be sporadic and less seasonal. Bacteria that commonly cause pulmonary infections in children include *Streptococcus* pneumonia, *Staphylococcus aureus* and *Haemophilus influenzae*. Although there is some overlap, viruses tend to produce an interstitial pattern while bacteria tend to produce alveolar consolidation.

Mycoplasma may produce an interstitial or alveolar pattern, or a combination of the two.

The most important question on the CXR of a child with a lower respiratory infection is therefore: 'Is alveolar consolidation present?' If the answer is 'No', then treatment will consist of supportive measures without the use of antibiotics. If the answer is 'Yes', then a bacterial aetiology is suspected and antibiotics may be required.

Patterns of viral infection

The child with a viral infection usually presents with a couple of days of malaise, tachypnoea and cough. The most common pattern seen with viral pulmonary infection is bilateral parahilar infiltration. This consists of irregular linear opacity extending into each lung from the hilar complexes, with bronchial wall thickening a prominent feature. Hilar lymphadenopathy may increase the amount of hilar opacification.

Atelectasis due to mucous plugs and bronchial inflammation will commonly complicate this pattern. Atelectasis may involve whole lobes, or it may be seen as linear opacities that may be multiple, and that may be transient and migratory on serial films. It is important to recognize the lung volume loss associated with atelectasis, as this will differentiate it from consolidation. Consolidation may rarely complicate viral infection. It is thought to be due to haemorrhagic bronchiolitis rather than a genuine exudate.

Bronchiolitis

Although caused by viral infection, bronchiolitis represents a distinct clinical entity. Affected children present with tachypnoea, dyspnoea, cough and cyanosis. Bronchiolitis is usually caused by the respiratory syncitial virus, with a peak incidence at around 6 months of age. The usual CXR pattern seen is overexpansion of the lungs due to bilateral air trapping. Severe cases may be complicated by atelectasis (*Fig. 16.4*). Where bronchiolitis is recurrent or prolonged, underlying asthma or cystic fibrosis should be considered.

Bacterial infection

Children with a bacterial pulmonary infection usually present with abrupt onset of malaise, fever and cough. The typical X-ray pattern of bacterial infection is alveolar consolidation. The appearance of alveolar consolidation is as described in Chapter 7, i.e. fluffy opacity with air bronchograms that may be lobar or patchy in distribution. A common pattern of early infection in children is round pneumonia. This is seen on CXR as a dense round opacity, which may be mistaken for a mass (*Fig. 16.5*). The clinical setting should provide the

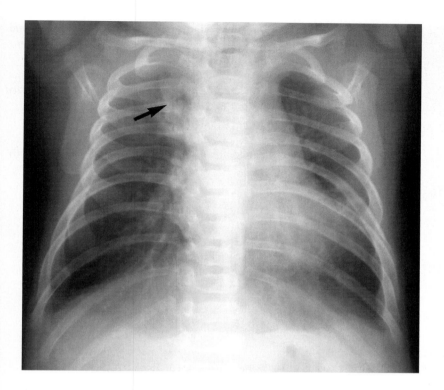

Figure 16.4 *Bronchiolitis complicated by atelectasis. Three-month-old male infant. The lungs are overexpanded with depression and flattening of the diaphragms. Note also atelectasis in the right upper lobe (arrow).*

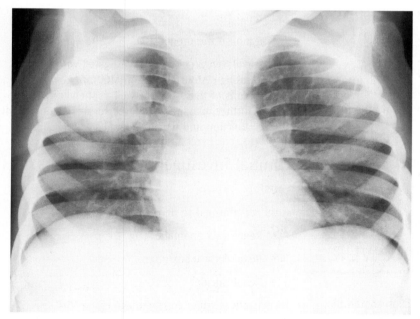

Figure 16.5 *Round pneumonia. A 6-year-old child presents with fever and cough. There is a dense round opacity in the right upper lobe. This is a typical appearance of round pneumonia, a pattern of lung infection more common in children. The opacity had resolved completely on a follow-up CXR after I week of antibiotic therapy.*

diagnosis and a follow-up CXR in 6–24 h will usually show evolution of the round opacity to a more lobar pattern. Round pneumonia is much less common in adults.

Established cases of bacterial infection are usually easily diagnosed on CXR. Difficulties may arise with early infections where the consolidation may be extremely subtle. Overlying structures may obscure

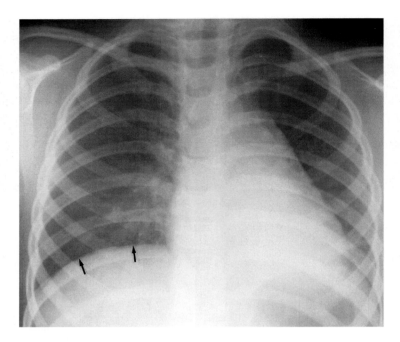

Figure 16.6 *Lower left lobe pneumonia. A 5-year-old child presented with fever and abdominal pain. The CXR was initially considered normal. On more careful scrutiny, however, it was realized that the left diaphragm is not visible. Compare this with the normal appearance of the right diaphragm (arrows). Note also the increased density behind the heart. These signs indicate consolidation of the left lower lobe, a commonly missed diagnosis.*

certain parts of the lung. Consolidation in these areas may be very difficult to see. Particular attention should be given to the following:

- Apical segments of the lower lobes, which are obscured by the hilar complexes.

- The lung bases, which are obscured by the diaphragms.

- The left lower lobe, which lies behind the heart (*Fig. 16.6*).

- The apical segments of the upper lobes, which are obscured by overlying ribs and clavicles.

For further notes on interpretation of CXRs, see Chapter 7.

Vesico-ureteric reflux (VUR)

All children with urinary tract infection should be investigated. The precise nature and sequence of investigations depends on local availability and expertise. The purposes of the investigations are to:

- Diagnose underlying anatomical abnormalities.

- Diagnose and grade severity of VUR.

- Document renal damage.

- Establish a baseline for subsequent evaluation of renal growth.

- Establish the prognosis.

Most children are initially investigated with US and micturating cystourethrogram (MCU). Depending on the results of these tests as well as the clinical situation, further imaging may be performed to document renal function and diagnose renal scars.

Initial investigations

US

US is performed to detect the following:

- Renal tract anomalies (*Fig. 16.7*).

- Renal cortical scarring.

- Renal calculi.

US is not sensitive for the diagnosis of VUR.

MCU

- Document site of insertion of ureter.

- Diagnose underlying anomalies, e.g. posterior urethral valves.

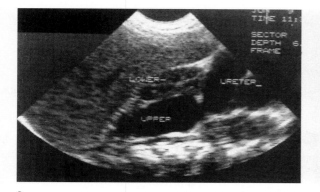
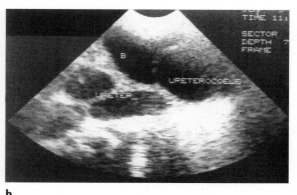

a **b**

Figure 16.7 *(a) Duplex kidney with ectopic ureterocele. Normal lower moiety. Dilated collecting system of upper moiety. Dilated tortuous ureter. (b) Ectopic ureterocele – US. The ureterocele is well seen projecting into the bladder. Note the dilated tortuous ureter posterior to the bladder.*

- Diagnose VUR and grade severity as below (*Fig. 16.8*).

VRU is graded as grades 1–5 as below:

- Grade 1: Reflux into non-dilated ureter.

- Grade 2: Reflux into non-dilated collecting system.

- Grade 3: Reflux into mildly dilated collecting system.

- Grade 4: Reflux into moderately dilated collecting system.

- Grade 5: Reflux into grossly dilated collecting system with dilated, tortuous ureter.

Further imaging studies

When moderate to severe reflux is diagnosed, or in the presence of underlying urinary tract anomalies, further imaging studies may be required.

Functional study by scintigraphy

- ^{99m}Tc-MAG3 or ^{99m}Tc-DTPA.

- Information on renal structure.

- Quantitate differential function.

- Differentiate obstructive from non-obstructive hydronephrosis.

Documentation of renal scars

- Scintigraphy with ^{99m}Tc-DMSA.

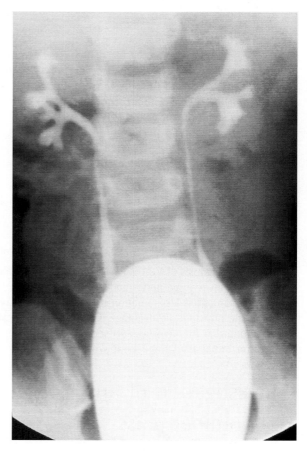

Figure 16.8 *Vesico-ureteric reflux – MCU.*
The bladder is well filled. There is bilateral vesico-ureter reflux with mild dilatation of the collecting systems, i.e. Grade III VUR.

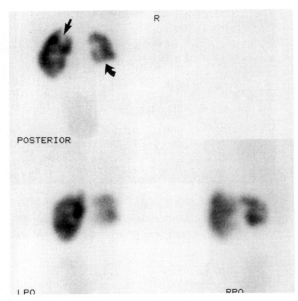

Figure 16.9 *Renal scars – DMSA scan.*
There is extensive scanning of the right kidney. The right kidney is much smaller than the left and in particular there is marked loss of cortex from its lower pole (curved arrow). There is also a scar in the upper pole of the left kidney (straight arrow).

- DMSA is taken up by cells of the proximal convoluted tubule and so outlines the renal cortex.

- More sensitive than US for documentation of renal scars (*Fig. 16.9*).

Scintigraphic reflux studies

Once the diagnosis of VUR is established, scintigraphic reflux studies may be performed for follow-up. The main advantage is less radiation dose than with X-ray MCU. The principal disadvantage is lack of anatomical resolution. For this reason, MCU should always be used for initial assessment as above.

Investigation of an abdominal mass

The essential roles of imaging for an abdominal mass are:

- Diagnosis of a mass.

- Define organ of origin.

- Characterize mass:
  (i)   Margins.
  (ii) Calcification, necrosis, cyst formation, fat.

- Diagnose complications and evidence of malignancy:
  (i)   Metastases.
  (ii) Lymphadenopathy.
  (iii) Invasion of surrounding structures.
  (iv) Vascular invasion.

- Pretreatment planning.

- Guidance of percutaneous biopsy or other interventional procedures such as nephrostomy.

- Follow-up: response to therapy, diagnosis of recurrent tumour.

US is the first investigation of choice in a child with a suspected abdominal mass. CT is then used to further define the mass and to diagnose complications as above. Plain films of the abdomen and chest are usually also performed in the initial work-up. Other imaging modalities such as scintigraphy, MRI and angiography are occasionally used in certain instances.

US

US is the first investigation for assessing the site of origin of a mass and as guidance for further investigations. It is an excellent screening tool in children where lack of mesenteric and retroperitoneal fat allows good definition of organs and blood vessels.

Plain films

Abdominal X-ray (AXR) and CXR are usually performed in the initial work-up of a child with an abdominal mass. Signs that may be seen on AXR include:

- Calcification.

- Displacement of bowel loops.

- Bone destruction in vertebral invasion.

Signs that may be seen on CXR include:

- Lymphadenopathy: mediastinal and paravertebral.

- Pulmonary metastases.

Although chest CT is more accurate for the detection of metastatic disease, an initial CXR is important to establish a baseline prior to treatment and follow-up.

CT

With its fast scanning times, helical CT is particularly advantageous in children. It provides accurate characterization of an abdominal mass and its organ of origin, and is highly sensitive for the presence of calcification and fat. CT is also used to diagnose complications of malignancy as follows:

- Invasion of surrounding structures.
- Lymphadenopathy.
- Liver metastases.
- Vascular encasement/invasion.

MRI

MRI has several advantages in children:

- No radiation.
- No iodinated contrast media.
- Multiplanar scanning:
  (i) Coronal scanning may be useful in hydronephrosis for detecting the level of obstruction.
  (ii) Coronal images also demonstrate liver, adrenal and renal tumours very well.
- Imaging of blood vessels:
  (i) Renal vein invasion by nephroblastoma can be detected without the use of iodinated contrast media.

Disadvantages of MRI include its high cost, lack of availability in some areas, and the relative difficulties of administering anaesthesia to uncooperative patients.

MRI is generally used for difficult cases to define specific clinical problems, such as spinal invasion by neuroblastoma.

Scintigraphy

Renal scintigraphy complements US in the assessment of benign renal conditions which may present as an abdominal mass, i.e. hydronephrosis, multicystic dysplastic kidney and polycystic conditions. ^{99m}Tc-DTPA or ^{99m}Tc-MAG3 may be used. MAG3 (mercaptoacetyl-

triglycine) is a newer agent with more efficient renal extraction than DTPA. It is gaining wide acceptance in renal imaging, particularly in paediatric and transplant patients. Renal scanning with DTPA or MAG3 provides physiological information such as differential renal function and diuretic 'wash-out', as well as anatomical information such as level of obstruction.

Bone scintigraphy with ^{99m}Tc-MDP is performed for suspected skeletal metastases.

^{123}I-MIBG (metaiodobenzylguanidine) is a specialized agent used for staging of neuroblastoma.

Other modalities

- MCU in hydronephrosis (see below).
- Angiography: done rarely to provide a surgical 'road map', especially in liver tumours.
- Cavography: sometimes required to assess the inferior vena cava (IVC) where US and CT are equivocal for the diagnosis of tumour invasion.

Common paediatric abdominal masses: imaging findings

A number of non-neoplastic renal conditions may present in childhood as an abdominal mass. These are outlined below followed by descriptions of the more common neoplastic abdominal masses found in children.

Hydronephrosis

The more common causes of hydronephrosis in children are:

- Pelvi-uretic junction (PUJ) obstruction.
- Vesico-ureteric reflux.
- Primary megaloureter.
- Duplex kidney with upper pole ureterocele.

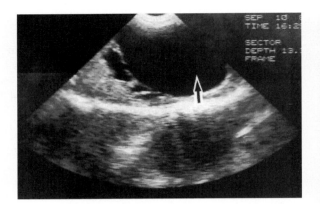

Figure 16.10 *Pelvi-uretic junction (PUJ) obstruction –
US.*
*Gross dilation of the renal pelvis (arrow). (Courtesy of Dr
J. Ratcliffe, Brisbane.)*

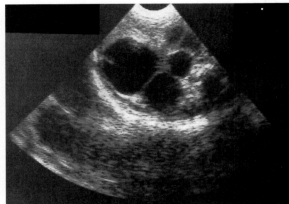

Figure 16.11 *Multicystic dysplastic kidney – US.*
*The kidney is replaced by a large number of cysts of
varying sizes. There is no recognizable renal tissue and
no obvious communication between the cysts is
demonstrated. (Courtesy of Dr J. Ratcliffe, Brisbane.)*

Hydronephrosis may present as a palpable abdominal
mass, with urinary tract infection (see below), or may
be detected on prenatal screening US. PUJ obstruction
and multicystic dysplastic kidney are the most
common benign renal conditions that present as an
abdominal mass. The advent of virtually universal
prenatal US screening has led to a marked increase in
the early diagnosis of hydronephrosis.

The roles of imaging of hydronephrosis in the neonate
are:

* Document severity of urinary tract dilatation.

* Define level of obstruction.

* Differentiate obstructive from non-obstructive
  causes.

* Diagnose underlying anatomical anomalies.

US

US is the initial imaging modality of choice in the
investigation of hydronephrosis. Signs that may be
seen include:

* Dilated renal pelvis and calyces.

* Round, markedly dilated renal pelvis in PUJ
  obstruction (*Fig. 16.10*).

* Thinned renal cortex.

* Underlying anomalies such as ureterocele or duplex
  collecting system (*see Fig. 16.7*).

Scintigraphy

Scintigraphy with ^{99m}Tc-MAG3 or ^{99m}Tc-DTPA will show
the dilated collecting system.

Diuretic scintigraphy is used to differentiate mechanical obstruction from other non-mechanical causes of
hydronephrosis. Furosemide injected after the renal
collecting system is filled with isotope. The rate of
'washout' of isotope is then assessed. With mechanical
obstruction such as PUJ obstruction, isotope continues
to accumulate in the collecting system following
diuretic injection. With non-mechanical obstruction
such as congenital megaloureter, isotope is rapidly
washed out of the dilated collecting system.

MCU

MCU is performed to document VUR and to diagnose
underlying anomalies such as posterior urethral valves.

Multicystic dysplastic kidney (MCDK)

US

* Kidney replaced by a lobulated collection of
  variably sized non-communicating cysts (*Fig. 16.11*).

* Anomalies in contralateral kidney in 15%, most
  commonly PUJ obstruction.

Scintigraphy

- ^{99m}Tc-MAG3 or ^{99m}Tc-DTPA.

- Non-function on early scans.

- Later scans may show minor peripheral activity with no evidence of central migration of isotope.

Polycystic renal conditions

Polycystic renal conditions are classified according to genetic inheritance, pathological findings and clinical presentation.

Autosomal recessive polycystic kidney disease (ARPKD)

ARPKD refers to a spectrum of disorders with associated liver disease, with infantile and juvenile forms described. In infantile cases, the renal disease tends to be more severe with less hepatic involvement; in older children the liver disease is the dominant feature.

US shows symmetrically enlarged kidneys which are markedly hyperechoic.

Autosomal dominant polycystic kidney disease (ADPKD)

ADPKD usually presents in middle age with enlarged kidneys and hypertension. At this time the kidneys are enlarged and contain cysts of varying size. ADPKD rarely presents in childhood with bilateral enlarged kidneys, which may be asymmetrical. On US examination, the kidneys are of increased echogenicity due to multiple cysts that are too tiny to be seen individually. Occasionally, separate small anechoic cysts are seen.

Glomerulocystic kidney disease

This is a rare, non-genetic condition with multiple glomerular cysts of around 2–3 mm diameter.

Hereditary syndromes associated with renal cysts

- Tuberous sclerosis.

- von Hippel–Lindau disease.

Nephroblastoma (Wilms' tumour)

Nephroblastoma is the most common solid intra-abdominal tumour in childhood. Fifteen per cent have associated congenital anomalies including:

- Non-familial aniridia.

- Congenital hemihypertrophy.

- Weidemann–Beckwith syndrome.

US

- Hyperechoic mass with hypoechoic areas due to necrosis.

- The mass tends to replace renal parenchyma with progressive enlargement and distortion of the kidney.

- Nephroblastoma may be bilateral, therefore must always image the contralateral kidney.

- Complications: lymphadenopathy, invasion of renal vein and IVC, liver metastases.

CT

- Renal mass with distortion of kidney.

- Mass is of equal or reduced attenuation compared with renal parenchyma and shows less contrast

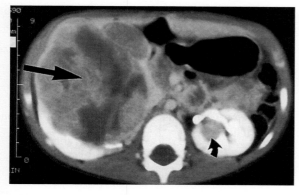

Figure 16.12 *Wilms' tumour – CT.*
Note:
- *large mass arising from the right kidney (straight arrow)*
- *low-attenuation areas within the mass due to necrosis*
- *small contralateral tumour in left kidney (curved arrow).*

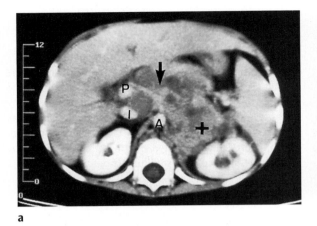

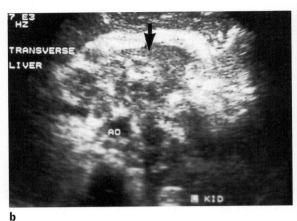

a   b

Figure 16.13 *Neuroblastoma.*
(a) US. US in the transverse plane shows a large mass (arrow) anterior to the aorta (AO), with posterolateral displacement of the left kidney.
(b) CT.
Note:
- *mass arising from the left adrenal gland (+) continuous across the midline with enlarged pre-aortic lymph nodes (arrow)*
- *contrast enhancement in aorta (A), IVC (I) and portal vein (P).*

enhancement than functioning renal tissue (*Fig. 16.12*).

- Invasion of surrounding structures.

- Vascular invasion: dilated renal vein with a filling defect that may extend into the right atrium.

Chest CT

- Chest CT is more accurate than CXR for the initial diagnosis of pulmonary metastases.

CXR

- Although less accurate than CT for initial diagnosis, a CXR should always be performed to establish a baseline for follow-up examinations.

Neuroblastoma

Neuroblastoma is a malignant childhood tumour arising from primitive sympathetic neuroblasts of the embryonic neural crest. Sixty per cent occur in the abdomen; of these two-thirds arise in the adrenal gland. Other common abdominal sites are the periaortic sympathetic ganglia, and ganglia at the aortic bifurcation. The peak age of incidence is 2 years with most occurring below 5 years.

A less common subgroup is congenital neuroblastoma in infants. This tumour has a better prognosis due to its tendency to spontaneous regression.

US

- Homogeneous hyperechoic mass, or heterogeneous texture due to areas of necrosis, haemorrhage and calcification.

- Tend to spread across midline to encase or displace major blood vessels.

CT

- Heterogeneous mass with displacement or invasion of the kidney (*Fig. 16.13*).

- Calcification is seen on CT in most cases.

- Invasion of surrounding structures including vertebral invasion.

- Lymphadenopathy; liver metastases.

- Pulmonary metastases.

AXR

- Soft tissue mass with displacement of bowel loops and loss of retroperitoneal fat planes.

- Calcification seen in 70%.

Bone scintigraphy

99mTc-MDP

- More accurate than plain films for detection of skeletal metastases.

MIBG scintigraphy

- 123I-MIBG.

- Localization of non-adrenal primary tumour.

- Staging: more sensitive than bone scintigraphy for detection of metastases.

Hepatoblastoma

Hepatoblastoma is the most common hepatic tumour in children. It has an increased incidence in Weidemann–Beckwith syndrome; it is not associated with cirrhosis.

US

- Well-circumscribed mass of higher echogenicity than surrounding liver.

- Hypoechoic areas due to necrosis.

- Invasion of portal vein or IVC may be seen.

CT

- Mass of equal or reduced attenuation compared with adjacent liver tissue.

- Less enhancement than normal liver tissue.

- Areas of necrosis, calcification and occasionally fat.

- Vascular invasion: filling defect within an enlarged portal vein or IVC.

Angiography

Still used in liver tumours for accurate demonstration of vascular anatomy prior to surgical resection (surgical 'road map'). Full angiographic assessment includes anatomical localization of the tumour, plus visualization of the portal vein, hepatic artery, and in doubtful cases the IVC.

Hepatocellular carcinoma

Hepatocellular carcinoma is uncommon in children, with an increased incidence in chronic liver diseases, e.g. biliary atresia, tyrosinaemia. US shows an ill-defined hypoechoic mass in the liver. CT may show a solitary low-attenuation mass or multiple confluent masses.

Haemangioendothelioma

Haemangioendothelioma is a highly vascular benign multicentric liver tumour, which may be associated with cutaneous haemangiomas. It usually presents in infancy with hepatomegaly, cardiac failure or acute haemorrhage.

US shows multiple discrete hyperechoic masses in the liver. CT shows multiple low-attenuation masses with occasional calcification.

Angiography reveals enlarged tortuous arteries with early filling of large draining veins, and pooling of contrast material.

Intussusception

Intussusception refers to prolapse or telescoping of a segment of bowel (referred to as the intussusceptum) into the lumen of more distal bowel (the intussuscepiens). The most common form of intussusception is ileo-colic, i.e. prolapse of distal small bowel into the colon. The ileo-ileal form is much less common. Intussusception occurs most commonly in young children, usually from 6 months to 2 years of age, with a peak incidence at around 9 months. At this age intussusception is usually regarded as idiopathic, although enlarged lymph nodes secondary to viral infection are thought to be responsible in most cases. In older children, a lead point should be strongly suspected. Such causes include Meckel diverticulum, mesenteric cyst and lymphoma. Intussusception may also occur in adults with underlying causes including benign small bowel tumours such as lipoma, Meckel diverticulum and foreign body.

Common signs and symptoms of intussusception include vomiting, bloodstained stool, colicky abdominal pain, listlessness and palpable abdominal mass.

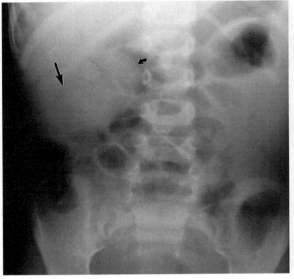 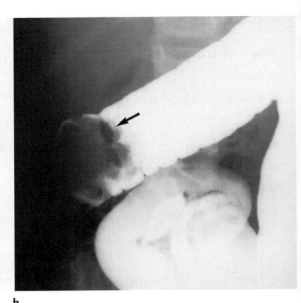

a   b

Figure 16.14 *Intussusception.*
(a) Plain film. Note:
- *apparent mass in right upper quadrant (straight arrow)*
- *intussusceptum shows as a convex opacity outlined by gas; this is the meniscus sign (curved arrow).*
(b) Contrast enema. The intussusceptum is seen as a filling defect in the transverse colon causing obstruction to the flow of contrast (arrow).

Imaging consists of an AXR followed by US. Contrast enema should no longer be required for diagnosis of intussusception. Confirmation of intussusception is followed in suitable cases by radiological reduction.

AXR

- 'Target' lesion in right upper quadrant due to swollen hepatic flexure seen end-on with layers of peritoneal fat within and surrounding the intussusception.

- Meniscus sign due to air outlining intussusceptum (*Fig. 16.14*).

- Relatively gasless right side of abdomen.

- Small bowel obstruction.

- Free air indicates intestinal perforation.

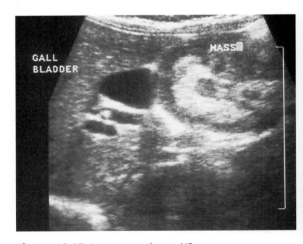

Figure 16.15 *Intussusception – US.*
The intussusception is well seen as a heterogeneous mass in the right upper abdomen, lying just to the left of the gallbladder. Note that the mass shows alternating hypoechoic and hyperechoic layers due to layers of oedematous bowel wall, mucosa and mesenteric fat.

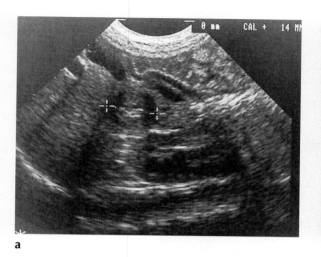 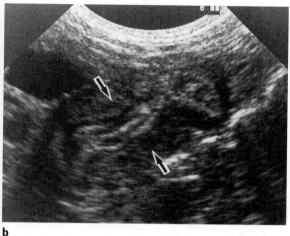

a   b

Figure 16.16 *(a) Pyloric stenosis – US. In transverse section pyloric stenosis appears as a 'target' lesion with an outer thick hypoechoic rim due to hypertrophied pyloric muscle, and a hyperechoic centre. (b) Pyloric stenosis – US. Longitudinal section of the pyloric canal showing the hypertrophied muscle wall (arrows).*

US

- Characteristic appearance with kidney-shaped mass longitudinally and 'target' lesion in cross-section (*Fig. 16.15*).

- Hypoechoic rim surrounding hyperechoic concentric rings due to layers of oedematous bowel wall and mesentery.

- May occasionally see a lead point such as lymphoma or duplication cyst, though in the majority of cases in children no lead point is seen.

Treatment of intussusception

Intussusception is a surgical emergency and early involvement of radiological and surgical teams is mandatory.

Contraindications to radiological reduction:

- Shock: the child must be adequately hydrated.

- Perforation, i.e. signs of peritonism and/or free air on AXR.

A duration of greater than 12 h or small bowel obstruction make radiological reduction more difficult

and so decrease the likelihood of success, but are not in themselves absolute contraindications.

Reduction

Reduction is most commonly performed under X-ray screening with various operators using a variety of contrast agents including barium, water-soluble contrast and gas. Gas reduction is now widely used and has several advantages. It is relatively quick and clean, and if perforation does occur it is safer than with barium. Some centres use US-guided liquid reduction.

Follow-up

A postevacuation film is performed to exclude early recurrence. Recurrences occur in 5–10% of cases and should lead to repeat enema reduction. With multiple recurrences or a suspected pathological lead point, surgical intervention is mandatory.

Hypertrophic pyloric stenosis

Hypertrophic pyloric stenosis refers to idiopathic hypertrophy of the circular muscle fibres of the

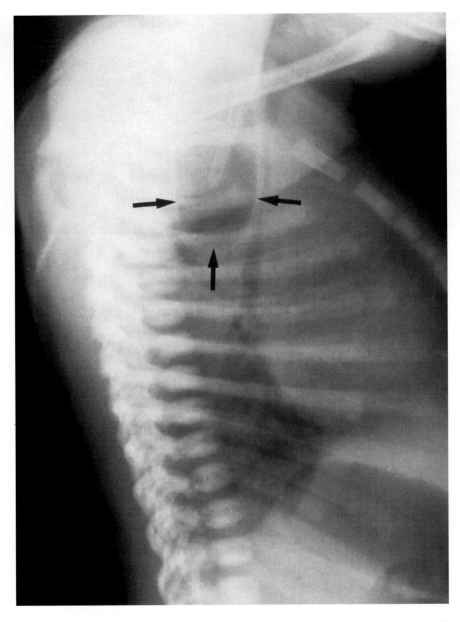

Figure 16.17 *Oesophageal atresia.*
The atretic oesophagus is well seen as a distended air-filled pouch posterior to the trachea (arrows). Note the nasogastric tube. Contrast is not required in this situation. Note that there is gas in the stomach and small bowel indicating the presence of a tracheo-oesophageal fistula.

pylorus, which produces progressive gastric outlet obstruction. The condition is most common in first-born male infants and the peak age of presentation is at around 6 weeks.

Palpation of a pyloric muscular mass in the right upper quadrant of an infant with a typical clinical history, i.e. forceful non-bile-stained vomiting leading to dehydration and hypokalaemic alkalosis is diagnostic of hypertrophic pyloric stenosis and imaging is not required in such cases.

Imaging is useful in infants with equivocal symptomatology, or with typical symptoms where a mass cannot be palpated.

US

US is highly accurate for the diagnosis of pyloric stenosis and has replaced X-ray imaging. The thickened pylorus is seen as a target lesion in cross-section. The target appearance is produced by a rim of hypoechoic thickened muscle with a hyperechoic centre. The thickened pylorus is measured with positive measurements as follows:

- Total pyloric diameter >13 mm.
- Pyloric muscle thickness >3 mm.
- Pyloric length >16 mm (*Fig. 16.16*).

The stomach is usually distended and no gastric contents are seen to pass through the thickened pylorus on real-time scanning.

Barium meal

Barium meal is now rarely used since implementation of US. Its main role is in the postoperative patient to diagnose incomplete pylomyotomy or to diagnose gastro-oesophageal reflux as a cause of persistent vomiting.

Persistent thickened pyloric muscle produces a long narrow pyloric canal with rounded margins associated with delayed gastric emptying.

Oesophageal atresia with or without tracheo-oesophageal fistula (TOF)

Classification:

- Oesophageal atresia with distal TOF: 85%.
- Oesophageal atresia without TOF: 10%.
- TOF without oesophageal atresia ('H-type' fistula): 5%.
- Oesophageal atresia with proximal TOF: very rare.

Plain films: CXR and AXR

Plain-film findings depend on the type of lesion present. The most common form, i.e. oesophageal atresia with distal TOF, shows the following plain film signs:

- Air in upper oesophageal pouch posterior to trachea.
- Nasogastric tube curled in pouch.

- Air in gastrointestinal tract implies a distal fistula (*Fig. 16.17*).

A gasless abdomen is seen with no TOF or a proximal TOF. In all forms, signs of aspiration pneumonia may be seen on the CXR.

Contrast studies are usually not needed except as below.

Prenatal US

With the widespread use of US in obstetric care, oesophageal atresia and TOF may be suspected prenatally. US findings include:

- Polyhydramnios.
- Absence of fluid-filled stomach.
- Distended pouch of atretic oesophagus may be identified in the neck or upper chest.

'H-type' TOF

In this uncommon variant, the oesophagus is formed normally, i.e. there is no oesophageal atresia. The upper oesophagus is joined to the trachea by a thin fistula. Plain films are often normal, apart from signs of aspiration pneumonia. Contrast studies are important as the fistula may be very small and difficult to image. Water-soluble contrast is injected through a feeding tube placed in the upper oesophagus.

Associated anomalies

Associated anomalies occur in approximately 25% of cases and include the following:

- Vertebral anomalies.
- Anorectal atresia.
- Duodenal atresia.
- Renal anomalies, e.g. MCDK, renal agenesis.
- Cardiac anomalies, e.g. VSD, ASD, PDA.
- Radial dysplasia and other limb anomalies.
- Right-sided aortic arch is seen in 5% of cases. It is important to diagnose preoperatively as the surgical approach may have to be amended.

Given the above, all patients with a TOF should have a renal US and an echocardiogram. The plain films of the chest and abdomen should be closely perused for vertebral anomalies.

Postoperative complications: plain films and contrast studies

- Oesophageal leak: pneumomediastinum, pneumothorax and pleural effusion.

- Oesophageal stricture.

- Tracheomalacia.

- Recurrent fistula.

Gut obstruction and/or bile-stained vomiting in the neonate

Neonatal gut obstruction with or without bile-stained vomiting is a common clinical problem with a wide differential diagnosis. In some cases such as duodenal obstruction, AXR alone is sufficient for diagnosis. In other cases, the AXR may be normal eg. malrotation, or may have non-specific appearances, e.g. Hirschsprung disease.

Contrast studies such as upper gastrointestinal (GI) series and contrast enema are often required for diagnosis, particularly for malrotation and large bowel disorders.

Duodenal obstruction

Duodenal atresia is the most common cause of congenital duodenal obstruction. Other causes include duodenal stenosis or web, and annular pancreas. Associated anomalies occur in 60% of cases as follows:

- Oesophageal atresia.

- Imperforate anus.

- Renal anomalies.

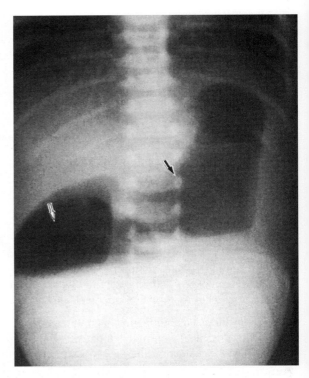

Figure 16.18 *Duodonal atresia.*
Classic 'double-bubble' appearance due to distended stomach (solid arrow) and duodenal cap (hollow arrow). Note lack of gas in distal bowel.

- Congenital heart disease.

- Down syndrome in 30%.

Prenatal US

Duodenal atresia may be suspected on prenatal ultrasound with polyhydramnios plus a fluid-filled double bubble in the upper abdomen due to dilated fluid-filled stomach and duodenal cap.

AXR

- Classic double-bubble sign due to gas in distended stomach and duodenal cap (*Fig. 16.18*).

- Absence of gas in distal bowel.

- 'Triple bubble' may be seen with gas in the gallbladder.

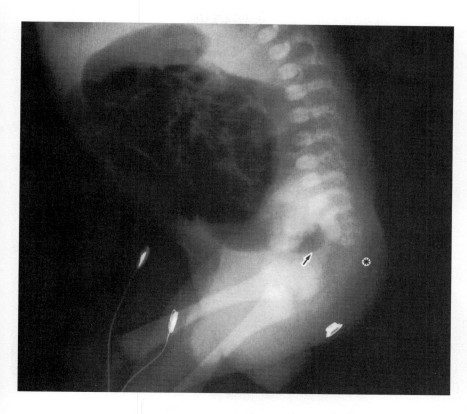

Figure 16.19 *Anorectal malformation.*
A high lesion with the most distal part of the bowel (arrow) well above the pelvic floor. Note:
- *absence of distal sacrum and coccyx (*)*
- *metal marker on perineum. (Courtesy of Dr M. Hendry, Edinburgh.)*

Jejuno-ileal atresia

AXR

- Dilated small bowel.
- Occasionally, widespread calcification due to meconium peritonitis may be seen.

Contrast enema

- Small colon.

Anorectal atresia

Anorectal atresia is classified as either a low or high anomaly. With a low anomaly the bowel ends below levator sling. With a high anomaly the bowel ends above levator sling and is usually associated with a fistula into the vagina or posterior urethra.

AXR

A lateral rectal view is performed to classify the lesion by assessing the relationship of the most distal part of the bowel to the pelvic floor (*Fig. 16.19*). Gas in the bladder or vagina indicates the presence of a fistula.

Associated sacral anomalies may also be seen:

- Failure of sacral segmentation.
- Sacral agenesis.

US

US of the perineum may determine the distance between the anal dimple on the perineal surface and the distal bowel end, and thus aid in surgical planning.

Hirschsprung disease

Hirschsprung disease refers to an aganglionic segment of distal large bowel. This occurs during embryological development due to arrest of normal craniocaudal migration of neuroblasts. A distal short aganglionic segment is the most common form. This causes distal obstruction with dilatation of normally innervated bowel proximal to the aganglionic segment. Total colonic aganglionosis occurs in 5%.

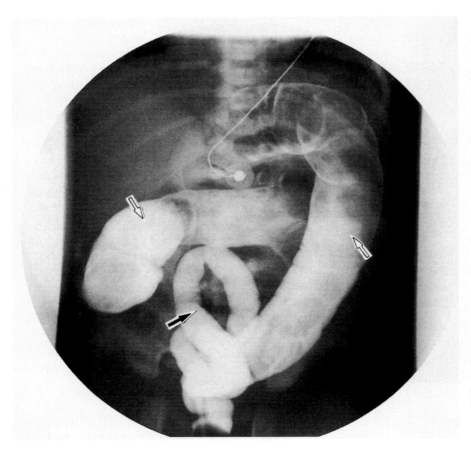

Figure 16.20
Hirschsprung disease. The rectum and sigmoid colon are of normal calibre (solid arrow). The remainder of the bowel was dilated and contains retained faecal material (hollow arrows). (Courtesy of Dr M. Hendry, Edinburgh.)

AXR

- Dilated bowel loops.

Contrast enema

- Abrupt transition zone from small aganglionic bowel distally to dilated innervated bowel (*Fig. 16.20*).

Meconium ileus

Meconium ileus occurs in association with cystic fibrosis (mucoviscidosis).

Prenatal US

- Polyhydramnios.

- Hyperechoic contents in small bowel.

AXR

- 'Soap bubble' appearance in right lower quadrant.

- Dilated small bowel loops of variable calibre with no fluid levels on the erect view (*Fig. 16.21*).

Contrast enema

- Microcolon.

- Large distal ileum with filling defects due to meconium.

Meconium plug syndrome

Meconium plug syndrome refers to inspissated meconium causing distal large bowel obstruction. It is not related to meconium ileus.

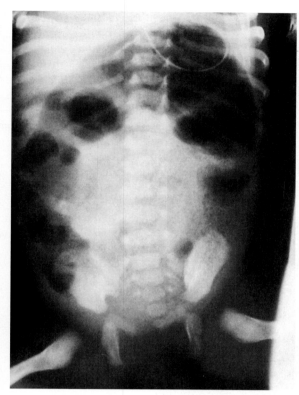

Figure 16.21 *Meconium ileus.
Grossly dilated small bowel loops contain a mixture of
air and viscous meconium giving the characteristic 'soap
bubble' appearance. (Courtesy of Dr M. Hendry,
Edinburgh.)*

AXR

Dilated small bowel loops.

Contrast enema

- Often therapeutic.
- Dilated rectum.
- Large filling defects in the colon.

Small left colon syndrome

AXR

- Dilated bowel loops.

Contrast enema

- Normal distensible rectum.
- Small sigmoid and descending colon.
- Transition to dilated colon at splenic flexure.

Malrotation and midgut volvulus

Malrotation refers to a wide spectrum of anatomical
variants, the common feature being abnormal rotation
of the gut. These anatomical variations include:

- Duodenum and duodenojejunal flexure to the right
  of midline.
- Colon to the left of midline.
- Caecum in the left upper abdomen.
- Transverse colon lying posterior to the superior
  mesenteric artery.
- Peritoneal (Ladd) bands, i.e. fibrous bands that
  cross the duodenum and may cause compression.
- Internal paraduodenal hernia.
- Shortened small bowel mesenteric attachment.

Complications, which occur secondary to these
anatomical variants include:

- Volvulus of the small bowel and duodenum.
- Intestinal obstruction due to Ladd bands or
  paraduodenal hernia.

These complications lead to two common types of
clinical presentation:

- Severe bile-stained vomiting in neonates.
- Intermittent symptoms in older children: vomiting,
  nausea and abdominal pain.

AXR

- Often normal, particularly when the child is asymptomatic.
- May show dilated duodenum.

Upper GI series

An upper GI contrast series to outline the stomach,
duodenum and small bowel is preferable to contrast

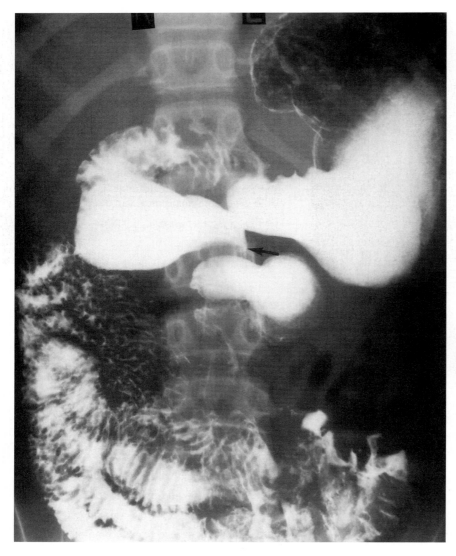

Figure 16.22 *Malrotation – barium meal.*
An 11-year-old child with repeated bile-stained vomiting. Note the features of volvulus of the duodenum:
- *dilated upper duodenum with 'beaked' ending (arrow)*
- *the duodenum has a 'twisted ribbon' or 'corkscrew' appearance.*
Note also that the jejunum lies in an abnormal position to the right of the midline.

enema as the initial investigation. Signs that may be seen with malrotation include:

- Duodenal obstruction.
- Proximal jejunum lies on the right with an abnormally positioned duodenojejunal flexure.
- 'Corkscrew' appearance of small bowel loops (*Fig. 16.22*).
- Abnormally high caecum on follow-through films.

US

- The positions of the superior mesenteric vessels are reversed, with the superior mesenteric vein lying abnormally to the left of the superior mesenteric artery.

Non-accidental injury (*Fig. 16.23*)

Non-accidental injury is a distressing condition for all involved. The importance of making an early diagnosis cannot be overstated and plain films of affected areas, plus skeletal survey, i.e. radiographs of the ribs, skull and long bones, are important in the diagnostic work-up. In considering the diagnosis of non-accidental injury, one should be alert for:

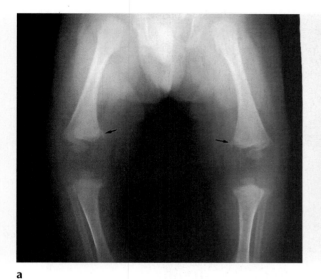

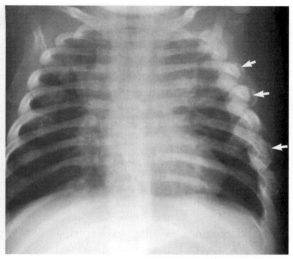

a

b

Figure 16.23 *Non-accidental injury.*
(a) Lower limb. There are metaphyseal corner fractures of the lower femora (arrows). (b) Chest. Note callous formation around multiple healing left rib fractures (arrows).

- Fractures inconsistent with the history.

- Multiple fractures at different stages of healing.

- Fractures at unusual sites such as sternum or scapula.

The following patterns may also be seen:

Long bones

- Periosteal new bone formation related to prior fractures.

- Metaphyseal or epiphyseal plate fractures.

- Spiral diaphyseal fractures.

Ribs

Up to 80% of rib fractures are occult and may only become visible with healing. Posterior rib fractures are particularly suspicious.

Skull

Accidental fractures tend to be linear. Non-accidental fractures tend to have the following features:

- Multiple/complex.

- Depressed fractures, especially in the occipital bone.

- Wide fractures, i.e. >5 mm.

Other

A wide range of soft tissue injuries may also occur, including hepatic, splenic and renal damage, as well as brain damage.

Subdural haematoma along the falx cerebri in the midline usually indicates severe shaking of the child.

Differential diagnosis of non-accidental injury includes birth-related trauma, and conditions causing abnormally fragile bones such as osteogenesis imperfecta.

Hip problems in children

Developmental dysplasia of the hip (DDH)

DDH occurs in 1–2 per 1000 births. It involves females more commonly than males by a ratio of 8:1. The left hip is much more commonly involved than the right. Previously known as congenital hip dislocation, the term DDH more accurately reflects the underlying disorder, i.e. dysplasia of the acetabulum, which may lead to varying degrees of hip joint subluxation, dislocation and dysfunction. Risk factors for the development of DDH include:

- Family history.
- Breech presentation.
- Neuromuscular disorders.
- Foot deformities.

Early diagnosis is essential, as conservative management such as splinting for a few weeks is usually successful in all but the most severe cases. Clinical tests such as Ortolani and Barlow manoeuvres may be helpful. Imaging assessment has in the past consisted of a pelvic X-ray. This has limited accuracy, however, especially below the age of 6 months as most of the essential structures such as the femoral head and acetabular rim are composed of cartilage and cannot be seen.

US is now the investigation of choice for suspected DDH. It has a number of advantages including:

- No radiation.
- Cartilage structures are well seen.
- Reproducible measurements of the angle of the acetabular roof and the position of the femoral head may be taken and used in follow-up examinations.
- Dynamic real-time examination may be used to assess hip stability.
- Position of the hip in a splint may be confirmed.

Plain-film assessment is used in children over 9 months of age. At this age US is less accurate due to ossification of the femoral head obscuring the deeper structures of the acetabulum.

The patient with missed DDH may present with a limp, late walking or asymmetry. Permanent acetabular dysplasia and delayed femoral head ossification may occur with long-term complications including:

- Limp.
- Early and severe osteoarthritis.
- Labral tear.

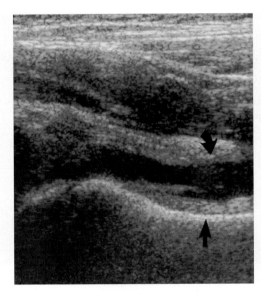

Figure 16.24 *Hip effusion – US.*
The scan is performed with the US probe parallel to the femoral neck. Note the surface of the femoral neck (straight arrow) and the joint capsule (curved arrow). The hip joint effusion is seen as anechoic fluid lifting the joint capsule off the femoral neck.

Septic arthritis of the hip

Septic arthritis of the hip usually presents before the age of 3 years. It is usually due to haematogenous spread from respiratory or urinary tract infection. Plain films are insensitive and early scintigraphy may be negative. US is the investigation of choice to diagnose the presence of a hip joint effusion (*Fig. 16.24*). Diagnostic aspiration may be safely performed under US control.

Transient synovitis (irritable hip)

Transient synovitis is a benign, self-limiting hip disorder. Peak age is 4–10 years, with males more commonly affected than females. A limp develops rapidly over 1–2 days. There is often a history of a recent viral illness and mild fever. Full blood count and ESR are performed followed by bed rest, with imaging usually not required. Plain films are usually normal with signs of joint effusion such as joint space widening being quite insensitive. If imaging is

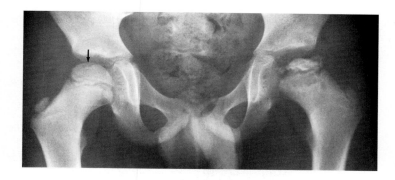

Figure 16.25 *Perthe's disease.*
Note the following changes of late Perthe's disease in the left hip:
- *sclerosis and irregular collapse of the femoral epiphysis*
- *widening of the medial joint space*
- *widening of the femoral neck*
- *cystic changes in the metaphysis.*
Note also the small subcapital fracture in the right femoral head indicating early Perthe's disease (arrow). This X-ray demonstrates that Perthe's disease is often bilateral, and stresses the importance of always examining both sides carefully.

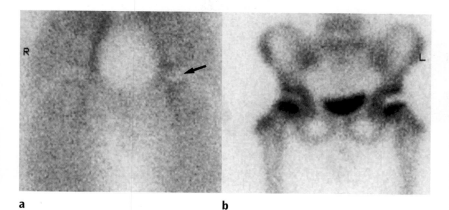

a   b

Figure 16.26 *Perthe's disease – scintigraphy.*
On the blood pool phase (a) of this study there is a subtle decrease in activity corresponding to the left femoral head (arrow). On the delayed bone phase (b) there is a more obvious defect indicating lack of blood flow to the upper epiphysis of the left femur. There is normal activity on the right side.

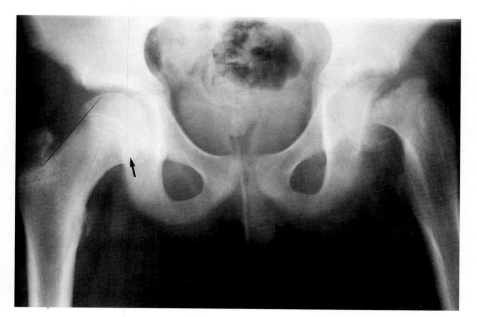

Figure 16.27 *Slipped capital femoral epiphysis. There is obvious and severe slip of the left capital epiphysis. Note the appearance of the normal right hip. A line drawn along the superior margin of the femoral neck should normally intersect part of the femoral head. Note also a triangular area of increased density where the acetabulum overlaps part of the femoral metaphysis – this is known as the metaphyseal overlay (arrow).*

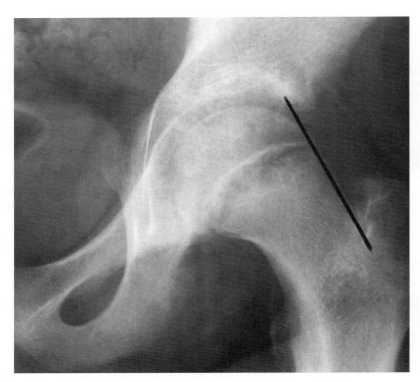

Figure 16.28 *Slipped capital femoral epiphysis.*
This is a less obvious case than in Fig. 16.27. *Compare with the normal right hip in* Fig. 16.27 *and note the following signs:*
- *loss of metaphyseal overlay*
- *widening and irregularity of the epiphyseal plate*
- *A line drawn along the superior margin of the femoral neck does not intersect the femoral head.*

required, US is the investigation of choice to diagnose a joint effusion.

Perthe's disease

Perthe's disease of the hip has a peak age of incidence of 4–7 years, with females more commonly affected than males. Ten per cent of cases are bilateral, with changes often being asymmetric. It is therefore important to carefully scrutinize both hip joints, even if only one is symptomatic (*Fig. 16.24*).

Early plain films are often normal. Scintigraphy may show a photopaenic spot due to ischaemia (*Fig. 16.25*). Increased uptake is seen later in the course of the disease due to revascularization.

Early X-ray signs include:

- Reduced size and sclerosis of the femoral epiphysis.
- Joint space widening.
- Subchondral fracture.

Late X-ray signs include:

- Delayed maturation of femoral head.

- Fragmentation.
- Metaphyseal cysts.
- Coxa plana, i.e. flattening of the femoral head.
- Coxa magna, i.e. widening of the femoral neck.

Slipped capital femoral epiphysis (SCFE)

SCFE is a disorder of adolescent males. It is bilateral in 20% of cases. Associations include obesity and avascular necrosis. The capital femoral epiphysis undergoes posteromedial slip, producing hip pain and a limp. Plain-film signs are best appreciated on a lateral projection where the slip of the femoral head is well seen. Signs on the AP film include:

- Widened irregular growth plate.
- Reduced height of epiphysis.
- Loss of metaphyseal overlay (*Figs 16.26 & 16.27*).

For notes on other skeletal disorders of childhood, plus notes on skeletal trauma, please see Chapter 13.

Index